PSYCHIATRIC NURSING CLINICAL GUIDE

PSYCHIATRIC NURSING CLINICAL GUIDE

Assessment Tools & Diagnosis

Elizabeth M. Varcarolis, RN, MA
Professor Emeritus
Formerly Deputy Chairperson, Department of Nursing
Borough of Manhattan Community College
New York, New York

Associate Fellow
Albert Ellis Institute for
Rational Emotive Behavioral Therapy (REBT)
New York, New York

W.B. SAUNDERS COMPANY
An Imprint of Elsevier Science
Philadelphia   London   New York   St. Louis   Sydney   Toronto

W.B. SAUNDERS COMPANY
An Imprint of Elsevier Science

The Curtis Center
Independence Square West
Philadelphia, Pennsylvania 19106

Library of Congress Cataloging-in-Publication Data

Varcarolis, Elizabeth M.
    Psychiatric nursing clinical guide : assessment tools and
diagnoses / Elizabeth M. Varcarolis.
        p. ; cm
    Includes bibliographical references.
    ISBN 0–7216–8336–3
    1. Psychiatric nursing. 2. Nursing assessment. I. Title.
    [DNLM: 1. Mental Disorders—nursing. 2. Nursing Assessment.
    3. Psychiatric Nursing—methods. WY 160 V278p 2000]
    RC440 .V374 2000
    610.73'68—dc21

99–049759

Vice President, Nursing Editorial Director: Sally Schrefer
Acquisitions Editor: Terri Wood

PSYCHIATRIC NURSING CLINICAL GUIDE   ISBN 0–7216–8336–3

Printed in the United States of America

Last digit is the print number   9   8   7   6   5   4

Dedicated to the memory of

SUZANNE LEGO, RN, PhD, CS, CGP, FAAN

Mentor, Teacher
1938–1999

Thanks for the good times

And to my dear husband

PAUL

Thanks for all times, always

PREFACE

I t is hoped that this clinical guide will help you plan realistic nursing care plans individualized to your client's present level of functioning and priority of needs. The interventions offered are designed for all levels of nursing, and are concretely stated and meant to be immediately useful.

About Outcomes and Long- and Short-Term Goals

Textbooks advocate identifying outcome criteria, then long-term, then short-term goals to help the client reach the outcome criteria. And that is appropriate. However, in the clinical setting, one client's short-term goal may be another's long-term goal. This is especially true for clients with biologically based psychiatric disorders. Therefore, there is not one set of goals, or series of goals (short-term, long-term, outcome criteria) that fits all clients.

Goals and interventions need always to be chosen according to your client's priority of needs, level of functioning, and level of present skills. Therefore, short-term goals in this text can be either long- or short-term depending upon the individual client.

Elizabeth M. Varcarolis

CONTRIBUTOR

Cherrill W. Colson, RN, EdD, CS
Consultant, Leake & Watts Children's Services,
Yonkers, New York

Mental Disorders of Childhood and Adolescence

ACKNOWLEDGMENTS

A huge thanks to Cherrill Colson, BSN, MS, EdD, for her outstanding child and adolescent chapter. This thorough and comprehensible work offers useful and concrete interventions for a wide variety of difficult and complex issues. These interventions can be easily adapted to any level nursing professional.

I am deeply grateful to my excellent reviewers whose backgrounds included both clinicians and educators. Their dedication and love for nursing was evident in their attention to detail and wide breadth of knowledge. Their contribution was invaluable and I thank each and every one.

Carol Alvarez, MS, RN, CS
Harborview Medical Center
University of Washington
Seattle, Washington

Vicki L. Britt, MSN, RN, CS
St. Francis College
Loretto, Pennsylvania

Patricia A. Goeden, RN, BSN, MSN
Assistant Professor
Mount Marty College
Staff Nurse
Mickelson Center for the Neurosciences
Yankton, South Dakota

Rebecca Crews Gruener, MSN, RN
Associate Professor
Louisiana State University
Alexandria, Louisiana

Betty J. Houser, MS, RN, CS
Clinical Specialist in Child Adolescent Psychiatric
    Mental Health Nursing
Missouri Southern State College
Joplin, Missouri

Catherine M. Lala, RN, CS
Psychiatric Home Care Nurse
Priority Home Care, Inc.
New York, New York

Barbara J. Michaels, EdD, EN, LMFT
Private Practice
Dallas, Texas

Linda Denise Oakley, RN, PhD
University of Wisconsin, Madison
Madison, Wisconsin

Terri Pensabene, RN, PhD
University of Texas at Arlington
Arlington, Texas

Patricia A. Rahe, RN, CAN, BSN, MS
Ivy Tech State College, Region II
Lawrenceburg, Indiana

Linda Sue Smith, DSN, RN
Assistant Professor
Oregon Health Sciences University
Klamath Falls, Oregon

Margaret Swisher, MSN, RN
Montgomery County Community College
Blue Bell, Pennsylvania

The support I receive from W.B. Saunders never falters. My
thanks to Terri Wood, my new editor, who generously offered
every assistance possible to help facilitate this project. To Catherine
Ott, Terri's editorial assistant, who courageously forges ahead in the
midst of manuscript chaos, and to all of the other fine and depend-
able production staff at Saunders.

CONTENTS

PART I

OVERVIEW

CHAPTER 1

Guidelines for Planning Psychosocial Nursing Care

MAXIMIZING THE NURSING PROCESS

The nursing process continues to be the basic framework for nursing practice with clients. A client can be an individual, a family, a group, or a community. The Standards of Psychiatric–Mental Health Clinical Nursing Practice (American Nurses Association [ANA], 1994) are authoritative statements that describe the responsibilities for which nurses are accountable, and provide direction for professional nursing practice and a framework for the evaluation of practice. The Psychiatric–Mental Health Clinical Nursing Practice standards define the nursing process within the context of six standards of care (see also Fig. 1–1):

Standard I—Assessment:	Gathering and organizing data
Standard II—Nursing diagnosis:	Identifying areas for intervention
Standard III—Outcome identification:	Setting outcome criteria (long/short-term goals)
Standard IV—Planning:	Planning actions to meet these goals
Standard V—Implementation:	Carrying out those actions
Standard VI—Evaluation:	Evaluating if long- and short-term goals (outcomes) are met

◆ ASSESSMENT

The assessment of a client's *psychosocial status* is a part of any nursing assessment, along with assessment of the client's physical

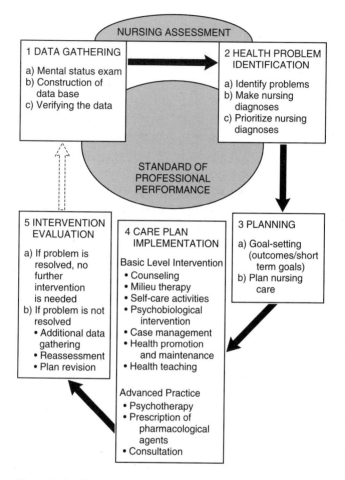

Figure 1–1 ◆ Standards of professional performance in the nursing process. (From Varcarolis, E. [1998]. *Foundations of Psychiatric Mental Health Nursing*, 3rd ed. Philadelphia: W.B. Saunders Company, p. 163; reprinted by permission.)

health. Depression, suicidal thoughts, anger, disorientation, delusions, and hallucinations may be encountered in medical-surgical wards, obstetrical and intensive care units, outpatient settings, extended care facilities, emergency departments, community centers, and home settings. The purpose of the assessment is to identify and clearly articulate specific problems in the individual's life that are causing physical or mental disequilibrium or harm. In order to help clients and their families, nurses define client problems/

processes that warrant intervention in very specific terms called *nursing diagnoses*. The assessment is the first step in identifying key nursing diagnoses.

The purpose of the *psychosocial assessment*, then, is to:

- **Establish a rapport**
- **Obtain an understanding of current illness**
- **Understand how this illness/process has affected the client's life** (self-esteem, loss of intimacy, role change, change in family dynamics, lifestyle change, employment issues)
- **Identify recent life changes or stressors** (refer to Chapter 15 for a useful tool)
- **Obtain information on previous psychiatric problems or disorder(s)**
- **Gather current lifestyle information** (social patterns, interests and abilities, how client handles stress, substance use and abuse, relationship issues)
- **Perform a mental status exam** (to identify dysfunctions in emotional, cognitive, or behavioral spheres) (See Chapter 12)
- **Formulate a plan of care**

A psychiatric nursing assessment contains both *subjective* and *objective* components. The basic components of the *psychosocial/ psychiatric nursing assessment* include a client's history (largely subjective) and a mental and emotional status evaluation (largely objective) (e.g., mental status exam). Because it is always preferable to verify one's data, family members should be a part of the assessment whenever possible. It is helpful for the nurse to know (1) if there is anything going on in the family, (2) how the family defines the problem(s), and (3) how the client's problems affect the family.

Friends and neighbors can also verify or contradict the client's self-perception and actions and may add data. If a police officer is the one who brought the client into the psychiatric emergency department, it is important for the nurse to know as much as possible about what the client was doing that warranted police intervention. Old charts and medical records can also offer background information. This is particularly important if the client is too psychotic, withdrawn, or agitated to provide a history. In many places this information may be easily available through the use of computer-based client records (CBRs). Laboratory reports also provide important information. When the body's chemistry is abnormal, personality changes and violent behaviors can result. For example, abnormal liver enzymes can explain irritability, depression, and lethargy.

The use of a standardized nursing assessment tool facilitates the assessment process. Many assessment forms are easily available;

for example, hospitals and clinics often have their own assessment tools. Even though an assessment tool is used, it is best to gather information from the client in an informal fashion, with the nurse clarifying, focusing, and exploring pertinent data with the client. This method allows clients to state their perceptions in their own words and enables the nurse to observe a wide range of nonverbal behaviors. When the order and the questions on the assessment tool are too rigidly applied, spontaneity is reduced. Assessment is a skill that is learned over time. Practice, supervision, and patience enhance the development of this skill. A personal style of interviewing congruent with the nurse's personality develops as comfort and experience increase.

Table 1–1 is an example of an assessment tool for use in the clinical area. Tables 1–2, 1–3, and 1–4 can help the nurse identify and define specific unfamiliar terms.

Another helpful tool that can give nurses and other health care workers important information about the client is the **multiaxial assessment** system of the American Psychiatric Association (APA) (1994) (Box 1–1).

❖　　　　　　B O X　　1 – 1　　　　　　❖
Multiaxial Assessment System

Axis I	Clinical Disorders
	Other Conditions That May Be a Focus of Clinical Attention
Axis II	Personality Disorders
	Mental Retardation
Axis III	General Medical Conditions
Axis IV	Psychosocial and Environmental Problems
Axis V	Global Assessment of Functioning

From American Psychiatric Association. (1994). Diagnostic and Statistical Manual of Mental Disorders, 4th ed. Washington, DC: American Psychiatric Press, p. 25; reprinted with permission. Copyright 1994 American Psychiatric Association.

Axes IV and V can give the nurse and others information that is important for setting realistic goals and planning effective care. **Axis IV—Psychosocial and Environmental Problems** identifies things going on in the client's life that may greatly impact the

---

Table 1–1 ◆ Comprehensive Nursing Assessment Tool

1. Client History

I. **GENERAL HISTORY OF CLIENT**
   Name _____ Age _____ Sex _____
   Racial and ethnic data _____
   Marital status _____
   Number and ages of children/siblings
   Living arrangements
   Occupation
   Education
   Spiritual beliefs and affiliations

II. **PRESENTING PROBLEM**
   A. Statement in the client's own words of why he or she is hospitalized or
      seeking help _____
      _____
      _____

   B. Recent difficulties/alterations in
      1. Relationships   3. Behavior
      2. Usual level of functioning   4. Perceptions or cognitive abilities

   C. Increased feelings of
      1. Depression   4. Being overwhelmed
      2. Anxiety   5. Suspiciousness
      3. Hopelessness   6. Confusion

   D. Somatic changes, such as
      1. Constipation   4. Weight loss or gain
      2. Insomnia   5. Palpitations
      3. Lethargy

III. **RELEVANT HISTORY—PERSONAL**
   A. Previous hospitalizations and illnesses _____

   B. Educational background _____

   C. Occupational background _____
      1. If employed, where? _____
      2. How long at that job? _____
      3. Previous positions and reasons for leaving _____
      4. Special skills _____

   D. Social patterns
      1. Describe friends _____
      2. Describe a usual day _____

   E. Sexual patterns
      1. Sexually active? _____
      2. Sexual orientation _____
      3. Sexual difficulties _____

   F. Interests and abilities
      1. What does the client do in his or her spare time? _____
      2. What is the client good at? _____
      3. What gives the client pleasure? _____

(Table continued on following page)

Table 1–1 ◆ Comprehensive Nursing Assessment Tool
(*Continued*)

    G. Substance use and abuse
       1. What nonprescription drugs does the client take? _____
         How often? _____ How much? _____
       2. How many drinks of alcohol does the client take per day? _____
         Per week? _____
       3. What meds (prescription and OTC) is the client taking? _____
         How often? _____ How much? _____

    H. How does the client cope with stress?
       1. What does the client do when he or she gets upset? _____
       2. Whom can the client talk to? _____
       3. What usually helps to relieve stress? _____
       4. What did the client try this time? _____

IV. RELEVANT HISTORY—FAMILY
    A. Childhood
       1. Who was important to the client growing up? _____
       2. Was there physical or sexual abuse? _____
       3. Did the parents drink or use drugs? _____
       4. Who was in the home when the client was growing up? _____

    B. Adolescence
       1. How would the client describe his or her feelings in adolescence? ____
         _____
       2. Describe the client's peer group at that time. _____

    C. Use of drugs
       1. Was there use or abuse of drugs by any family member? _____
         Prescription _____ Street _____ By whom? _____
       2. What was the effect on the family? _____

    D. Family physical or mental problems
       1. Who in the family had physical or mental problems? _____
       2. Describe the problems. _____
       3. How did it affect the family? _____

    E. Was there an unusual or outstanding event the client would like to
       mention? _____

2. Mental and Emotional Status
    A. Appearance
       Physical handicaps _____
       Dress appropriate _____ Sloppy _____
       Grooming neat _____ Poor _____
       Eye contact held _____ Describe posture _____

    B. Behavior*
       Restless _____ Agitated _____ Lethargic _____
       Mannerisms _____ Facial expressions _____ Other _____

    C. Speech
       Clear _____ Mumbled _____ Rapid _____ Slurred _____
       Constant _____ Mute or silent _____ Barriers to communication _____
       Specify (e.g., client has delusions or is confused, withdrawn, or
       verbose) _____

    D. Mood
       What mood does the client convey? _____

E. Affect
   What is the client's affect? (bland, apathetic, dramatic, bizarre, or appropriate?)
   Describe _____

F. Thought process*
   1. Characteristics
      Describe the characteristics of the person's responses:
      Looseness of association _____ Blocking _____ Concrete _____
      Confabulation _____ Tangential _____ Flights of ideas _____
      Describe _____
   2. Cognitive ability
      Proverbs: Concrete _____ Abstract _____
      Serial sevens: How far does the client go? _____
      Can the client do simple math? _____
      What seems to be the reason for poor concentration? _____
      _____

G. Thought content*
   1. Central theme: What is important to the client? _____
      Describe _____
   2. Self-concept: How does the client view him- or herself? _____
      What does the client want to change about him- or herself? _____
   3. Insight? Does the client realistically assess his or her symptoms? _____
      Realistically appraise his or her situation? _____
   4. Suicidal or homicidal ideation? _____ What is suicide potential? _____
      Family history of suicide or homicide attempt or successful completion? _____
      _____
      Explain _____
      Preoccupations*: does the client have hallucinations? _____
      Delusions _____ Obsessions _____ Rituals _____ Phobias _____
      Grandiosity _____ Religiosity _____ Worthlessness _____
      Describe _____

H. Reality orientation
   Time: _____
   Place: _____
   Person: _____
   Memory: _____

I. Level of anxiety
   Mild   Data _____
   Moderate   Data _____
   Severe   Data _____
   Panic   Data _____

OTC, over the counter.
Adapted from Varcarolis, E. (1998). Foundations of Psychiatric Mental Health
Nursing, 3rd ed. Philadelphia: W.B. Saunders Company, p. 996–998; reprinted with
permission.

client's life, or may in themselves be the primary focus of clinical
attention. Examples of Axis IV problems include (APA, 1994):

- **Problems with primary support groups** (deaths, illness, divorce, sexual/physical abuse, neglect of child, discord with siblings, birth of a sibling)
- **Problems related to the social environment** (death or loss of friends, inadequate social support, living alone, difficulty with

Table 1–2 ◆ Abnormal Motor Behaviors

BEHAVIOR	DEFINITION	EXAMPLE
Echopraxia	Repeating the movements of another person.	Every time the nurse would move or gesture with her hands, the client would copy her gestures.
Echolalia	Repeating the speech of another person.	The nurse said to the client, "Tell me your name." The client responded, "Tell me your name, tell me your name."
Waxy Flexibility	Having one's arms or legs placed in a certain position and holding that same position for hours.	The nurse lifted the client's arm to check the pulse, and the client left his arm extended in the same position.
Parkinson-like Symptoms	Making mask-like faces, drooling, and having shuffling gait, tremors, and muscular rigidity. Seen in people who are on antipsychotic medication, such as phenothiazines.	The nurse noticed that the client's face held no emotion. He walked very stiffly, leaning forward, almost robot-like.
Akathisia	Displaying motor restlessness, feeling of muscular quivering; at its worst, patient is unable to sit still or lie quietly.	The client's leg kept jiggling up and down when he talked to the nurse. When his feet were still, his arm would jiggle constantly during the interview.
Dyskinesia	Having distortion of voluntary movements, such as involuntary muscular activity (e.g., tic, spasm, or myoclonus).	The client had a marked facial tic around his mouth, which was distracting to the nurse during the interview.

From Varcarolis, E. (1998). Foundations of Psychiatric Mental Health Nursing, 3rd ed. Philadelphia: W.B. Saunders Company, p. 999; reprinted with permission.

acculturation, discrimination, adjustment to life-cycle transition [e.g., retirement])
- **Educational problems** (illiteracy, academic problems, discord with teachers or classmates, inadequate school environment)
- **Occupational problems** (unemployment, threat of job loss, stressful work schedule, difficult work conditions, job dissatisfaction, job change, discord with boss or co-workers)
- **Economic problems** (extreme poverty, inadequate finances, insufficient welfare support)
- **Problems with access to health care services** (inadequate health care services, transportation to health care facilities unavailable, inadequate health insurance)
- **Problems related to interaction with the legal system/crime** (arrest, incarceration, litigation, victim of crime)

Axis V—Global Assessment of Functioning is the clinician's judgment of the client's overall level of functioning. This information helps the health care team plan treatment and predict outcomes. (See Box 1–2 for the Global Assessment of Functioning Scale.)

❖   B O X   1 – 2   ❖
Global Assessment of Functioning (GAF) Scale

Consider psychological, social, and occupational functioning on a hypothetical continuum of mental health–illness. Do not include impairment in functioning due to physical (or environmental) limitations.

Code   (**Note:** Use intermediate codes when appropriate, e.g., 45, 68, 72.)

100   **Superior functioning in a wide range of activities, life's problems never seem to get out of hand, is sought out by others because of his or her many**
91   **positive qualities. No symptoms.**

90   **Absent or minimal symptoms** (e.g., mild anxiety before an exam), **good functioning in all areas, interested and involved in a wide range of activities, socially effective, generally satisfied with life, no more than everyday problems or concerns** (e.g., an
81   occasional argument with family members).

Continued

| 80 | **If symptoms are present, they are transient and expectable reactions to psychosocial stressors** (e.g., difficulty concentrating after family argument); **no more than slight impairment in social, occupational, or school functioning** (e.g., temporarily falling |
| 71 | behind in schoolwork). |

| 70 | **Some mild symptoms** (e.g., depressed mood and mild insomnia) **OR some difficulty in social, occupational, or school functioning** (e.g., occasional truancy, or theft within the household), **but generally functioning pretty well, has some meaningful inter-** |
| 61 | **personal relationships.** |

| 60 | **Moderate symptoms** (e.g., flat affect and circumstantial speech, occasional panic attacks) **OR moderate difficulty in social, occupational, or school functioning** (e.g., few friends, conflicts with peers or |
| 51 | co-workers). |

| 50 | **Serious symptoms** (e.g., suicidal ideation, severe obsessional rituals, frequent shoplifting) **OR any serious impairment in social, occupational, or school** |
| 41 | **functioning** (e.g., no friends, unable to keep a job). |

| 40 | **Some impairment in reality testing or communication** (e.g., speech is at times illogical, obscure, or irrelevant) **OR major impairment in several areas, such as work or school, family relations, judgment, thinking, or mood** (e.g., depressed man avoids friends, neglects family, and is unable to work; child frequently beats up younger children, is defiant at |
| 31 | home, and is failing at school). |

| 30 | **Behavior is considerably influenced by delusions or hallucinations OR serious impairment in communication or judgment** (e.g., sometimes incoherent, acts grossly inappropriately, suicidal preoccupation) **OR inability to function in almost all areas** |
| 21 | (e.g., stays in bed all day; no job, home, or friends). |

| 20 | **Some danger of hurting self or others** (e.g., suicide attempts without clear expectation of death; frequently violent; manic excitement) **OR occasionally fails to maintain minimal personal hygiene** (e.g., smears feces) **OR gross impairment in communica-** |
| 11 | **tion** (e.g., largely incoherent or mute). |

Continued

10 1	**Persistent danger of severely hurting self or others** (e.g., recurrent violence) **OR persistent inability to maintain minimal personal hygiene OR serious suicidal act with clear expectation of death.**
0	Inadequate information.

After the nurse has conducted the initial assessment, it is useful to summarize pertinent data with the client. This summary provides clients with reassurance that they have been heard, and it allows them the opportunity to clarify any misinformation. They should then be told what will happen next. For example, if the initial assessment takes place in the hospital, the nurse should tell the client whom else the client will be seeing. If a psychiatric nurse in a mental health clinic conducts the initial assessment, the nurse will let the client know when and how often they will meet to work on the client's problems. If the nurse thinks a referral is necessary (e.g., to a psychiatrist, social worker, or medical physician), he or she will discuss this with the client.

Assessment of a Non–English-Speaking Client

More and more English-speaking nurses are caring for clients who are non–English speaking. If a nurse does not speak a given client's language, data gathering can be extremely difficult. It is to a nurse's benefit, when working with a majority of clients who speak a specific language (e.g., Spanish), to learn at the very least relevant words, phrases, and questions in that language. The Americans with Disabilities Act (ADA) has established federal standards that ensure that communication does not interfere with equal access to health care for all people. All health care establishments are to establish systems for identifying available language interpreters, interpreters trained in sign language, telecommunication devices for the deaf (TDDs), closed-caption decoders for televisions, and amplifiers on phones (Gorman et al., 1996).

Therefore, nurses must often rely on interpreters. Interpreters may be family members, friends or neighbors, employees within the health care institution who have other responsibilities, or professional interpreters. Each group may have their drawbacks. For

Text continued on page 18

Table 1–3 ◆ Summary of Abnormal Thought Processes

THOUGHT PROCESS	DEFINITION	EXAMPLE
Tangentiality	Association disturbance in which the speaker goes off the topic. When it happens frequently and the speaker does not return to the topic, interpersonal communication is destroyed.	The nurse asked the client to talk more about his family. The client continuously left the topic and talked about boats, animals, his apartment, and so forth. Each time the nurse tried to help the client to focus, he would go off on another topic.
Neologisms	Words a person makes up that have meaning only for the person himself, often part of a delusional system.	"I am afraid to go to the hospital because the *norks* are looking for me there."
Looseness of Association	Thinking is haphazard, illogical, and confused. Connections in thought are interrupted. Seen mostly in schizophrenic disorders.	"Can't go to the zoo, no money, Oh . . . I have a hat, these members make no sense, man . . . What's the problem?"
Flights of Ideas	Constant flow of speech in which the person jumps from one topic to another in rapid succession. There is a connection between some topics, although it is sometimes hard to identify. Characteristically seen in manic states.	"Say babe, how's it going . . . Going to my sister's to get money . . . money, honey, you got any bread . . . bread and butter, staff of life, ain't life grand?"
Blocking	Sudden cessation of a thought in the middle of a sentence. Person is unable to continue his train of thought. Often sudden new thoughts crop up unrelated to the topic. Can be disturbing to the individual.	"I was going to get a new dress for the . . . I forgot what I was going to say."

Circumstantiality	Before getting to the point or answering a question, the person gets caught up in countless details and explanations.	"Where are you going for the weekend, Harry?" "Well I first thought of going to my mother's, but that was before I remembered that she was going to my sister's. My sister is having a picnic. She always has picnics at the beach. The beach that she goes to is large and gets crowded. That's why I don't like that beach. So I decided to go someplace else. I thought of going to by brother's house. He has a large house on a quiet street. . . . I finally decided to stay home."
Perseveration	Involuntary repetition of the same thought, phrase, or motor response to different questions or situations. Associated with brain damage.	N: How are you doing, Harry? H: Fine, nurse, just fine. N: Did you go for a walk? H: Fine, nurse, just fine. N: Are you going out today? H: Fine, nurse, just fine.
Confabulation	Filling in a memory gap with detailed fantasy believed by the teller. The purpose is to maintain self-esteem; seen in organic conditions, such as Korsakoff's psychosis	The nurse asked Harry, who spent the weekend at home, what he did for the weekend. "Well, I just came back from California after signing a contract with MGM for a film on the life of Roosevelt. We had the most marvelous tour of the studio . . . went to lunch with the director . . ."
Word Salad	Mixture of words and phrases that have no meaning.	"I am fine . . . apple pie . . . no sale . . . furniture store . . . take it slow . . . cellar door . . ."

From Varcarolis, E. (1998). Foundations of Psychiatric Mental Health Nursing, 3rd ed. Philadelphia: W.B. Saunders Company, p. 1000; reprinted with permission.

Table 1–4 ◆ Preoccupation in Thought Content

THOUGHT CONTENT	DEFINITION	EXAMPLE
Hallucinations	A sense of perception for which no external stimuli exist. Hallucinations can have an organic or a functional etiology.	
	Visual: Seeing things that are not there.	During alcohol withdrawal he kept shouting, "I see snakes on the walls."
	Auditory: Hearing voices when none are present.	"I keep hearing my mother's voice telling me I am bad. She died a year ago."
	Olfactory: Smelling smells that do not exist.	"I smell my stomach rotting."
	Tactile: Feeling touch sensations in the absence of stimuli. (Also referred to as haptic.)	A paranoid man feels electrical impulses "from outer space" entering his body and controlling his mind.
	Gustatory: Experiencing taste in the absence of stimuli.	A paranoid woman tastes poison in her food while eating at her son's wedding.
Delusions	A false belief held to be true even with evidence to the contrary. Three common delusions follow:	
	Persecution: The thought that one is being singled out for harm by others.	An intern believes that the chief of staff is plotting to kill him to prevent the intern from becoming too powerful.
	Grandeur: The false belief that one is a very powerful and important person.	A newly admitted patient told the nurse that he was God, and he was here to save the world.
	Jealousy: The false belief that one's mate is going out with other people. The person may take everyday occurrences for "proof."	Sally "knew" that her husband, Jim, was being unfaithful. Even when Sally's brother swore he and Jim really did play pool Friday nights, Sally declared Jim's not being home then was her "proof."

Obsessions	An idea, impulse, or emotion that a person cannot put out of his or her consciousness. Can be mild or severe.	A young mother, Jane, told the nurse that she was hounded by constant thoughts that something terrible was going to happen to her baby. She knew that this was crazy, but she could not get the thought to stop.
Rituals	Repetitive actions that people must do over and over until either they are exhausted or anxiety is decreased. Often done to lessen the anxiety triggered by an obsession.	Jane stated to the nurse the only way she could temporarily get these obsessions to cease was to say three "Hail Marys" and knock on wood twice to reassure herself that "nothing terrible was happening."
Phobias	An intense irrational fear of an object, situation, or place. The fear persists even though the object of the fear is perfectly harmless and the person is aware of the irrationality.	Although she was aware that cats would not harm her, Mary was deathly afraid of cats and refused to visit her sister and friends who had cats.

From Varcarolis, E. (1998). Foundations of Psychiatric Mental Health Nursing, 3rd ed. Philadelphia: W.B. Saunders Company. p. 1001; reprinted with permission.

example, a family interpreter may want to protect the client and filter out information given to the client. Conversely, the family member may want to filter out information about a problem or crisis in the family, and not clearly relay the information back to the nurse. It is best to avoid a family member acting as an interpreter. Family members acting as interpreters should be avoided altogether when the client is a child. Employees with other jobs who speak English as a second language may have difficulty understanding the information you wish to convey. Friends and neighbors may find it embarrassing to discuss private and personal matters. The nurse can explore the use of the AT&T Interpreter Service.

Gorman and associates (1996) make the following suggestions when working through an interpreter:

- **Address the client directly** rather than speaking to the interpreter. Maintain eye contact with the client to ensure client involvement and strengthen personal contact.
- **Avoid interrupting the client and interpreter.** At times their interaction may take longer because of the need to clarify issues. Descriptions may require more time because of dialect differences, or the interpreter's awareness that the client needs more preparation before being asked a particular question.
- **Instruct the interpreter to give you verbatim translations.**
- **Avoid using medical jargon** that the interpreter, or the client for that matter, may not understand.
- **Avoid talking or commenting to the interpreter at length;** the client may feel left out and distrustful.
- **Always ask for permission to discuss intimate or emotionally laden topics** first, and prepare the interpreter for the content of the interview.
- **Be aware that asking intimate or emotionally laden questions may be difficult for the client as well as for the interpreter.** Lead up to these questions slowly.
- **Whenever possible, arrange for the interpreter and the client to meet each other ahead of time** to establish some rapport.
- **Try to use the same interpreter** for succeeding interviews with the client.

When an interpreter is not immediately available, aids such as picture charts or flash cards can help the nurse and the client communicate important basic information about the client's immediate needs (e.g., degree of pain or need for elimination).

Because of cultural backgrounds or wanting to be helpful, some clients with limited English may tend to appear agreeable and nod "yes" even though they do not understand. Asking questions that require more than a yes-or-no answer can give you a better idea of the client's level of understanding.

◆ NURSING DIAGNOSIS

A nursing diagnosis is a clinical judgment about individual, family, or community responses to actual or potential health problems/life processes (North American Nursing Diagnosis Association [NANDA], 1999). This clinical judgment is derived through a deliberate, systematic process of data collection and analysis. A nursing diagnosis provides the basis for selection of nursing interventions chosen to achieve outcomes for which the nurse is accountable (NANDA, 1999). A nursing diagnosis is expressed concisely and includes the etiology ("Related To's") of the condition and is supported by objective and subjective data ("As Evidenced By's"). (See Appendix B for current nursing diagnoses in use.) Nursing diagnoses are updated every 2 years by NANDA in the *Nursing Diagnosis: Definitions and Classifications.* Nursing diagnoses are added and updated based on research and clinical evaluation.

Physicians and researchers also have formulated clear and accurate guidelines for identifying and categorizing clinical psychiatric disorders and syndromes. The APA provides specific criteria that must be met before a medical psychiatric diagnosis is arrived at. The most current of these criteria is found in the ***Diagnostic and Statistical Manual of Mental Disorders, Fourth Edition*** (**DSM-IV**) (APA, 1994). In each clinical chapter in this manual, the DSM-IV criteria will be provided as well as the appropriate nursing diagnosis. The classification system used for medical diseases and medical treatments is found in the ***International Classification of Diseases, Tenth Edition*** (**ICD-10**) (World Health Organization, 1992).

Therefore, the psychiatric–mental health nurse uses nursing diagnoses and standard classifications of mental disorders (DSM-IV), as well as the standard international classification of diseases (ICD-10), to develop a treatment plan based on assessment data and theoretical premises.

A nursing diagnosis has three structural components: (1) problem/process, (2) etiology (Related To's), and (3) supporting data (As Evidenced By's).

Problem/Process

The nursing diagnostic title states what should change, for example:

Risk for injury

Etiology (Related To's)

The etiology includes probable cause or factors that contribute to or are *related to* the development or maintenance of a nursing diagnosis title. Stating the etiology or probable cause tells what needs to be done to effect change, and identifies causes that the nurse can treat through interventions. Etiology is linked to the diagnostic title with the words "related to." Therefore, the "related to" component of the nursing diagnosis needs to be defined as clearly as possible, because it tells you what needs to be targeted. Take the following two examples:

Risk for injury: *related to extreme agitation and constant, uncontrollable motor activity*

This activity is a probable nursing diagnosis for a client in the manic phase of bipolar disorder. In this case the potential for injury is *related to* uncontrollable hyperactivity in a person who is unable to use his or her usual problem-solving skills to avoid harm. Contrast this with the same nursing diagnostic title for a woman who is being constantly battered by her mate:

Risk for injury: *related to mate's poor impulse control and rage reaction*

In this case probable cause for injury is *related to* a woman living with a physically violent partner, in a situation that she believes she cannot leave (fear for her life, no way to support herself financially, fear for her children).

Supporting Data (As Evidenced By's)

Supporting signs and symptoms (As Evidenced By's) are the defining characteristics that cluster in patterns and support the validity of the diagnosis (NANDA, 1994). Therefore, one can assume that, after interventions have been made and are successful, these signs and symptoms would no longer be present or a problem for the client.

For example, using the situation above, manic clients may have observable signs and symptoms that alert the medical staff that injury or potential for injury is present and requires nursing/

medical interventions. The client may have bruises or wounds resulting from falls, may suffer from lack of sleep as a result of constant physical activity, may have dehydration from not drinking or eating related to hyperactivity or an inability to concentrate on the task of eating/drinking, and may be near exhaustion or even cardiac collapse. A complete nursing diagnostic statement would then read:

> Risk for injury: related to extreme agitation and constant, uncontrollable motor activity *as evidenced by less than 2 hours' rest a night, poor skin turgor, and abrasions on hands and arms.*

Members of the health team would expect to see the client obtain adequate rest or sleep (e.g., 6 hours per night), good skin turgor, and an ability on the client's part to rest and refrain from agitated physical activity for frequent periods during the day as the final outcome of effective medical and nursing interventions.

Summary

From data, nurses make clinical judgments about an individual's, family's, or community's response to actual or potential health problems/life processes and formulate nursing diagnoses accordingly. The nurse then plans and provides nursing actions that target the client's health problem or life process.

◆ OUTCOME IDENTIFICATION

Outcome criteria describe in behavioral or measurable terms the desired results of nursing interventions planned for a client. Outcome criteria also provide the basis for evaluating the effectiveness of care. Outcome criteria are essentially *goals* stated in behavioral or measurable terms and may have time factors (in 1 week, by discharge, within 2 days) or may be end results, or hoped-for results. They may also indicate a future steady state, for example:

- Client will function independently in the community with aid of social support, or
- Client will refrain from self-harm.

so that they can be evaluated and revised as the client progresses. These goals are always client centered (not staff centered) and can be short term or long term. Goals are only useful if they are reasonable and attainable within a specified time period. The short-term goals for each nursing diagnosis can include a variety of steps leading to the final outcome criteria. Some of these goals will be attained in varying amounts of time by different clients. Because each client and situation is unique, a goal that takes a long time to reach by one client may be quickly reached by another. For some clients, the final outcome criteria may not be realistic goals, whereas for other clients the goals may be not only realistic but easily attainable. Goals that are difficult to attain for one client may be readily attainable for others. For these reasons, the nurse needs to use good judgment based on the client's database to identify realistic outcome criteria, and select appropriate goals to reach the final long-term goal (outcome criteria).

For example, for the above-stated nursing diagnosis:

Risk for injury: related to extreme agitation and constant, uncontrollable motor activity as evidenced by less than 2 hours' rest a night, poor skin turgor, and abrasions on hands and arms.

Possible outcome criteria:

- By discharge, client will be sleeping 6 to 8 hours per night.
- Client will willingly maintain an adequate diet (1500 to 2000 cal) and fluids by the time of discharge.
- Client will be free from infections and abrasions/wounds will be in final healing stages by time of discharge.
- Client will continue attendance at support group within the community.
- Client will adhere to medication regimen.

Possible short-term goals (outcomes) might include:

- Client will sleep 3 to 4 hours per night within 2 days with the aid of medication.
- Client will drink 8 oz of fluid (juice, milk, milkshake) every hour with the aid of nursing intervention.
- Client's skin turgor will be within normal limits within 24 hours.
- Client will spend 10 minutes in a quiet, nonstimulating area with nurse each hour during the day.

◆ PLANNING

Each stated goal should include nursing interventions, which are instructions for all people working with the client. These written plans aid in the continuity of care for the client and are points of information for all members of the health team. More and more units, in both inpatient and community-based facilities, use standardized care plans or clinical/critical pathways for clients with specific diagnoses. However, even standardized care plans and critical pathways need to be tailored to specific clients, and there are often places on the standardized forms for client-centered revisions. Nursing interventions planned for meeting a specific goal need to be:

Safe: They must be safe for the client as well as for other clients, staff, and family.

Appropriate: They must be compatible with other therapies and with the client's personal goals and cultural values, as well as with institutional rules.

Effective: They should be based on scientific principles.

Individualized: They should be realistic: (1) written within the capabilities of the client's age, physical strength, condition, and willingness to change; (2) based on the number of staff available; (3) reflective of actual available community resources; and (4) within the student's or nurses' capabilities.

◆ IMPLEMENTATION

Implementation is the actions the nursing staff takes to carry out the nursing measures identified in the care plan in order to achieve the expected outcome criteria. Nursing interventions may be called actions, approaches, nursing orders, or nursing prescriptions. When carrying out the nursing interventions, additional data may be gathered and further refinements of the care plan may be made.

The Standards of Psychiatric–Mental Health Clinical Nursing Practice (ANA, 1994) identified 10 areas for intervention for psychiatric nurses. Recent graduates and practitioners new to the psychiatric setting will participate in many of these activities. Interventions at the *basic level* include:

1. Counseling
2. Milieu therapy
3. Self-care activities
4. Psychobiological interventions
5. Health teaching
6. Case management
7. Health promotion and health maintenance

The psychiatric–mental health advanced practice registered nurse is prepared at the master's level or beyond. *Advanced practice interventions* include:

8. Psychotherapy
9. Prescription of pharmacological agents (in several but not all states)
10. Consultations and referrals

♦ EVALUATION

Evaluation is often the most neglected part of the nursing process. Ideally, evaluation should be part of each phase in the process. Evaluation of the outcome criteria (long- and short-term goals) can have three possible outcomes: The goal is either met, not met, or partially met. Using our original example from above for the nursing diagnosis:

> Risk for injury: related to extreme agitation and constant, uncontrollable motor activity as evidenced by less than 2 hours' rest a night, poor skin turgor, and abrasions on hands and arms.

For the short-term goal (outcome):

• Client will drink 8 oz of fluid (juice, milk, milkshake) every hour during the day with the aid of nursing intervention.

In evaluation, the nurse might chart:

> *Goal met*: Client takes frequent sips of fluid equaling 8 oz an hour provided in portable containers with lid, during the hours of 9 AM to 4 PM with reminders from nursing staff.

For the short-term goal (outcome):

• Client will spend 10 minutes in a quiet, nonstimulating area with nurse each hour during the day.

In evaluation, the nurse might chart:

> *Goal partially met*: After 2 days client continues restless and purposeless pacing up and down the halls, and is only able to stay quiet with nurse for 4 to 6 minutes an hour.

For the short-term goal (outcome):

• Client's skin turgor will be within normal limits within 24 hours as evidenced by skin pinched over sternum and released, raised—area disappears in 3 seconds or less.

In evaluation, the nurse might chart:

> *Goal not met*: At 8:00 AM this morning client's skin turgor still poor. Pinched skin over sternum disappeared 4 seconds post-release. Evaluate need for increasing daytime fluids from 9 AM to 9 PM.

The chapters in Parts II and III of this book present specific psychiatric clinical disorders and phenomena that may require nursing interventions. Under each disorder or phenomenon, the most common nursing diagnoses are presented. Suggested outcomes and short-term goals are offered for each nursing diagnosis. Outcome criteria are the final long-term goals that signal that the nursing diagnosis should no longer be a target for intervention.

Keep in mind that all goals are tailored to each client's current level of functioning and realistic potential. For that reason one person's short-term outcome might be appropriately another's long-term outcome.

For each nursing diagnosis, specific nursing actions are suggested with supporting rationales. This clinical reference guide is intended to help nurses formulate well-stated nursing diagnoses, set realistic outcome criteria with suggested steps (short-term goals) to reach the final outcome. Realistic and appropriate nursing interventions are provided and nurses identify which are appropriate to their clients. Some of the interventions are well within the student's realm; others may be better suited to a more advanced practitioner. They are all included to help give a more thorough overview of what constitutes nursing interventions. This clinical nursing guide is intended for students in planning care, as a guide to staff new to a psychiatric unit, and for clinicians as a quick clinical reference.

◆ INTERNET SITES OF INTEREST

Nursing Net
Information and web links for students as well as seasoned nurses
http://www.nursingnet.org

Lesson: Nursing Process
A lesson in the online class NUR301: Perspectives in Professional Nursing, on the Northern Arizona University Web site
http://jan.ucc.nau.edu/~erw/nur301/practice/process/lesson.html

American Nurses Association
http://www.nursingworld.org

CHAPTER 2

Communication and Counseling Tools

Peplau (1952) identified two main principles that guide the communication process during the nurse-client interview. Those two main principles are (1) clarity and (2) continuity. *Clarity* means that the meaning of the message is accurately understood by both parties. *Continuity* promotes the connection among ideas "and the feelings, events, or themes conveyed in those ideas." This chapter offers a way to use and categorize your communication techniques, and it is hoped it will help you to enhance your ability to follow both of these principles.

Communication and interviewing techniques are acquired skills. Nurses learn to increase their ability to use communication and interviewing skills through practice and supervision. Communication is a complex process that can involve a variety of personal and environmental factors that may distort the sending and receiving of messages. Example include:

Personal Factors: emotions (mood), knowledge level, language use, attitudes, and bias

Social Factors: previous experience, culture, language, health beliefs and practice

Environmental Factors: physical factors (background noise, lack of privacy, uncomfortable accommodations) and societal factors (presence of others, expectations of others)

Communication consists of *verbal* and *nonverbal* elements. Communication is roughly 10% verbal and 90% nonverbal (Shea, 1998). Nonverbal communication consists of an amalgam of feelings, feedback, local wisdom, cultural rhythms, ways to avoid confrontation, and unconscious views of how the world works. When we try to communicate only in words, the results range from the humorous to the destructive (Hall, 1983).

◆ VERBAL COMMUNICATION

Verbal communication consists of all words a person speaks. Talking is our most common activity. Talking links us with others, it is our primary instrument of instruction, and one of the most personal aspects of our private life. When we speak, we:

- Communicate our beliefs, values, attitudes, and culture
- Communicate perceptions and meanings
- Convey interests and understanding *or* insult and judgment
- Convey messages clearly or convey conflicting *or* implied messages
- Convey clear, honest feelings *or* disguised, distorted feelings

Verbal communication can become misunderstood and garbled even among people with the same primary language and/or from the same cultural background. In our multiethnic society, keeping communication clear and congruent takes thought and insight. Communication styles, eye contact, and touch all have different meanings and are used and interpreted very differently among cultures. Ensuring that your verbal message is what you mean to convey, and that the message you send is the same message that the other person receives, is a complicated skill.

At times people convey conflicting messages. A person will say one thing verbally, but convey the opposite in their nonverbal behavior. This is called a **double message** or **mixed message**. As in the saying, "actions speak louder than words," actions are often interpreted as the true meaning of a person's intent, whether that intent is conscious or unconscious. For example:

> A young man came to counseling because he was not making good grades in school and feared that he wouldn't be able to get into medical school. He appears bright and resourceful, and states he has good study habits. In the course of the session, he tells the nurse that he is a star on the tennis team, is president of his fraternity, and has an active and successful social life, "If you know what I mean." Implied in this exchange appears to be a double message. The verbal message is "I want good grades to get into medical school." The nonverbal message is that what is important to him is spending a great deal of time excelling at a sport, heading a social club, and in dating activities.

Dee (1991) suggests that one way a nurse can respond to verbal and nonverbal incongruity (double messages) is to reflect and validate the individual's thoughts and feelings. For example:

> "You say you are unhappy with your grades and as a consequence may not be able to get into medical school. Yet, from

what I hear you say, you seem to be filling up your time excelling in so many other activities that there is very little time left for adequate preparation for excelling in your main goal, that of getting into medical school. I wonder what you think about this apparent contradiction in priorities?"

◆ NONVERBAL COMMUNICATION

Nonverbal communication consists of the behaviors displayed by an individual. Tone of voice and manner in which a person paces speech are example of nonverbal communication. Other common examples of nonverbal communication (called *cues*) are facial expressions, body posture, amount of eye contact, eye cast (emotion expressed in the eyes), hand gestures, sighs, fidgeting, and yawning. Table 2–1 identifies some key components of nonverbal communication.

Sometimes gestures and other nonverbal cues can have opposite meanings depending on culture and context. For example, eye contact can be perceived as comforting and supportive or as invasive and intimidating. Touching a client gently on the arm can be experienced as supportive and caring, or threatening or sexual. Facial expressions such as a smile can appear to convey warmth and interest, or hide feelings of fear or anger.

Many nonverbal cues have cultural meaning. For example, in some Asian cultures, avoiding eye contact shows respect. Conversely, in many people with French, British, and African American backgrounds, avoidance of eye contact by another person may be interpreted as disinterest, not telling the truth, avoiding the sharing of important information, or dictated by social order.

There are numerous ways to interpret verbal and nonverbal communications for each cultural and subcultural group. Even if a nurse is aware of how a specific cultural group responds to, say, touch, the nurse could still be in error when dealing with an individual within that cultural group. Sustaining effective and respectful communication is very complex. It is the task of nurses to identify and explore the meaning of clients' nonverbal and verbal behaviors. Listed at the end of the chapter are Internet sites that provide further cultural information for health care professionals.

◆ EFFECTIVE COUNSELING AND COMMUNICATION TECHNIQUES
Degree of Openness

Any question or statement can be classified as (1) an open-ended verbalization, (2) a focused question, or (3) a closed-ended verbal-

Table 2–1 ◆ Nonverbal Behaviors

TYPE	POSSIBLE BEHAVIORS	EXAMPLE
Body Behaviors	Posture, body movements, gestures, gait	The client is slumped in a chair, puts her face in her hands, and occasionally taps her right foot.
Facial Expressions	Frowns, smiles, grimaces, raised eyebrows, pursed lips, licking lips, tongue movements	The client grimaces when speaking to the nurse; when alone, he smiles and giggles to himself.
Eye Cast	Angry, suspicious, and accusatory looks	The client squints his eyes, the pupils dilated.
Voice-Related Behaviors	Tone, pitch, level, intensity, inflection, stuttering, pauses, silences, fluency	The client talks in a loud, sing-song voice.
Observable Autonomic Physiologic Responses	Increase in respirations, diaphoresis, pupil dilation blushing, paleness	When the client mentions discharge, she becomes pale, her respirations increase, and her face becomes diaphoretic.
General Appearance	Grooming, dress, hygiene	The client is dressed in a wrinkled shirt and his pants are stained; his socks are dirty and he wears no shoes.
Physical Characteristics	Height, weight, physique, complexion	The client appears grossly overweight for his height and his muscle tone appears flabby.

From Varcarolis, E. (1998). Foundations of Psychiatric Mental Health Nursing, 3rd ed. Philadelphia: W.B. Saunders Company, p. 185; reprinted with permission.

ization. Furthermore, any question or statement can be classified along the *continuum of openness*. There are three variables that influence where any given verbalization sits on this openness continuum (Shea, 1998):

1. The degree to which the verbalization tends to produce spontaneous and lengthy response
2. The degree to which the verbalization does not limit the client's answer set
3. The degree to which the verbalization opens up a moderately resistant client

Refer to Table 2–2 during the following discussion.

Open-Ended Questions

Open-ended questions require more than one-word answers (e.g., a "yes" or "no"). Even with a client who is sullen, resistant, or guarded, open-ended questions can encourage lengthy information on experiences, perceptions of events, or responses to a situation. Examples of an open-ended question are: "What are some of the stresses you are grappling with?" "What do you perceive to be your biggest problem at the moment?" "Tell me something about your family."

Shea (1998) encourages the use of frequent open-ended questions or gentle inquiries (e.g., "Tell me about . . ."; "Share with me . . ."). This is especially helpful when beginning a relationship and in the early interviews. Although the initial responses may be short, after time the responses often become more informative as the client becomes more at ease. This is an especially valuable technique for clients who are resistant or guarded, but is a good rule for opening phases of any interview and especially in the early phase of establishing a rapport with an individual.

Closed-Ended Questions

Closed-ended questions, in contrast, are questions that ask for specific information (dates, names, numbers, "yes" or "no" information). These are closed-ended questions because they limit the client's freedom of choice. For example:

"Is your mother alive?"
"When were you born?"
"Did you seek therapy after your first suicide attempt?"
"Do you think the medication is helping you?"

Closed-ended questions give specific information when needed, such as during an initial assessment or intake interview, or to as-

Table 2–2 ◆ Degree of Openness Continuum

VERBALIZATION	EXAMPLE
Open ended	These questions are to be stated with a gentle tone of voice while expressing a genuine interest. They invite the client to share personal experiences. They cannot be answered with a "yes" or "no."
1. Open-ended questions (giving broad openings)	1. What would you like to discuss? 2. What are your plans for the future? 3. How will you approach your father? 4. What are some of your thoughts about the marriage?
2. Gentle commands (encouraging descriptions of perceptions)	1. Tell me something about your home life? 2. Share with me some of your hopes about your future. 3. Describe for me the problem with your boss.
Focused	These questions represent a middle ground with regard to openness. When the relationship is strong, these questions can result in spontaneous lengthy speech. Used with a resistant client, these questions may be answered tersely.
1. Exploring/focusing	1. Can you describe your feelings? 2. Can you tell me a little about your boss? 3. Can you say anything positive about your marriage? 4. Can you tell me what the voices are saying?
2. Qualitative questions	1. How's your appetite? 2. How's your job going? 3. How's your mood been?
3. Statements of inquiry (restating, reflecting, paraphrasing, clarifying)	1. You say you were fifth in your class? 2. So you left the marriage after 3 years? 3. So when she cries you feel guilty? 4. You seem to be saying that you're viewed as the bad guy in the family? 5. Give me an example of your being "no good."
4. Empathetic statements (making observations, sharing perceptions, seeking clarification)	1. It sounds like a troubling time for you. 2. It's difficult to end a marriage after 10 years.

(Table continued on following page)

Table 2–2 ◆ Degree of Openness Continuum (*Continued*)

VERBALIZATION	EXAMPLE
	3. It looks like you're feeling sad.
	4. You seem very disappointed about . . .
5. Facilitatory statements (accepting, offering general leads)	1. Uh-huh.
	2. Go on.
	3. I see.
Closed ended	**These techniques tend to decrease a client's response length. However, they can be effective in focusing a wandering client. Closed-ended questions help obtain important facts or ask for specific details. Closed-ended statements give information or explanations, or have an educational slant.**
1. Closed-ended questions (seeking information)	1. How long have you been hearing voices?
	2. Are you feeling happy, sad, or angry?
	3. What medications are you taking?
2. Closed-ended statements (giving information)	1. Anxiety can be helped with behavioral therapies.
	2. This test will determine. . . .
	3. I read in your chart that you tried suicide once before.
	4. We will begin by taking a blood sample to check your medication level.

Adapted from Shea, S.C. (1998). Psychiatric Interviewing: The Art of Understanding, 2nd ed. Philadelphia: W.B. Saunders Company, p. 82; reprinted with permission.

certain results, as in "Are the medications helping you?" They are usually answered by a "yes," "no," or short answer. When closed-ended questions are used frequently during a counseling session, or especially during an initial interview, they can close an interview down rapidly. This is especially true with a guarded or resistant client.

Other useful tools for nurses when communicating with their clients are (1) clarifying/validating techniques, (2) the use of silence, and (3) active listening.

Clarifying/Validating Techniques

Understanding depends on clear communication, which is aided by verifying with a client the nurse's interpretation of the client's messages. The nurse must request feedback on the accuracy of the message received from verbal and nonverbal cues. The use of clarifying techniques helps both participants to identify major differences in their frames of reference, giving them the opportunity to correct misperceptions before they cause any serious misunderstandings. The client who is asked to elaborate on or clarify vague or ambiguous messages needs to know that the purpose is to promote mutual understanding. For example, "I hear you saying that you are having difficulty trusting your son after what happened. Is that correct?"

Paraphrasing

For clarity, the nurse might use paraphrasing, which means to restate in different (often fewer) words the basic content of a client's message. Using simple, precise, and culturally relevant terms, the nurse may readily confirm interpretation of the client's previous message before the interview proceeds. By prefacing statements with a phrase such as "I am not sure I understand" or "In other words, you seem to be saying . . . ," the nurse helps the client form a clearer perception of what may be a bewildering mass of details. After paraphrasing, the nurse must validate the accuracy of the restatement and its helpfulness to the discussion. The client may confirm or deny the perceptions through nonverbal cues or by directly responding to a question such as "Was I correct in saying . . .?" As a result, the client is made aware that the interviewer is actively involved in the search for understanding.

Restating

With restating, the nurse mirrors the client's overt and covert messages; thus this technique may be used to echo feeling as well as content. Restating differs from paraphrasing in that it involves repetition of the same key words the client has just spoken. If a client remarks "My life has been full of pain," additional information may be gained by restating, "Your life has been full of pain." The purpose of this technique is to explore more thoroughly subjects that may be significant. However, too-frequent and indiscriminate use of restating might be interpreted by clients as inattention or disinterest. It is very easy to overuse this tool and become mechanical. Inappropriately parroting or mimicking what another has said may be perceived as poking fun at the person, making this nondirective approach a definite drawback to communication. To avoid overuse of restating, the nurse can combine restating with use of other clarifying techniques that encourage descriptions. For example:

"Tell me about how your life has been full of pain."
"Give me an example of how your life has been full of pain."

Exploring

A technique that enables the nurse to examine important ideas, experiences, or relationships more fully is exploring. For example, if a client tells the nurse that he does not get along well with his wife, the nurse will want to further explore this area. Possible openers might include:

"Tell me more about your relationship with your wife."
"Describe your relationship with your wife."
"Give me an example of you and your wife not getting along."

Asking for an example can greatly clarify a vague or generic statement made by a client:

Mary: No one likes me.
Nurse: *Give an example* of one person who doesn't like you.
Jim: Everything I do is wrong.
Nurse: *Give me an example* of one thing you do that you think is wrong.

Use of Silence

In many cultures in our society, including nursing, there is an emphasis on action. In communication, we tend to expect a high level of verbal activity. Many students and practicing nurses find that, when the flow of words stops, they become uncomfortable. The effective use of silence, however, is a helpful communication technique.

Silence is not the absence of communication. Silence is a specific channel for transmitting and receiving messages. The practitioner needs to understand that silence is a significant means of influencing and being influenced by others.

In the initial interview, the client may be reluctant to speak because of the newness of the situation, the strangeness of the nurse, self-consciousness, embarrassment, shyness, or anger. Talking is highly individualized: some find the telephone a nuisance, whereas others believe they cannot live without it. The nurse must recognize and respect individual differences in styles and tempos of responding.

Although there is no universal rule concerning how much silence is too much, silence has been said to be worthwhile only as long as it is serving some function and not frightening the patient. Knowing when to speak during the interview is largely dependent on the nurse's perception about what is being conveyed through the silence. Icy silence may be an expression of anger and hostility. Being ignored or "given the silent treatment" is recognized as an insult and is a particularly hurtful form of communication. Ingram (1991) points out that silence among some African American clients may relate to anger, insulted feelings, or acknowledgment of a nurse's lack of cultural sensitivity.

Silence can also convey acceptance, being comfortable in someone's company sharing time together, that a person is pondering an idea or forming a response to what has just been said, or feeling comfortable when there is nothing more to say at that moment. Successful interviewing may be largely dependent on the nurse's "will to abstain"—that is, to refrain from talking more than necessary. Silence may provide meaningful moments of reflection for both participants. It gives each an opportunity to contemplate thoughtfully what has been said and felt, to weigh alternatives, to formulate new ideas, and to gain a new perspective of the matter under discussion. If the nurse waits to speak and allows the client to break the silence, the client may share thoughts and feelings that could otherwise have been withheld. Nurses who feel compelled to fill every void with words often do so because of their own anxiety, self-consciousness, and embarrassment. When this occurs, the nurse's need for comfort tends to take priority over the needs of the client.

Conversely, prolonged and frequent silences by the nurse may hinder an interview that requires verbal articulation. Although the untalkative nurse may be comfortable with silence, this mode of communication may make the client feel like a fountain of information to be drained dry. Moreover, without feedback, clients have no way of knowing whether what they said was understood.

In naturally evolving interviews, open-ended techniques are interwoven with empathetic and facilitatory statements and closed-ended statements, all of which serve to clarify issues and demonstrate the interviewer's interest (Shea, 1998).

Active Listening

People want more than just physical presence in human communication. Most people are looking for the other person to be there for them psychologically, socially, and emotionally (Egan, 1994). Active listening includes:

- Observing and paraphrasing the client's nonverbal behaviors
- Listening to and seeking to understand clients in the context of the social setting of their lives
- Listening for the "false notes" (e.g., inconsistencies or things the client says that need more clarification)

We have already noted that effective interviewers need to become accustomed to silence. It is just as important, however, for effective interviewers to learn to become active listeners when the client is talking, as well as when the client becomes silent. During active listening, nurses carefully note what the client is saying verbally and nonverbally, as well as monitoring their own nonverbal responses (Parsons and Wicks, 1994). Using silence effectively and learning to listen on a deeper, more significant level to both the client and your own thoughts and reactions are key ingredients in effective communications. Both these skills take time, profit from guidance, and can be learned.

A word of caution about listening. It is important for all of us to recognize that it is impossible to listen to people in an unbiased way. In the process of socialization, we develop cultural filters through which we listen to ourselves, others, and the world around us (Egan, 1994). Cultural filters are a form of cultural bias or cultural prejudice.

> One of the functions of culture is to provide a highly selective screen between us and the outside world. In its many forms, culture therefore designates what we pay attention to and what we ignore. This screening provides structure for the world. (Hall, 1977, p. 85)

Egan (1994) states that we need these cultural filters to provide structure for ourselves and to help us interpret and interact with the world. However, unavoidably, these cultural filters also introduce various forms of bias in our listening, because they are bound to influence our personal, professional, familial, and sociological values and interpretations.

Active listening helps strengthen the client's ability to solve personal problems. By giving the client undivided attention, the nurse communicates that the client is not alone; rather, the nurse is working along with the client, seeking to understand and help. This kind of intervention enhances self-esteem and encourages the client to direct energy toward finding ways to deal with problems. Serving as a "sounding board," the nurse listens as the client tests thoughts by voicing them aloud. This form of interpersonal interaction often enables the client to clarify thinking, link ideas, and tentatively decide what should be done and how best to do it (Collins, 1983).

◆ TECHNIQUES TO MONITOR AND AVOID

Some techniques health care workers may employ are not useful and can negatively affect the interview and threaten rapport between the nurse and client. Using ineffective techniques that set up barriers to communication is something we all have done, and will do again. However, with thoughtful reflection, finding appropriate alternative therapeutic behaviors and methods, your communication skills will become more effective, and you will gain confidence in your abilities. Most importantly, you will improve your ability to work with clients, even those clients who present the greatest challenges. Supervision and peer support are immensely valuable in identifying techniques to target and change.

Some of the most common approaches that can cause problems and are especially noticeable in the nurse new to psychosocial nursing are (1) asking excessive questions, (2) giving advice, (3) giving false reassurance, (4) requesting an explanation, and (5) giving approval.

Asking Excessive Questions

Excessive questioning, especially *closed-ended* questions, puts the nurse in the role of interrogator, demanding information without respect for the client's willingness or readiness to respond. This approach conveys lack of respect and sensitivity to the client's needs. Excessive questioning controls the range and nature of response, and can easily result in a therapeutic stall or a shut-down interview. It is a controlling tactic and may reflect the interviewer's lack of security in letting the client tell his or her own story. It is better to ask more open-ended questions and follow the client's lead. For example:

Excessive questions:
　"Why did you leave your wife?" "Did you feel angry at her?"
　"What did she do to you?" "Are you going back to her?"

Better to say:
　"Tell me about the situation between you and your wife."

Giving Advice

When a nurse offers clients "solutions," they eventually begin to think that the nurse does not view them as capable of making effective decisions. Giving people advice undermines their feelings of adequacy and competence. It can foster dependence on the advice giver, and shifts the problem from client to nurse. Giving constant advice to clients (or others for that matter) devalues the other individual and prevents the other person from working through and thinking through other options either on their own or with the nurse. It keeps the "advice giver" in control and feeling like the strong one, although this might be unconscious on the nurse's part. This is very different from giving information to people. People need information to make informed decisions.

Giving advice:

> **Client**: "I don't know what to do about my brother. He is so lost."
>
> **Nurse**: "You should call him up today and explain to him you can't support him any longer, and he will have to go on welfare." (If I were you. . . . Why don't you . . . It would be best . . .)

Better to say:

> **Client**: "I don't know what to do about my brother. He is so lost."
>
> **Nurse**: "What do you see as some possible actions you can take?" (encourages problem solving)
>
> *or*
>
> **Nurse**: "Have you thought about discussing this with the rest of your family?" (offering alternatives the client can consider)

Clients often ask nurses for solutions. It is best to avoid this trap.

Giving False Reassurance

Giving false reassurance underrates a person's feelings and belittles a person's concerns. This usually causes people to stop sharing feelings because they feel they are not taken seriously, or are being ridiculed. Therefore, the person's real feelings remain undisclosed and unexplored. False reassurance in effect invalidates the client's experience and can lead to increased negative affect.

False reassurance:

> "Everybody feels that way."
> "Don't worry, things will get better."
> "It's not that bad."
> "You're doing just fine."

Better to say:

> "What specifically are you worried about?"
> "What do you think could go wrong?"
> "What do you see as the worst thing that could happen?"

Requesting an Explanation: "Why" Questions

A "why" question from a person in authority (nurse, doctor, teacher) can be experienced as intrusive and judgmental. "Why" questions may put people on the defensive, and serve to close down communication. It is much more useful to ask, "What is happening?" rather than why it is happening. People often have no idea why they did something, although most everyone can make up a ready answer on the spot. Unfortunately, the answer is mostly defensive and not useful for further exploration.

Why questions:

"Why don't you leave him if he is so abusive?"
"Why didn't you take your medications?"
"Why didn't you keep your appointment?"

Better to say:

"What are the main reasons you stay in this relationship?"
"Tell me about the difficulties you have regarding taking your medications."
"I notice you didn't keep your appointment even though you said that was a good time for you. What's going on?"

Giving Approval

We often give our friends and family approval when we believe they have done something well. Even when what they have done is not *that* great, we make a big point of it. It is natural to bolster up friends' and loved ones' egos when they are feeling down.

You may wonder what is wrong with giving a person a pat on the back once in a while. The answer is nothing, as long as it is done without involving a judgment (positive or negative) by the nurse. "Giving approval" in the nurse-client relationship is a much more complex matter than giving approval or "a pat on the back" to one's friends or colleagues. Often people coming into the psychiatric setting are feeling overwhelmed and alienated, and may be down on themselves. During this time, clients are vulnerable and may be needy for recognition, approval, and attention. Yet, when people are feeling vulnerable, a value comment may be misinterpreted. For example:

Value judgment:

"You did a great job of holding your temper when Sally started screaming at you. You are really getting good at maintaining your 'cool.'"

Implied in this message is that the nurse was pleased by the way the client kept his temper in a volatile situation. In many instances, the client may see this as a way to please the nurse, or get recognition from others. Therefore, the behavior becomes a way to gain approval. This may be a much healthier and more useful behavior for the client, but, when the motivation for any behavior starts to focus on getting recognition and approval from others, it stops coming from the individual's own volition or conviction. In addition, when the people the client wants approval from are not around, the motivation for the new behavior might not be there either. Thus it really is not a change in behavior as much as a ploy to win approval and acceptance from another person(s).

Better to say:

"I notice that you kept your temper when Sally screamed at you. You seem to be acting more even-tempered lately. How does it feel to be more in control of your emotions?"

This response opens the door to finding out how the client was feeling. Is this new behavior becoming easier? Was this situation of holding back anger difficult? Does the client want to learn more assertiveness skills? Was it useful for the client? Was there more to this situation the client wants to discuss? The above response by the nurse also makes it clear that this was a self-choice the client made. The client is given recognition for the change in behavior, and the topic is also open for further discussion.

◆ ASSESSING YOUR COMMUNICATIONS SKILLS

Gaining communication and counseling skills is a process that takes time. It is helpful to assess oneself over time and to note areas of improvement and areas to target for the future. Table 2–3 is a communication self-assessment checklist. It is helpful to check yourself frequently over time and note your progress.

◆ INTERNET SITES

EthnoMed Ethnic Medical Guide
http://healthlinks.washington.edu/clinical/ethnomed/

Transcultural Nursing Society
http://www.tcns.org

JAMARDA Resources, Inc.
Cultural diversity in the health care field
http://www.jamardaresources.com

Natural Health Village
Alternative systems of health practice
http://www.naturalhealthvillage.com/

Table 2–3 ◆ Nurse's Communication Self-Assessment Checklist

Instructions: Periodically during your clinical experience, use this checklist to identify areas needed for growth and progress made. Think of your clinical patient experiences. Indicate the extent of your agreement with each of the following statements by marking the scale: SA, strongly agree; A, agree; NS, not sure; D, disagree; SD, strongly disagree.

Statement	SA	A	NS	D	SD
1. I maintain appropriate eye contact.	SA	A	NS	D	SD
2. Most of my verbal comments follow the lead of the other person.	SA	A	NS	D	SD
3. I encourage others to talk about feelings.	SA	A	NS	D	SD
4. I ask open-ended questions.	SA	A	NS	D	SD
5. I restate and clarify a person's ideas.	SA	A	NS	D	SD
6. I paraphrase a person's nonverbal behaviors.	SA	A	NS	D	SD
7. I summarize in a few words the basic ideas of a long statement made by a person.	SA	A	NS	D	SD
8. I make statements that reflect the person's feelings.	SA	A	NS	D	SD
9. I share my feelings relevant to the discussion when appropriate to do so.	SA	A	NS	D	SD
10. I give feedback.	SA	A	NS	D	SD
11. At least 75% or more of my responses help enhance and facilitate communication.	SA	A	NS	D	SD
12. I assist the person to list some alternatives available.	SA	A	NS	D	SD
13. I assist the person to identify some goals that are specific and observable.	SA	A	NS	D	SD
14. I assist the person to specify at least one next step that might be taken toward the goal.	SA	A	NS	D	SD

Adapted from Myrick, D., and Erney, T. (1984). Caring and Sharing. Educational Media Corporation, p. 154; reprinted by permission. Copyright © 1984 by Educational Media Corporation.

CHAPTER 3

Guidelines for the Clinical Interview

RESPONSIBILITIES OF NURSES WHO COUNSEL CLIENTS

The foundation of nursing practice is the ability of the nurse to engage in interpersonal interactions in a goal-directed manner for the purpose of assisting clients with their emotional or physical health needs (Hagerty, 1984). This relationship between the nurse and client is a professional relationship, and as such implies certain responsibilities. Responsibilities inherent in the nurse-client relationship for all levels of nursing include:

- **Accountability**—The nurse assumes responsibility for the conduct and consequences of the assignment and for nurses' actions.
- **Focus on client needs**—The interest of the client, *not* that of other health care workers or the institution, is given first consideration. *The nurse's role is that of client advocate.*
- **Clinical competence**—The criteria on which the nurse bases his or her conduct are principles of knowledge and appropriateness to the specific situation. This involves awareness and incorporation of the latest knowledge made available from research.
- **Supervision**—Validation of performance quality is through regularly scheduled supervisory sessions. Supervision is conducted either by a more experienced clinician or through discussion with the nurse's peers in professionally conducted supervisory sessions.

◆ PHASES OF THE COUNSELING PROCESS

Many disciplines describe the phases of a therapeutic relationship during counseling. These phases are the same, although different disciplines may have their own names for these phases. We will use the names that are generally recognized in the practice of nursing, which are (1) the orientation phase, (2) the working phase, and (3) the termination phase.

In some situations, the nurse may only meet with the client once, or for only a few sessions. Even though the time spent together may be brief, the relationship or encounter(s) may be substantial, useful, and important to the client. This limited relationship is often referred to as a *therapeutic encounter.* Many of the following principle and practices still apply even to a limited encounter (e.g., issues of confidentiality, goals, tasks), although the working phase is brief and adapted to the brief encounter. Termination per se may not apply; however, the nurse may wish to find out what the client thought was helpful, or if there is an issue the client wishes to pursue that was discussed during the encounter, and may refer the client to appropriate staff or to members of the treatment team.

There are certain tasks and phenomena that are specific to each phase, although they may overlap. For example, the issue of confidentiality, first addressed in the orientation phase, may be discussed and reiterated throughout all phases of the nurse-client relationship. The following discussion highlights important aspects and responsibilities of the nurse during each phase.

◆ ORIENTATION PHASE

The orientation phase can last for a few meetings or can extend over a longer period of time. The first time the nurse and client meet, they are strangers to each other. When strangers meet for the first time, they interact according to their own backgrounds, standards, values, and experiences. This fact underlies the need for self-assessment and self-awareness on the part of the nurse.

Goals of the Orientation Phase

1. **To establish trust.** Establishing trust is essentially establishing a sound engagement with the client in a therapeutic alliance. Trust is something that will or will not develop between the two parties. Establishing an atmosphere in which trust can grow is the responsibility of the nurse. Trust is nurtured by demonstrating genuineness (congruence) and empathy, developing a positive regard for the client, demonstrating consistency, and offering assistance in alleviating the client's emotional pain or problems.
2. **To effect some degree of anxiety reduction in the client.**
3. **To instill hope and ensure that the client will remain compliant with treatment.**

4. **To develop an assessment from which nursing diagnoses can be formulated,** if a nursing assessment has not already been done.
5. **To develop appropriate treatment goals (outcome criteria) and a plan of care.**

Tasks of the Orientation Phase

During the orientation phase, the nurse addresses four specific issues: (1) the parameters of the relationship, (2) the formal or informal contract, (3) confidentiality, and (4) termination.

Parameters of the Relationship

Clients have the right to know about the nurse or counselor with whom they will be working. For example, who is this nurse and what is the nurse's background? They also need to know the stated purpose of the meetings. For a student, this information-giving might go something like:

> Hello, Mrs. Gonzalas, I am Sylvia Collins from Sullivan College. I am in my senior year and I am doing my psychiatric rotation. I will be coming to City College for the next eight Thursdays, and I would like to meet with you each Thursday if you are still here. I am here to be a support person for you as you work on your treatment goals.
>
> *or*
>
> Hello, Mrs. Gonzalas. I am Jim Santos from Ohio State College. Since I am here only once this week, we will have today to discuss your most important issues.

For an RN working in the clinical setting, the parameters may be altered:

> Hello, Mrs. Gonzalas, I am John Horton. I am an advanced practice psychiatric nurse and I have been counseling clients for about 4 years now. Dr. Sharp referred you to me and stated that you wished to work out some issues in counseling/therapy.

Formal or Informal Contract

A contract emphasizes the client's participation and responsibilities. It implies that the nurse does something *with* the client, not just for the client. The contract, either stated or written, includes the time, place, date, and duration of the meetings as well as mutual agreement as to goals. If a fee is to be paid, the client is told how much that will be and when the fee is due.

For a student, the statement of the contract might sound something like the following:

> Mr. Snyder, we will meet at 10:00 AM each Monday in the consultation room at the clinic for 45 minutes from September 15th to October 27th. We can use that time to further discuss your feelings of loneliness, and explore some things you could do to make things better for yourself.

For a psychiatric advanced practice nurse working in the clinical setting, the contract might be:

> Mrs. Lang, we will meet on Thursdays at 10:00 AM in my office at the clinic. Our sliding scale fee is $45.00 a session. Our policy states that, if you can't make a session, it is important to let us know 24 hours in advance, otherwise we will charge you for the session. We can use our time together to explore further your feelings of loneliness and anger with your husband and any other issues you wish to work on.

Confidentiality

The client has the right to know who else knows about the information being shared with the nurse. He or she needs to know that the information may be shared with specific people, such as a clinical supervisor, the physician, the treatment team, or other students in conference. The client also needs to know that the information will *not* be shared with the client's family, friends, or others outside the treatment team, except in extreme situations. Extreme situations include:

- When the client reveals information that may be harmful to the client or others (child abuse, elder abuse)
- When the client threatens self-harm
- When the client does not intend to follow through with the treatment plan

When information must be given to others, it is usually done by the physician according to legal guidelines. The nurse must be aware of the client's right to confidentiality, and must not violate that right. Refer to Box 3–1 for guidelines for confidentiality.

A student might phrase the issue of confidentiality something like:

> Mrs. Martin, I will be sharing some of what we discuss with my nursing instructor, and at times I may discuss certain concerns with my peers in conference, or with the staff. However, I will not be sharing this information with your husband

❖   B O X   3 – 1   ❖
Ethical Guidelines for Confidentiality

1. Keep all client records secure.
2. Consider carefully the content to be entered into the record.
3. Release information only with written consent and full discussion of the information to be shared, except when release is required by law.
4. Use professional judgment deliberately regarding confidentiality when the client is a danger to self or others.
5. Use professional judgment deliberately when deciding how to maintain the confidentiality of a minor. The rights of the parent/guardian must also be considered deliberately.
6. Disguise clinical material when used professionally for teaching and writing.
7. Maintain confidentiality in consultation and peer review situations.
8. Maintain anonymity of research subjects.
9. Safeguard the confidentiality of the student in teaching/learning situations.

From Colorado Society of Clinical Specialists in Psychiatric Nursing. (1990). Ethical guidelines for confidentiality. Journal of Psychosocial Nursing 28(3):42–44; reprinted with permission.

or any other members of your family or your friends without your permission.

For a psychiatric nurse specialist, the issue may be broached in the following manner:

Mr. Shapero, I may share some of what we discuss with Dr. Lean during bimonthly supervision or in peer-group supervision here at the clinic. I will not be discussing this information outside the clinic setting, or with any members of your family or friends, without your permission, unless I am concerned that your life or someone else's life is in danger.

Termination

The issue of termination is always discussed in the first interview. It may also be brought up during the working phase as well. In some cases the termination date may be known, such as in a student rotation, or short-term therapy, where sessions are specifically limited, or when insurance issues dictate only a specific number of sessions. At other times, when the nurse-client relationship is open-ended, the termination date may not be known.

A student may address termination by saying:

> Mrs. Tacinelli, as I mentioned earlier, our last clinical day is October 27th. We will have three more meetings after today.

A clinical specialist may broach termination by saying something like:

> Mr. Middelstaedt, you are here to work on your phobia of using public transportation. Many people become more comfortable with their phobias in 12 to 14 sessions. At the end of 14 sessions, we can evaluate your goals and/or see if there is anything else you wish to work on.

In summary, the initial interview includes the following elements:

1. The nurse's role is clarified and the responsibilities of both the client and the nurse are defined.
2. The contract containing the time, place, date, and duration of the meetings is discussed.
3. Confidentiality is discussed and assumed.
4. The terms of termination are introduced.

♦ WORKING PHASE

During the working phase, the nurse and client together identify and explore areas in the client's life that are causing problems. Some of the specific tasks of the working phase of the nurse-client relationship include (Moore and Hartman, 1988):

1. Maintaining the relationship
2. Gathering further data
3. Promoting the client's problem-solving ability
4. Facilitating behavior change
5. Overcoming resistance
6. Evaluating problems and goals, and redefining them as necessary
7. Practicing and experiencing alternative adaptive behaviors

It is important, however, to keep in mind that chronically ill clients, particularly those with schizophrenia, frequently are unable to define problem areas or goals. The illness impairs their cognitive functioning and ability to establish relationships. It is important to recognize that establishing trust with a chronically ill client, and even temporarily relieving the client's feelings of isolation and social withdrawal that accompany the illness, are significant goals to pursue.

During the orientation and working phase, clients often unconsciously employ "testing behaviors" that may be used to test the nurse. The client may want to know if the nurse will:

- Be able to set limits
- Still show concern if the client gets angry, babyish, unlikable, or dependent
- Still be there if the client is late, leaves early, refuses to speak, or is angry

Table 3–1 gives examples of common testing behaviors clients employ, and some suggested nursing responses.

◆ TERMINATION PHASE

Termination has been discussed in the first interview; it may also have been broached during the working phase of the relationship. Reasons for terminating include:

- Symptom relief
- Improved social functioning
- Greater sense of identity
- More adaptive behaviors in place
- Accomplishment of the client's goals
- An impass in therapy
- End of student rotation
- End of health maintenance organization contract
- Discharge or death

Termination is an integral part of the nurse-client relationship, and without it the relationship remains incomplete. Summarizing the goals and objectives achieved in the relationship is part of the termination process. Reviewing situations that occurred during the time spent together and exchanging memories can help validate the experience for both the nurse and the client, and can facilitate closure of the relationship.

During the termination process, old feelings of loss, abandonment, or loneliness may be reawakened in the client. Therefore, the termination phase may offer the client an opportunity to express these feelings, perhaps for the first time. These feelings may also be reawakened in the nurse, perhaps to a different degree or intensity, if he or she still has strong issues of loss. Nurses can benefit from discussing these feelings with more experienced nurses, supervisors, trusted instructors, and their mature peers. Because loss is an integral part of life, it is also an integral part of the human condition. Many feelings may be reawakened at termination, so clients may feel vulnerable and at a loss. Although many clients are able to talk about their feelings, client behaviors vary widely. For example, a client may respond with anger toward the nurse, or demonstrate symptoms thought to be resolved. In addition, a client may withdraw from the nurse during the last session, or refuse to spend time with the nurse at all. It is always a good idea to acknowledge what seems to be going on, and explore this with the client:

> "You seem very quiet today, and haven't made eye contact with me. Good-byes often stir up memories of past separations. Do you remember any past separations that were painful?"

Throughout the entire process (introduction, working, termination) pertinent clinical information is recorded in the client's record and verbally passed along to members of the treatment team.

◆ THE CLINICAL INTERVIEW

Anxiety during the first clinical interview is to be expected, as in any meeting between strangers. Clients may be anxious about their problems, about the nurse's reaction to them, or about their treatment. Shea (1998) identifies some common client fears and concerns during the first interview:

- Who is this nurse/clinician?
- Is he or she competent?
- Is this person understanding?
- What does he or she already know about me?
- Am I going to be hurt?
- Do I have any control in this matter?

Students and clinicians new to psychosocial nursing may have other concerns:

- What should I say?
- What should I do?
- Will the client like me?
- How will the client respond to me?
- Can I help this person?
- Can I hurt the client if I say the wrong thing?
- What will the instructor/supervisor think of what I am doing?
- How will I do compared to my peers?

Table 3–1 ◆ Testing Behaviors Used by Clients

CLIENT BEHAVIOR	CLIENT EXAMPLE	NURSE RESPONSE	RATIONALE
Shifts focus of interview *to* the nurse, *off* the client.	"Do you have any children?" or "Are you married?"	"This time is for you." If appropriate, the nurse should add: 1. "Do you have any children" or "What about your children?" 2. "Are you married?" or "What about your relationships?"	The nurse refocuses back to the client and client's concerns. The nurse sticks to the contract.
Tries to get the nurse to take care of him or her.	"Could you tell my doctor . . ."	"I'll leave a message with the ward clerk that you want to see him." or "You know best what you want him to know. I'll be interested in what he has to say."	1. The nurse validates that the client is able to do many things for him- or herself. This aids in increasing self-esteem. 2. The nurse always encourages the person to function at the highest level, even if he or she doesn't want to.
	"Should I take this job . . ."	"What do you see as the pros and cons of this job?"	
Makes sexual advances toward the nurse, e.g., touching the nurse's arm, wanting to hold hands or kiss nurse.	"Would you go out with me? . . . Why not?" or "Can I kiss you? . . . Why not?"	"I am not comfortable having you touch (kiss) me." The nurse briefly reiterates the nurse's role: "This time is for you to focus on your problems and concerns."	1. The nurse needs to set clear limits on expected behavior. 2. Frequently restating the nurse's role throughout the relationship can help maintain boundaries.

| Continues to arrive late for meetings. | "I'm a little late because (excuse)." | If the client stops: "I wonder what this is all about?" 1. Is the client afraid the nurse won't like him or her? 2. Is the client trying to take the focus off of problems? If the client continues: "If you can't cease this behavior, I'll have to leave. I'll be back at (time) to spend time with you then." The nurse arrives on time and leaves at the scheduled time. (The nurse does not let the client manipulate him or her or bargain for more time.) After a couple of times, the nurse can explore behavior, e.g.: "I wonder if there is something going on you don't want to deal with?" or "I wonder what these latenesses mean to you?" | 3. Whenever possible, the meaning of the client's behavior should be explored. 4. Leaving gives the client time to gain control. The nurse returns at the stated time. 1. The nurse keeps the contract. Clients feel more secure when "promises" are kept, even though clients may try to manipulate the nurse through anger, helplessness, and so forth. 2. The nurse doesn't tell the client what to do, but the nurse and client need to explore what the behavior is all about. |

From Varcarolis, E. (1998). Foundations of Psychiatric Mental Health Nursing, 3rd ed. Philadelphia: W.B. Saunders Company, p. 161; reprinted with permission.

How to Begin the Interview

Helping a person with an emotional or medical problem is rarely a straightforward task. The goal of assisting a client to regain psychological or physiological functional normality can be difficult to reach. Extremely important to any kind of counseling is permitting the client to set the pace of the interview, no matter how slow the progress happens to be (Parsons and Wicks, 1994).

Setting

Effective communication can take place almost anywhere. However, because the quality of the interaction—whether in a clinic, a ward, an office, or the client's home—depends on the degree to which the nurse and client feel safe, establishing a setting that enhances feelings of security can be important to helping the relationship. A health care setting, a conference room, or a quiet part of the unit that has relative privacy but is within view of others is ideal. Home visits offer the nurse a valuable opportunity to assess the person in the context of everyday life.

Seating

In all settings, chairs need to be arranged so that conversation can take place in normal tones of voice and eye contact can be comfortably maintained, or avoided. For example, a nonthreatening physical environment for nurse and client would involve:

- Assuming the same height—either both sitting or both standing.
- Avoiding a face-to-face stance when possible—a 90-degree angle or side by side may be less intense.
- Leaving plenty of space between client and nurse.
- Making sure that the door is easily accessible to both client and nurse. This is particularly important if the client is paranoid or has a history of violence.
- Avoiding a desk barrier between nurse and client.

Introductions

In the orientation phase, nurses tell the client who they are, the purpose of the meetings, and how long and at what time they will be meeting with the client. The issue of confidentiality is also covered at some point during the initial interview. The nurse can then ask the client how he or she would like to be addressed. This question accomplishes a number of tasks (Shea, 1998); for example:

- It conveys respect.
- It gives the client direct control.

How To Start

Once introductions have been made, the nurse can turn the interview over to the client by using one of a number of open-ended statements:

"Where should we start?"
"Tell me a little about what has been going on with you."
"What are some of the stresses you have been coping with recently?"
"Tell me a little about what has been happening in the past couple of weeks."
"Perhaps you can begin by letting me know what some of your concerns have been recently."
"Tell me about your difficulties."

The appropriate use of offering leads (e.g., "Go on"), statements of acceptance (e.g., " Uh-huh"), or other conveyances of the nurse's interest can facilitate communication.

Tactics To Avoid

The nurse needs to avoid some behaviors (Moscato, 1988):

- Do not argue with, minimize, or challenge the client.
- Do not praise the client or give false reassurance.
- Do not interpret to the client or speculate on the dynamics of the client's problem.
- Do not question the client about sensitive areas until trust is established.
- Do not try to "sell" the client on accepting treatment.
- Do not join in attacks the client launches on his or her mate, parents, friends, or associates.
- Do not participate in criticism of another nurse or any other staff member with the client.
- Do not barrage the client with many questions, especially closed-ended questions.

Helpful Guidelines

Some guidelines for conducting the initial interviews are offered by Meier and Davis (1989):

- Speak briefly.
- When you don't know what to say, say nothing.
- When in doubt, focus on feelings.
- Avoid advice; rather, look at how the client feels about the situation and what he or she wants to change.

- Avoid relying on questions.
- Pay attention to nonverbal cues.
- Keep the focus on the client.

Guidelines for Specific Client Behaviors

There are a number of common client behaviors that arise during the process of the nurse-client relationship in mental health settings. New nurses may not know how best to handle these situations. These behaviors include clients who (1) cry, (2) ask the nurse to keep a secret, (3) leave before the session is over, (4) say they want to kill themselves, (5) do not want to talk, (6) seek to prolong the interview, (7) give the nurse a present, and (8) ask personal questions. Table 3–2 identifies common nursing reactions to these situations and offers the nurse useful responses.

Table 3–2 ◆ Common Client Behaviors and Nurse Responses

CLIENT BEHAVIOR	POSSIBLE REACTIONS BY NURSE	USEFUL RESPONSES BY NURSE
The client cries	The nurse may feel uncomfortable and experience increased anxiety or feel somehow responsible for making the person cry.	The nurse should stay with the client and reinforce that it is all right to cry. Often, it is at that time that feelings are closest to the surface and can be best identified. "You seem ready to cry." "What are you thinking right now?" The nurse offers tissues when appropriate.
The client asks the nurse to keep a secret	The nurse may feel conflict because the nurse wants the client to share important information but is unsure about making such a promise.	The nurse *cannot* make such a promise. This information may be important to the health and safety of the client or others. "I cannot make that promise. It might be important for me to share it with other staff." The client then decides whether to share the information or not.
Another client interrupts during time with your selected client	The nurse may feel a conflict. The nurse does not want to appear rude. Sometimes the nurse tries to engage both clients in conversation.	The time the nurse had contracted with a selected client is that client's time. By keeping their part of the contract, nurses demonstrate that they mean what they say and that they view the sessions as important. "I am with Mr. Rob for the next 20 minutes. At 10 AM, after our time is up, I can talk to you for 5 minutes."

(Table continued on following page)

Table 3–2 ◆ Common Client Behaviors and Nurse Responses (*Continued*)

CLIENT BEHAVIOR	POSSIBLE REACTIONS BY NURSE	USEFUL RESPONSES BY NURSE
The client says he wants to kill himself	The nurse may feel overwhelmed or responsible to "talk the client out of it." The nurse may pick up some of the client's feelings of hopelessness.	The nurse tells the client that this is serious, that he or she does not want harm to come to the client, and that this information needs to be shared with other staff. "This is very serious, Mr. Lamb. I do not want any harm to come to you. I will have to share this with the other staff." The nurse can then discuss with the client the feelings and circumstances that led up to this decision. (Refer to Chapter 13 for strategies in suicide intervention.)
The clients says she does not want to talk	The nurse new to this situation may feel rejected or ineffective.	At first, the nurse might say something to this effect: "It's all right. I would like to spend time with you. We don't have to talk." The nurse might spend short, frequent periods (e.g., 5 minutes) with the client throughout the day. "Our 5 minutes is up. I'll be back at 10 AM and stay with you 5 more minutes." This gives the client the opportunity to understand that the nurse means what he or she says and is back on time consistently. It also gives the client time between visits to assess the nurse and perhaps feel less threatened.

The client gives the nurse a present	The nurse may feel uncomfortable when offered a gift. The meaning needs to be examined. Is the gift: 1. A way of getting better care? 2. A way to maintain self-esteem? 3. A way to making the nurse feel guilty? 4. A sincere expression of thanks? 5. A cultural expectation?	*Possible guidelines:* If the gift is expensive, the best policy is to perhaps graciously refuse. If it is inexpensive and 1. given *at the end* of hospitalization when a relationship has developed, graciously accept. 2. given *at the beginning* of hospitalization, graciously refuse and explore the meaning behind the present. "Thank you, but it is our job to care for our clients. Are you concerned that some aspect of your care will be overlooked?" If the gift is money, it may be best to graciously refuse.
The client asks you a personal question	The nurse may think it is rude not to answer the client's question. *or* A new nurse might feel relieved to put off having to start the interview. *or* The nurse may feel put on the spot and want to leave the situation. New nurses are often manipulated by a client to change roles. This keeps the focus off the client and prevents the building of a relationship.	The nurse may or may not answer the client's query. If the nurse decides to answer a natural question, he or she answers in a word to two, then refocuses back on the client. P: Are you married? N: Yes, do you have a spouse? P: Do you have any children? N: This time is for you—tell me about yourself. P: You can tell me if you have any children. N: This is your time to focus on your concerns. Tell me something about your family.

From Varcarolis, E. (1998). Foundations of Psychiatric Mental Health Nursing, 3rd ed. Philadelphia: W.B. Saunders Company, pp. 200–201; reprinted with permission.

PART II

Clinical Syndromes

CHAPTER 4

Mental Disorders of Childhood and Adolescence

The risk factors for mental disorders in childhood or adolescence are genetic, biochemical, and pre- and postnatal influences, individual temperament; and personal psychosocial development. The vulnerability to risk factors is the result of a complex interaction among many factors (e.g., constitutional endowment, trauma, disease, and interpersonal experiences). Vulnerability changes over time as children/adolescents grow, and as the emotional and physical environment changes. As children and adolescents mature, they develop competencies that enables them to communicate, remember, reality test, problem solve, make decisions, control drives and impulses, modulate affect, tolerate frustration, delay gratification, adjust to change, establish satisfying interpersonal relationships, and develop healthy self-concepts. These competencies reduce the risk for developing emotional, mental, or health problems. Children and adolescents who are missing any of these competencies, or are "at risk" for other reasons, need to be monitored so that early detection and intervention can help eradicate or at least minimize developing problems.

◆ ASSESSING FOR CHILD AND ADOLESCENT DISORDERS

Data are collected from the parent/caregiver, and whenever possible from the child/adolescent and siblings. Methods for collecting data include interviewing, screening questionnaires or checklists, testing (neurological, psychological, intelligence), and observing and interacting with the child or adolescent. Table 4–1 lists types of assessment data that should be collected for each client. Areas to

Table 4–1 ◆ Types of Assessment Data

History of Present Illness
- Chief complaint
- Development and duration of problems
- Help sought and tried
- Effect of problem on child's life at home and school
- Effect of problem on family and sibling's life

Developmental History
- Pregnancy, birth, neonatal data
- Developmental milestones
- Description of eating, sleeping, elimination habits, and routines
- Attachment behaviors
- Types of play
- Social skills and friendships
- Sexual activity

Developmental Assessment
- Psychomotor
- Language
- Cognitive
- Interpersonal-social
- Academic achievement
- Behavior (response to stress, changes in the environment)
- Problem solving and coping skills (impulse control, delay of gratification)
- Energy level and motivation

Neurological Assessment
- Cerebral functions
- Cerebellar functions
- Sensory functions
- Reflexes
- Cranial nerves
  Functions can be observed in developmental assessment and while playing games involving a specific ability (e.g., "Simon Says, touch your nose.")

Medical History
- Review of body systems
- Trauma, hospitalization, operations, and child's response
- Illnesses or injuries affecting the central nervous system
- Medications (past and current)
- Allergies

Family History
- Illnesses in related family members (e.g., seizures, mental disorders, mental retardation, hyperactivity, drug and alcohol abuse, diabetes, cancer)
- Background of family members (occupation, education, social, activities, religion)
- Family relationships (separation, divorce, deaths, contact with extended family, support system)

Mental Status Assessment
- General appearance
- Activity level
- Coordination/motor function
- Affect
- Speech
- Manner of relating
- Intellectual functions
- Thought processes and content
- Characteristics of child's play

assess under presenting problem(s) are identified under "History of Present Illness." Information about particular problems helps to focus later questions in collecting data about the "Developmental," "Medical," and "Family History."

The observation/interaction part of a mental health assessment begins with a semistructured interview in which the child or adolescent is asked about life at home with parents and siblings, and life at school with teachers and peers. Because the interview is not structured, children are free to describe their current problems, even giving information about their own developmental history. Play activities such as games, drawing, puppets, and free play are used for younger children who cannot respond to a direct approach. An important part of the first interview is observing interactions among the child, the caregiver, and the siblings (if available).

The following group of disorders most commonly seen in children and adolescents are presented in this chapter: **Pervasive Developmental Disorders, Attention Deficit** and **Disruptive Behavior Disorders**. Anxiety Disorders are covered in Chapter 6; however, currently accepted psychopharmacological agents used in treatment of anxiety disorders in children and adolescents are included in Table 4–4.

Assessment Tools

The **developmental assessment** in Table 4–1 provides information about the child/adolescent's current maturational level. This can help the nurse identify current lags or deficits. Table 4–2, the **Mental Status Assessment,** provides information about the child/adolescent's current mental state. The developmental and mental status assessment have many areas in common, and for this reason any observation and interaction will provide data for both assessments.

◆ PERVASIVE DEVELOPMENTAL DISORDERS

Pervasive developmental disorders are characterized by their severe and pervasive impairment in reciprocal social interaction and communication skills. The four subtypes of pervasive developmental disorders are autistic, Asperger's, Rett's, and childhood disintegrative disorders. They are described in the following sections.

Autistic Disorder

Autistic disorder is a syndrome resulting from abnormal left brain function. The left hemisphere abnormality causes problems in language, logic, and reasoning, whereas right brain functions involving music and visual-spatial activities may be enhanced. Oversensitivity or indifference to stimuli are characteristics of abnormal arousal in the affected individual.

Etiology for the abnormal brain function is largely undetermined. There appears to be a familial pattern, with autism being more common in siblings than in the general population. The prevalence is 2 to 5/10,000; and the male-to-female ratio is 4:1 or 5:1.

Table 4–2 ♦ Child/Adolescent Mental Status Assessment

General Appearance
- Size—height and weight
- General health and nutrition
- Dress and grooming
- Distinguishing characteristics
- Gestures and mannerisms
- Looks/acts younger or older than chronological age

Speech
- Rate, rhythm, intonation
- Pitch and modulation
- Vocabulary and grammar appropriate to age
- Mute, hesitant, talkative
- Articulation problems
- Other expressive problems
- Unusual characteristics (pronoun reversal, echolalia, gender confusion, neologisms)

Intellectual Functions
- Fund of general information
- Ability to communicate (follow directions, answer questions)
- Memory
- Creativity
- Sense of humor
- Social awareness
- Learning and problem solving
- Conscience (sense of right and wrong, accepts guilt and limits)

Characteristics of Child's Play
- Age appropriate use of toys
- Themes of play
- Imagination and pretend play
- Role and gender play
- Age-appropriate play with peers
- Relationship with peers (empathy, sharing, waiting for turns, best friends)

Activity Level
- Hyper/hypoactivity
- Tics, other body movements
- Autoerotic and self-comforting movements (thumb sucking, ear/hair pulling, masturbation)

Coordination/Motor Function
- Posture
- Gait
- Balance
- Gross motor movement
- Fine motor movement
- Writing and drawing skills
- Unusual characteristics (bizarre postures, tiptoe walking, hand flapping, head banging, hand biting)

Manner of Relating
- Eye contact
- Ability to separate from caregiver, be independent
- Attitude toward interviewer
- Behavior during interview (ability to have fun/play, low frustration tolerance, impulsive, aggressive)

Thought Processes and Content
- Orientation
- Attention span
- Self-concept and body image
- Sex role, gender identity
- Ego-defense mechanisms
- Perceptual distortions (hallucinations, illusions)
- Preoccupations, concerns, and unusual ideas
- Fantasies and dreams

Adapted from Goodman, J.D., and Sours, J. (1987). The Child Mental Status Examination, 2nd ed. New York: Basic Books; reprinted with permission.

Autistic disorder is usually recognized before the age of 3, but its behavioral symptoms in infancy can be subtle and difficult to distinguish. The symptoms become more obvious after the age of 2. Some children will experience improvement in social and/or language skills, but these can improve or decline independently of each other. Puberty brings change in either direction.

The prognosis is generally poor. However, improvement depends on the IQ level and the development of social and language skills. A very small percentage are able to live and work independently, and about one third can achieve partial independence.

Presenting Symptoms

IMPAIRMENT IN SOCIAL INTERACTIONS

- Lack of responsiveness to and interest in others
- Lack of eye-to-eye contact and facial responses
- Indifference to or aversion to affection and physical contact
- Failure to cuddle or be comforted
- Lack of seeking or sharing enjoyment, interest, or achievement with others
- Failure to develop cooperative play or imaginative play with peers
- Lack of friendships

IMPAIRMENT IN COMMUNICATION AND IMAGINATIVE ACTIVITY

- Language delay or total absence of language
- Immature grammatical structure, pronoun reversal, inability to name objects
- Stereotyped or repetitive use of language (echolalia, idiosyncratic words, inappropriate high-pitched squealing/giggling, repetitive phrases, sing-song speech quality)
- Lack of spontaneous make-believe play or imaginative play
- Failure to imitate

MARKEDLY RESTRICTED, STEREOTYPED PATTERNS OF BEHAVIOR, INTERESTS, AND ACTIVITIES

- Rigid adherence to routines and rituals with catastrophic reactions to minor changes in them or changes made in the environment (moving furniture)
- Stereotyped and repetitive motor mannerisms (hand/finger flapping, clapping, rocking, dipping, swaying, spinning, dancing around and walking on toes, head banging or hand biting)
- Preoccupation with certain objects (buttons, parts of the body, wheels on toys) that is abnormal in intensity or focus
- Preoccupation with certain repetitive activities (pouring water/sand, spinning wheels on toys, twirling string) that is abnormal in intensity or focus

Asperger's Disorder

This disorder differs from autistic disorder in that it appears to have a later onset and there is no significant delay in cognitive and language development (APA, 1994). The exact prevalence is unknown, and it affects more males than females. There appears to be a familial pattern to the disorder.

Presenting Symptoms

- Recognized later than autistic disorder.
- No significant delays in cognitive and language development.
- Severe and sustained impairment in social interactions.
- Development of restricted, repetitive patterns of behaviors, interests, and activities resembling autistic disorder.
- May have delayed motor developmental milestones with clumsiness noted in preschool.
- Social interaction problems more noticeable when child enters school.
- Problems with empathy and modulating social relationships may continue into adulthood.

Rett's Disorder

This disorder differs from autistic and Asperger's disorders in that it has been observed only in females, with the onset before the age of 4 (APA, 1994). The exact etiology is unknown, but the disorder is associated with electroencephalographic abnormalities, seizure disorder, and severe or profound mental retardation.

Presenting Symptoms

- Development of multiple deficits after a normal prenatal and postnatal period of development
- Head circumference is normal at birth but growth rate slows between the 5th and 48th months of life
- Persistent and progressive loss of previously acquired hand skills between the 5th and 30th months of life
- Development of stereotyped hand movements (hand-wringing and hand-washing)
- Problems with coordination of gait and trunk movements
- Severe psychomotor retardation
- Severe problems with expressive and receptive language
- Loss of interest in social interactions but may develop this interest later in childhood or adolescence

Childhood Disintegrative Disorder

This disorder is rare and occurs in both sexes, but is more common in males (APA, 1994). Onset is between 2 and 10 years, with most cases occurring between the ages of 3 and 4. The onset can be abrupt or insidious. The etiology is unknown, although the disorder is thought to be related to an insult to the central nervous system.

Presenting Symptoms

- Marked regression in multiple areas of function after at least 2 years of normal development
- Loss of previously acquired skills in at least two areas (communication, social relationships, play, adaptive behavior, motor skills, and bowel/bladder control)
- Deficits in communication and social interactions (same as autistic disorder)
- Stereotyped behaviors (same as autistic disorder)
- Loss of skills reaches a plateau, then there may be limited improvement

Sample Questions (for the Parent or Caregiver)

The nurse uses a variety of therapeutic techniques to obtain the answers to the following questions. Use your discretion and decide which questions are appropriate to complete your assessment.

1. "Describe the child's temperament and adjustment as a newborn."
2. "Describe any unusual responses to stimuli." (sounds, lights, or being touched)
3. "When did the child develop a social smile? Become responsive to words and physical contact?"
4. "Can the child be comforted? How does the child comfort self?"
5. "Does the child show interest in others? Concern when others are hurt?"
6. "When did speech develop? Unusual characteristics?" (in rate, rhythm, tone, inflection pattern, echolalia, made-up words)
7. "Describe any unusual behaviors." (hand/finger flapping, clapping, rocking, dipping, swaying, spinning, dancing around, and walking on toes)
8. "What, if any, behaviors cause self-injury?" (head banging, slapping, or hand biting)
9. "What are the child's favorite toys? Any preoccupation with round or shiny objects, objects that can spin or move, or parts of the body?"
10. "What is the child's favorite activity? Any preoccupation with repetitive activities?" (pouring water/sand, spinning/twirling objects, chewing or eating inedibles)

11. "How does the child respond to limit setting? Tantrum behaviors?"
12. "How does the child respond to changes?" (routines, schedules, activities or rituals, changes in furniture arrangements)
13. "How well does the child do at self-care activities?" (dressing, toileting, eating)
14. "Have previously learned skills or abilities changed or been lost?"

$\equiv$	ASSESSMENT ALERTS

1. Assess for developmental spurts, lags, uneven development, or loss of previously acquired abilities. (Use baby books/diaries, photographs, films/videotapes. First-time mothers may not be aware of development lags and family members may need to be consulted.)
2. Assess the quality of the relationship between the child and parent/caregiver for evidence of bonding, anxiety, tension, and difficulty-of-fit between the parents' and child's temperament.
3. Be aware that children with behavioral and developmental problems are at risk for abuse.

Nursing Diagnoses with Interventions

The child with pervasive developmental disorders has severe impairments in social interactions and communications skills. Often these are accompanied by stereotyped behavior, interests, and activities. The severity of the impairment is demonstrated by the child's lack of responsiveness to or interest in others, lack of empathy or sharing with peers, and lack of cooperative or imaginative play with peers. Therefore, **Impaired Social Interaction** is almost always present. Language delay or absence of language and the unusual stereotyped or repetitive use of language is another area for nursing interventions. Therefore, **Impaired Communication** and **Altered Growth and Development** (language delay) are useful nursing diagnoses. Stereotyped and repetitive motor behaviors can include behaviors like head banging, face slapping, and hand biting. The child's apparent indifference to pain can result in serious self-injury, so **Risk for Self-Mutilation** and/or **Risk for Injury** can become a priority. If the child's rigid adherence to specific routines and rituals is disrupted, the child may have a catastrophic reaction such as a severe temper tantrums or rage reactions, leading to **High Risk for Violence.** The child's lack of interest in activities outside of self and the frequent disregard for bodily needs interfere with the development of a personal identity, so **Personal Identity Disturbance** may be an appropriate nursing diagnosis.

OVERALL GUIDELINES FOR NURSING INTERVENTIONS

Help the child reach his or her full potential by fostering developmental competencies and coping skills:

1. Increase the child's interest in reciprocal social interactions.
2. Foster the development of social skills.
3. Facilitate the expression of appropriate emotional responses, including the development of trust, empathy, shame, remorse, anger, pride, independence, joy, and enthusiasm.
4. Foster the development of reciprocal communication, especially language skills.
5. Provide for the development of psychomotor skills in play and activities of daily living (ADLs).
6. Facilitate the development of cognitive skills (attention, memory, cause and effect, reality testing, decision making, and problem solving).
7. Foster the development of self-concepts (identity, self-awareness, body image, and self-esteem).
8. Foster the development of self-control, including impulse control, tolerating frustration, and the delay of gratification.

Impaired Social Interaction

A state in which an individual participates in an insufficient or excessive quantity or ineffective quality of social exchange

---

Related To (Etiology)

◆ Self-concept disturbance [immaturity or developmental deviation]
◆ Absence of available significant others/peers
● Impaired neurological development or dysfunction
● Disturbance in response to external stimuli
● Disturbance in attachment/bonding with the parent/caregiver

---

◆ NANDA accepted; ● In addition to NANDA.

As Evidenced By (Assessment Finding/Diagnostic Cues)

◆ Dysfunctional interaction with peers
● Lack of responsiveness to or interest in others (eye contact, facial expressions, verbalizations)
● Lack of bonding or affectional ties to parental figures (indifference or aversion to physical contact)
● Lack of interest or ability to play and share with peers
● Lack of empathy or concern for others

Outcome Criteria

Child will:

• Participate in at least four activities that reflect reciprocal social interactions within 1 year
• Initiate interactions with peers and trusted adults

Short-Term Goals

Child will:

• Seek out nurse/caregiver for activities/ADLs and for comfort when distressed within 1 to 3 months
• Show interest and begin to participate in play activities with others, especially peers, within 2 to 6 months
• Use at least two social skills to initiate contact with peer(s) at the same developmental level within 6 to 12 months

Interventions and Rationales

Intervention	Rationale
1. Use one-to-one interaction to engage the client in a working alliance.	1. Assigning the same primary nurse who will be a parental surrogate can promote attachment.
2. Monitor for signs of anxiety/distress. Intervene early to provide comfort.	2. Anticipating need for help in managing stress enhances the client's feelings of security.
3. Provide emotional support and guidance for ADLs and other activities; use a system of rewards for attempts and successes.	3. Learning occurs through meaningful social interactions involving imitation, modeling, feedback, and reinforcement.

◆ NANDA accepted; ● In addition to NANDA.

4. Set up play situations with peers starting with parallel play and moving toward cooperative play.

4. Learning to play with peers is sequential.

5. Help the client find a special friend.

5. Having a special friend enhances learning experience.

6. Role model social inter-action skills (interest, empathy, sharing, waiting, and required language).

6. Facilitates the development of needed social/emotional skills.

7. Reward attempts to interact and play with peers and the use of appropriate emotional expressions.

7. Behaviors that are rewarded are repeated.

8. Role play situations that involve conflicts in social interactions to teach reality testing, cause and effect, and problem solving.

8. These cognitive skills are needed for successful social/emotional reciprocity.

Impaired Verbal Communication

The state in which an individual experiences a decreased, de-layed, or absent ability to receive, process, transmit, and use a system of symbols—anything that has meaning (i.e., transmits meaning).

Related To (Etiology)

◆ Physiological conditions
◆ Alteration of central nervous system
● Impaired neurological development or dysfunction
● Disturbance in attachment/bonding with the parent/caregiver

As Evidenced By (Assessment Finding/Diagnostic Cues)

● Language delay or total absence of language
● Immature grammatical structure, pronoun reversal, inability to name objects

---

◆ NANDA accepted; ● In addition to NANDA.

- Stereotyped or repetitive use of language (echolalia, idiosyncratic words, inappropriate high-pitched squealing/giggling, repetitive phrases, sing-song speech quality)
- Lack of response to communication attempts by others

Outcome Criteria

Child will:

- Communicate at least four basic needs (hunger, thirst, fatigue, pain) verbally and/or through gestures and body language with parents/caregiver and peers
- Communicate in words/gestures that are understood by others

Short-Term Goals

Child will:

- Communicate through eye contact, facial expressions, and other nonverbal gestures within 1 month
- Attempt to use language and begin to communicate with words within 5 to 6 months
- Increase language skills needed for social and emotional reciprocal interactions within 6 to 8 months
- Use language or gestures to identify self, others, objects, feelings, needs, plans, and desires within 12 months

Interventions and Rationales

Intervention	**Rationale**
1. Use one-to-one interactions to engage the client in non-verbal play.	1. The nurse enters the client's world in a nonthreatening interaction to form a trusting relationship.
2. Recognize subtle cues indicating the client is attending or attempting to communicate.	2. Cues are often difficult to recognize (glancing out of the corner of the eye).
3. Describe for the client what is happening, and put into words what the client might be experiencing.	3. Naming objects and describing action, thoughts, and feelings helps the client use symbolic language.
4. Encourage vocalizations with sound games and songs.	4. Children learn through play and enjoyable activities.

◆ NANDA accepted; ● In addition to NANDA.

5. Identify desired behaviors and reward them (e.g., hugs, treats, tokens, points, or food).

5. Behaviors that are rewarded will increase in frequency. Desire for food is a powerful incentive in modifying behavior.

6. Use names frequently, and encourage the use of correct pronouns (e.g., I, me, he).

6. Problems with self-identification and pronoun reversal are common.

7. Encourage verbal communication with peers during play activities using role modeling, feedback, and reinforcement.

7. Play is the normal medium for learning in a child's development.

8. Increase verbal interaction with parents, and siblings by teaching them how to facilitate language development.

8. Education and emotional support helps parents and siblings be more therapeutic in their interactions with the client.

Risk for Self-Mutilation

A state in which an individual is at risk to perform an act upon the self to injure, not kill, which produces tissue damage and tension relief

Related To (Etiology)

- Impaired neurological development or dysfunction
- Need for painful stimuli to increase opiate levels and reduce tension
- Rage reactions and aggression turned toward self
- Lack of impulse control and the ability to tolerate frustration

As Evidenced By (Assessment Finding/Diagnostic Cues)

- History of self-injuries (head banging, biting, scratching, hair pulling) when frustrated or angry
- Old scars or new areas of tissue damage
- Self-injurious tantrums when changes are made in routines, rituals, or the environment, or when asked to end a pleasurable activity

◆ NANDA accepted; ● In addition to NANDA.

Outcome Criteria

Child will:

- Be free of self-inflicted injury
- Demonstrate new behaviors and skills to cope with anxiety and feelings

Short-Term Goals

Child will:

- Respond to a parent or surrogate's limits on self-injurious behaviors within 1 to 6 months
- Seek help when anxiety and tension rise within 1 to 6 months
- Express feelings and describe tensions verbally and/or with non-injurious body language within 6 months to 1 year
- Use appropriate play activities for the release of anxiety and tension within 1 to 6 months

Interventions and Rationales

Intervention	Rationale
1. Monitor the client's behavior for cues of rising anxiety.	1. Behavioral cues signal increasing anxiety.
2. Determine emotional and situational triggers.	2. Knowledge of triggers is used in planning ways to prevent or manage outbursts.
3. Intervene early with verbal comments or limits, and/or removal from the situation.	3. Potential outbursts can be defused through early recognition, verbal interventions, or removal.
4. Give plenty of notice when having to change routines or rituals or end pleasurable activities.	4. Children often react to change with catastrophic reactions and need time to adjust.
5. Provide support for the recognition of feelings, reality testing, impulse control.	5. These competencies are often underdeveloped in these children.
6. If the client does not respond to verbal interventions, use therapeutic holding.	6. Therapeutic holding reassures the client that the adult is in control; feelings of security can

Some may need special restraints (helmets, mittens, special padding).

7. Help the client connect feelings and anxiety to self-injurious behaviors.

8. Help the client develop ways to express feelings and reduce anxiety verbally and through play activities. Use various types of motor and imaginative play (e.g., swinging, tumbling, role playing, drawing, singing).

become feelings of comfort and affection.

7. Self-control is enhanced through understanding the relationship between feelings and behaviors.

8. Methods for modulating and directing the expression of emotions and anxiety need to be learned in order to control destructive impulses.

Personal Identity Disturbance

Inability to distinguish between self and nonself

Related To (Etiology)

◆ Biochemical imbalance
● Impaired neurological development or dysfunction
● Failure to develop attachment behaviors resulting in fixation at autistic phase of development
● Interrupted or uncompleted separation/individuation process resulting in extreme separation anxiety

As Evidenced By (Assessment Finding/Diagnostic Cues)

● Seemingly unaware of or uninterested in others or their activities
● Unable to identify parts of the body or bodily sensations (enuresis, encopresis)
● Fails to imitate others or not able to stop imitating other's actions or words (echolalia, echopraxis)
● Fails to distinguish parent/caregiver as a whole person, instead relates to body parts (e.g., takes person's hand and places it on doorknob)

◆ NANDA accepted; ● In addition to NANDA.

- Becomes distressed by bodily contact with others
- Spends long periods of time in self-stimulating behaviors (self-touching, sucking, rocking)
- Needs ritualistic behaviors and sameness to control anxiety
- Has extreme distress reactions to changes in routines or the environment
- Cannot tolerate being separated from parent/caregiver

Outcome Criteria

Child will:

- Demonstrate recognition of self-boundaries and being separate from others

Short-Term Goals

Child will:

- Seek comfort and physical contact from others within 1 to 2 months
- Relate to caregiver by name with eye contact and verbal requests within 6 months
- Recognize body parts, body boundaries, and sexual identity within 6 months
- Show an interest in the activities of others and tolerate their presence within 3 to 6 months
- Spend more time in purposeful activities rather than rituals and self-stimulating activities in 2 to 6 months
- Recognize body sensations (pain, hunger, fatigue, elimination needs) within 2 to 6 months
- Express a full range of feelings within 4 to 6 months
- Recognize the feelings and activities of others as separate within 6 months
- Adjust to changes in activities and the environment within 5 to 9 months

Interventions and Rationales

Intervention	Rationale
1. Use one-to-one interaction to engage the client in a safe relationship with nurse/caregiver.	1. A consistent caregiver provides for the development of trust needed for a sense of safety and security.

◆ NANDA accepted; ● In addition to NANDA.

2. Use names and descriptions of others to reinforce their separateness.

2. Consistent reinforcement will help break into the client's autistic world.

3. Draw the client's attention to the activities of others and events that are happening in the environment.

3. Interrupts the client's self-absorption and stimulates outside interests.

4. Limit self-stimulating and ritualistic behaviors by providing alternative play activities, or providing comfort when stressed.

4. Redirecting the client's attention to favorite or new activities, or giving comfort, reduces anxiety.

5. Foster self-concept development; reinforce identity, sexual identity, and body boundaries through drawing, stories, and play activities.

5. Learning body parts and sexual identity is necessary and fun in play activities.

6. Help client distinguish body sensations and how to meet bodily needs by picking up on cues and using ADLs to teach self-care.

6. The lack of self-awareness contributes to problems with self-care, especially toileting.

7. Provide play opportunities for the client that identify the feelings of others (stories, puppet play, peer interactions).

7. Consistent feedback about the feelings of others helps with self-differentiation and the development of empathy.

◆ ATTENTION-DEFICIT AND DISRUPTIVE BEHAVIOR DISORDERS

The majority of children and adolescents receiving treatment for mental disorders have behaviors that disrupt their lives at home and at school. The distinguishing characteristics for these disorders, **attention-deficit/hyperactivity disorder**, **oppositional defiant disorder**, and **conduct disorder**, are presented in the following sections.

Attention-Deficit/Hyperactivity Disorder (ADHD)

Attention-deficit/hyperactivity disorder (**ADHD**) is a behavioral syndrome characterized by an inappropriate degree of inattention, impulsiveness and hyperactivity (APA, 1994). ADHD occurs in 3% to 5% of schoolchildren and is four to nine times more common in boys than girls. ADHD children have a higher incidence of problems with temper outbursts, labile moods, poor school performance, rejection by peers, low self-esteem, and enuresis and/or encopresis. ADHD is often dually diagnosed with **oppositional defiant disorder** or **conduct disorder,** and may precede the development of **Tourette's syndrome**.

Presenting Symptoms

INATTENTION

- Has difficulty paying attention in tasks or play.
- Does not seem to listen, follow through, or finish tasks.
- Does not pay attention to details and makes careless mistakes.
- Dislikes activities that require sustained attention.
- Is easily distracted, loses things, and is forgetful in daily activities (symptoms worsen in situations requiring sustained attention).

HYPERACTIVITY

- Fidgets, unable to sit still or stay seated in school.
- Runs and climbs excessively in inappropriate situations.
- Had difficulty in playing in leisure activities quietly.
- Acts as if "driven by a motor," constantly "on the go."
- Talks excessively.

IMPULSIVITY

- Blurts out answer before question is completed.
- Has difficulty waiting for turns.
- Interrupts, intrudes in others' conversations and games.

OTHER

- Some hyperactivity, impulsiveness, or inattention present before age 7.
- Clear evidence of impairment in social, academic, or occupational functioning.
- Impairment from symptoms in at least two settings (home, school, work).

Oppositional Defiant Disorder

Oppositional defiant disorder is a recurrent pattern of negativistic, disobedient, hostile, defiant behavior toward authority figures without the serious violations of the basic rights of others (APA, 1994). The behavior is usually evident before 8 years of age and no later than early adolescence. It is more common in males until puberty, when the male-to-female ratio may become equal. The behavior is evident at home and may not be elsewhere. The behavior persists for at least 6 months and may be a precursor of a **conduct disorder**.

Presenting Symptoms

- Often loses temper.
- Often argues with adults.
- Often actively defies or refuses to comply with requests.
- Deliberately annoys others and is easily annoyed by others.
- Blames other for his or her mistakes.
- Is often angry, resentful, spiteful, and vindictive.

Other behaviors that often accompany this disorder are low self-esteem, labile moods, low frustration tolerance, swearing, early use of alcohol and illicit drugs, and conflicts with parents, teachers, and peers.

Conduct Disorder

Conduct disorder is a persistent pattern of behavior in which the rights of others and age-appropriate societal norms or rules are violated (APA, 1994). It is one of the most frequently diagnosed disorders, with rates for males 6% to 16% and for females 2% to 9%.

Childhood-onset type occurs prior to age 10 and mainly in males who are physically aggressive, have poor peer relationships with little concern for others, and lack guilt or remorse. Although they try to project a "tough" image, they have low self-esteem, low frustration tolerance, irritability, and temper outbursts. They are more likely to have their conduct disorder persist through adolescence and develop into **antisocial personality disorder**.

In the **adolescent-onset type,** no conduct problems occurred prior to age 10. These children are less likely to be aggressive, have more normal peer relationships, and act out their misconduct with their peer group. Males are more apt to fight, steal, vandalize, and have school discipline problems, whereas girls lie, are truant, run away, abuse substances, and engage in prostitution.

Complications associated with conduct disorders are school failures, suspension and dropout, juvenile delinquency, and the need for the juvenile court system to assume responsibility for youths who cannot be managed by their parents. Psychiatric disorders that frequently coexist with conduct disorder are anxiety, depression, ADHD, and learning disabilities.

Presenting Symptoms

AGGRESSION TOWARD PEOPLE AND ANIMALS

- Often bullies, threatens, and intimidates others.
- Often initiates physical fights.
- Has used a weapon that could cause serious injury.
- Has been physically cruel to others and/or animals.
- Has stolen while confronting a victim.
- Has forced someone into sexual activity.

DESTRUCTIVE OF PROPERTY

- Has deliberately set fires intending to cause damage.
- Has deliberately destroyed another's property.

DECEITFULNESS OR THEFT

- Has broken into a house, building, or car.
- Often lies to obtain goods or favors.
- Has stolen items of nontrivial value (shoplifting).

SERIOUS VIOLATIONS OF RULES

- Often stays out at night despite parental prohibition before age 13.
- Has run away from home at least twice, or once for a lengthy period of time.
- Often truant from school before age 13.

Sample Questions for Attention Deficit and Disruptive Disorders (for the Parent or Caregiver)

The nurse uses a variety of therapeutic techniques to obtain the answers to the following questions. Use your discretion and decide which questions are appropriate to complete your assessment.

1. "Describe the child's temperament." (easy, highly reactive, difficult)
2. "Describe the child's overall activity level." (high energy, hyperactive)
3. "Who is/was the primary caregiver? Any disruptions in that relationship?"
4. "Problems going to sleep or staying asleep?" (nightmares, sleepwalking) "Describe the child's adjustment to feeding schedules or new foods." (food refusal, food fetishes)

5. "Any difficulty separating from you if left in the care of others?"

6. "How does the child show affection toward you, siblings, peers?"

7. "What comforts the child when stressed?"

8. "Does the child express concern when others are injured or distressed? Express remorse or guilt when hurtful to others?"

9. "How does the child respond to limits? Being told "no"? Having to wait, share, or end a favorite activity?" (protests, tantrums)

10. "How motivated is the child to learn new skills? (persistence, patience, response to frustration)

11. "How long will the child attend to an activity? Easily distracted?"

12. "Can the child follow 1, 2, and 3-part directions?"

13. "Does the child have difficulty organizing or completing tasks? Lose personal belongings?"

14. "Does the child have friends? How well do they play together?"

15. "Does the child frequently seek attention? Talk a lot? Interrupt or intrude on other's activities or body space?"

16. "At what grade level is the child? How is the child's academic progress?"

17. "Describe any problematic behaviors." (impulsive or dangerous acts, physically aggressive, hostile, cruel to people and animals, manipulative, lies and cheats, steals, destroys property, sets fires, swears, skips school, runs away from home, uses drugs or alcohol, sexually acts out)

ASSESSMENT ALERTS

1. Assess the quality of the relationship between the child and parent/caregiver for evidence of bonding, anxiety, tension, and difficulty-of-fit between the parents' and the child's temperament, which can contribute to the development of disruptive behaviors.

2. Assess the parent/caregiver's understanding of growth and development, parenting skills, and handling of problematic behaviors, because lack of knowledge contributes to the development of these problems.

3. Assess cognitive, psychosocial, and moral development for lags or deficits, because immature developmental competencies result in disruptive behaviors.

Continued

For Attention-Deficit/Hyperactivity Disorder

1. Observe the child for level of physical activity, attention span, talkativeness, and the ability to follow directions and control impulses. Medication is often needed to ameliorate these problems.
2. Assess for difficulty in making friends and performing in school. Academic failures and poor peer relationships lead to low self-esteem, depression, and further acting out.
3. Assess for problems with enuresis and encopresis.

For Oppositional Defiant Disorder

1. Identify issues that result in power struggles, when they began, and how they are handled.
2. Assess the severity of the defiant behavior and its impact on the child's life at home, at school, and with peers.

For Conduct Disorder

1. Assess the seriousness of the disruptive behavior, when it started, and what has been done to manage it. Hospitalization or residential placement may be necessary, as well as medication.
2. Assess the child's levels of anxiety, aggression, anger, and hostility toward others, and the ability to control destructive impulses.
3. Assess the child's moral development for the ability to understand the impact of the hurtful behavior on others, to empathize with others, and to feel remorse.

Nursing Diagnoses and Interventions

Children and adolescents with attention-deficit/hyperactivity disorder, oppositional defiant disorder, and conduct disorder have disruptive behaviors that are impulsive, angry/aggressive, and often dangerous (**Risk for Violence**). These children and adolescents are often in conflict with parents and authority figures, refuse to comply with requests, do not follow age-appropriate social norms, or have inappropriate ways of getting needs met (**Defensive Coping**). When their behavior is disruptive or aggressive and hostile, they have difficulty making or keeping friends (**Impaired Social Interaction**). Their problematic behaviors can impair learning and result in academic failure. Interpersonal and academic problems lead to high levels of anxiety, low self-esteem, and blaming others for one's troubles (**Self-Esteem Disturbance**). Parents/caregivers have difficulty handling disruptive behaviors and being effective parents, so their participation in the therapeutic program is essential (**Altered Parenting**).

OVERALL GUIDELINES FOR NURSING INTERVENTIONS

Help the child reach his or her full potential by fostering developmental competencies and coping skills:
1. Protect the child from harm and provide for biological and psychosocial needs while acting as a parental surrogate.
2. Increase the child's ability to trust, control impulses, modulate the expression of affect, tolerate frustration, concentrate, remember, reality test, recognize cause and effect, make decisions, problem solve, use interpersonal skills to maintain satisfying relationships, form a realistic self-identity, and play with enjoyment and creativity.
3. Foster the child's identification with positive role models so that positive attitudes and moral values can develop that enable the child to experience feelings of empathy, remorse, shame, and pride.
4. Provide support, education, and guidance for the parents/caregivers.

Risk for Violence: Self-Directed or Directed at Others

Behaviors in which an individual demonstrates that he or she can be physically, emotionally, and/or sexually harmful to self or to others

Related To (Etiology)

◆ Impaired neurological development or dysfunction
◆ Cognitive impairment (e.g., learning disabilities, attention-deficit disorder, decreased intellectual functioning)
● Birth temperament
● Disturbance or immaturity in the competencies of normal growth and development result in lack of impulse control, poor frustration tolerance, and lack of empathy toward others

---

◆ NANDA accepted; ● In addition to NANDA.

- Disturbances in attachment or bonding with the parent/caregiver
- Identification with aggressive and abusive role models

As Evidenced By (Assessment Finding/Diagnostic Cues)

- ◆ Bullies, threatens, and has physical fights with others.
- ◆ Physically cruel to people and animals.
- ◆ Sets fires and/or destroys property.
- ◆ Forces someone into sexual activity (attempted rape, rape, sexual molestation).
- History of aggressive behavior (e.g., mugs or robs others).

Outcome Criteria

Child/adolescent will:

- Control aggressive, impulsive behaviors
- Demonstrate respect for the rights of others

Short-Term Goals

Child/adolescent will:

- Respond to limits on aggressive and cruel behaviors within 2 to 4 weeks
- Identify at least three situations that trigger violent behaviors within 1 to 2 months
- Channel aggression into constructive activities and appropriate competitive games within 2 to 4 weeks
- State the effects of his or her behavior on others within 2 to 4 weeks
- Demonstrate the ability to control aggressive impulses and delay gratification within 2 to 8 weeks

Interventions and Rationales

Intervention

1. Use one-on-one or appropriate level of observation to monitor rising levels of anxiety; determine emotional and situational triggers.
2. Intervene early to calm the client and defuse a potential incident.

Rationale

1. External controls are needed for ego support and to prevent acts of aggression and violence.

2. Learning can take place before the client losses control; new ways to cope can be discussed and role modeled.

◆ NANDA accepted; ● In addition to NANDA.

3. Use graduated techniques for managing disruptive behaviors (Table 4–3).

3. Techniques such as signals/warnings, proximity and touch control, humor, and attention may be all that is needed.

4. Set clear, consistent limits in a calm, nonjudgmental manner; remind client of consequences of acting out.

4. A child gains a sense of security with clear limits and calm adults who follow through on a consistent basis.

5. Avoid power struggles and repeated negotiations about rules and limits.

5. When limits are realistic and enforceable, manipulation can be minimized.

6. Use strategic removal if the client cannot respond to limits (time out, quiet room, therapeutic holding).

6. Removal allows the client to express feelings and discuss problems without losing face in front of peers.

7. Process incidents with the client to make it a learning experience.

7. Reality testing, problem solving, and testing new behaviors are necessary to foster cognitive growth.

8. Use a behavior modification program that rewards the client for seeking help with handling feelings and controlling impulses to act out.

8. Rewarding the client's efforts can increase positive behaviors and foster development of self-esteem.

9. Redirect expressions of disruptive feelings into nondestructive, age-appropriate behaviors; channel excess energy into physical activities.

9. Learning how to modulate the expression of feelings and use anger constructively is essential for self-control.

10. Help the client see how acting out hurts others; appeal to the child's sense of "fairness" for all.

10. These children are insensitive to the feelings of others. However, they can understand the concept of "fairness" and generalize it to other persons.

11. Encourage feelings of concern for others and remorse for misdeeds.

11. Development of empathy is a therapeutic goal with these children.

12. Use medication if indicated to reduce anxiety and aggression or to modulate moods.

12. A variety of medications are effective in children who experience behavioral dyscontrol.

Defensive Coping

The state in which an individual repeatedly projects falsely positive self-evaluation based on a self-protective pattern that defends against underlying perceived threats to positive self-regard

---

Related To (Etiology)

◆ Disturbance in pattern of tension release (problems in impulse control, and frustration tolerance)
● Impaired neurological development or dysfunction
● Birth temperament (highly reactive, difficult to comfort, high motor activity)
● Disturbed relationship with parent/caregiver (lack of trust, abuse, neglect, conflicts, inadequate role models, disorganized family system)

As Evidenced By (Assessment Findings/Diagnostic Cues)

◆ Use of forms of coping that impede adaptive behavior (defiant, negativistic, and/or hostile toward authority figures)
● Refuses to follow directions or comply with limits set on behaviors
● Persistent testing of limits
● Argumentative, stubborn, and unwilling to give in or negotiate
● Temper tantrums and rage reactions when unable to get his or her own way
● Refusing to accept responsibility for misbehavior, often blames others

Outcome Criteria

Child/adolescent will:

• Comply with requests and limits on behaviors in the absence of arguments, tantrums, or other acting-out behaviors
• Question the requests or limits that seem unreasonable and negotiate a settlement

Short-Term Goals

Child/adolescent will:

• Demonstrate increased impulse control within 2 weeks using a scale of 1 to 10 (1 being the most controlled)

◆ NANDA accepted; ● In addition to NANDA.

Table 4–3 ◆ Techniques for Managing Disruptive Behaviors in Children

1. Planned ignoring	1. Evaluate surface behavior and intervene when the intensity is becoming too great.
2. Use of signals or gestures	2. Uses a word, gesture, or eye contact to remind child/adolescent to use self-control.
3. Physical distance and touch control	3. Move closer to the child/adolescent for a calming effect, maybe put arm around child/adolescent.
4. Increase involvement in the activity	4. Redirect child/adolescent's attention to the activity and away from a distracting behavior by asking a question.
5. Additional affection	5. Ignore the provocative content of the behavior and give the child emotional support for the current problem.
6. Use of humor	6. Use well-timed kidding as a diversion to help the child/adolescent save face and relieve feelings of guilt or fear.
7. Direct appeals	7. Appeal to the child/adolescent's developing self-control (e.g., "Please, . . . not now.").
8. Extra assistance	8. Give early help to the child/adolescent who "blows up" and is easily frustrated when trying to achieve a goal; do not overuse this technique.
9. Clarification as intervention	9. Help child/adolescent understand the situation and his or her own motivation for the behavior.
10. Restructuring	10. Change the activity in ways that will lower the stimulation or the frustration (e.g., shorten a story or change to a physical activity).
11. Regrouping	11. Use total or partial changes in the group's composition to reduce conflict and contagious behaviors.
12. Strategic removal	12. Remove child/adolescent who is disrupting or acting dangerously, but consider whether it gives too much status or makes the child a scapegoat.
13. Physical restraint	13. Use "therapeutic holding" to control, give comfort, and assure a child that he or she is protected from his or her own impulses to act out.

(Table continued on following page)

Table 4–3 ◆ Techniques for Managing Disruptive Behaviors in Children (*Continued*)

14. Setting limits and giving permission	14. Use sharp, clear statements about what behavior is not allowed and give permission for the behavior that is expected.
15. Promises and rewards	15. Use very carefully and very infrequently to avoid situations in which the child/adolescent bargains for a reward.
16. Threats and punishment	16. Use very carefully; the child/adolescent needs to internalize the frustration generated by the punishment and use it to control impulses rather than externalizing the frustration in further acting out.

Adapted from Redl, F., and Wineman, D. (1957). The Aggressive Child. Glencoe, IL: The Free Press; reprinted with permission.

- Demonstrate the ability to tolerate frustration and delay gratification within 2 to 6 weeks
- Demonstrate an absence of tantrums, rage reactions, or other acting-out behaviors within 4 to 8 weeks
- Discuss requests and behavioral limits and understand their rationale with the authority figure within 4 weeks
- Accept responsibility for misbehaviors within 2 to 6 weeks

Interventions and Rationales

Intervention	Rationale
1. Use one-on-one or appropriate level of observation to monitor rising levels of frustration; determine emotional and situational triggers.	1. External controls are needed for emotional support and to prevent tantrums and rage reactions.
2. Intervene early to calm the client, problem solve, and defuse a potential outburst.	2. Learning can take place before the client loses control; new solutions and compromises can be proposed.
3. Avoid power struggles and "no-win" situations.	3. Therapeutic goals are lost in power struggles.
4. Use a behavior modification program to reward	4. Rewarding the client's efforts will increase the

tolerating frustration, delaying gratification, and responding to requests and behavioral limits.

5. Allow the client to question the requests or limits *within reason*; give simple, understandable rationale for requests or limits.

5. Discussion allows the client to maintain some sense of autonomy and power. (Rationale is tailored to the developmental age and promotes socialization.)

6. When feasible, negotiate an agreement on the expected behaviors. Avoid giving bribes or allowing the client to manipulate the situation.

6. An agreement on expected behavior will result in better compliance. However, constant negotiations can result in increased manipulation and testing of limits.

7. Use medication if indicated to reduce anxiety, rage, aggression; to modulate moods.

7. A variety of medications are effective in children who experience behavioral and emotional dyscontrol.

Impaired Social Interaction

The state in which an individual participates in an insufficient or excessive quantity or ineffective quality of social exchange

---

Related To (Etiology)

- Impaired neurological development or dysfunction
- Disturbance in the development of impulse control, frustration tolerance, or empathy for others
- Disturbed relationship with parents/caregiver (lack of trust, abuse, neglect, conflicts, disorganized family system)
- Lack of appropriate role models and/or identification with aggressive/abusive models
- Loss of friendships due to disruptions in family life and living situations

---

◆ NANDA accepted; ● In addition to NANDA.

As Evidenced By (Assessment Finding/Diagnostic Cues)

◆ Dysfunctional interaction with peers (teases, taunts, bullies, and fights with others)
● Difficulty making friends because of immature, disruptive, destructive, cruel, or manipulative behaviors
● Isolated, having few or no friends, and/or poor sibling relationships
● Blames others for poor peer relationships
● Sad/depressed about not being liked by peers
● Low self-esteem, or unrealistic, inflated esteem as the aggressor

Outcome Criteria

Child/adolescent will:

• Use age-appropriate interpersonal skills to establish genuine, satisfying, and equal-status friendship with at least one peer

Short-Term Goals

Child/adolescent will:

• Participate in one-to-one and group activities without attempts to interrupt, intimidate, or manipulate others within 4 to 6 weeks
• Use age-appropriate skills in play activities and interpersonal exchanges within 4 to 8 weeks
• Describe a realistic sense of self using feedback from adults and peers within 4 to 8 weeks

Interventions and Rationales

Intervention	Rationale
1. Use one-to-one relationship to engage the client in a working relationship.	1. The client needs positive role models for healthy identification.
2. Monitor for negative behaviors and identify maladaptive interaction patterns.	2. Negative behaviors are identified and targeted to be replaced with age-appropriate social skills.
3. Intervene early, give feedback and alternative ways to handle the situation.	3. Children learn from feedback; early intervention prevents rejection by peers and provides immediate ways to cope.

◆ NANDA accepted; ● In addition to NANDA.

4. Use therapeutic play to teach social skills such as sharing, cooperation, realistic competition, and manners.

5. Use role playing, stories, therapeutic games, and the like to practice skills.

6. Help client find and develop a special friend; set up one-to-one play situations; be available for problem solving peer relationship conflicts; role mode social skills.

7. Help the client develop equal-status peer relationships with reciprocity for honest, appropriate expression of feelings and needs.

4. Learning new ways to interact with others through play allows for the development of satisfying friendships and self-esteem.

5. Solidifies new skills in safe environment.

6. The abilities to reality test, problem solve, and resolve conflicts in peer relationships are important competencies needed for interpersonal skills.

7. When people can identify personal feelings and needs, they are better prepared to use more direct communication rather than manipulation and/or intimidation.

Self-Esteem Disturbance

Negative self-evaluation and feelings about self or self-capabilities, which may be directly or indirectly expressed

---

Related To (Etiology)

- Disturbances in development of self-concept formation
- Disturbed relationship with parent/caregiver (lack of trust, abuse, neglect, conflicts, inadequate role models, disorganized family system)
- Negative feedback for failure to perform expected roles (academic, work related, interpersonal) or achieve desired skills
- Being targeted by peers for rejection or abuse

As Evidenced By (Assessment Findings/Diagnostic Cues)

- ◆ Self-negating verbalization.
- ◆ Lacks initiative to try new things and fearful in new situations.
- ◆ Expresses feelings of shame, doubt, and/or guilt.

◆ NANDA accepted; ● In addition to NANDA.

- Has unrealistic, overvalued appraisal of self-worth (grandiosity).
- Uses defense mechanisms (denial, rationalization, projection, reaction formation) to protect against threats to self-esteem.
- Uses manipulation or intimidation.
- Presents self as dependent and/or helpless.
- Discounts positive feedback.
- Overly sensitive to negative feedback

Outcome Criteria

Child/adolescent will:

- Develop cognitive and emotional competencies needed for self-concept development
- Participate in new activities and new situations with relative comfort
- Identify positive personal attributes
- Develop genuine, positive self-regard based on a more realistic appraisal of personal abilities/talents

Short-Term Goals

Child/adolescent will:

- Recognize when feeling threatened in unfamiliar situations and seek adult help in reducing anxiety and enhancing self-esteem within 2 to 4 weeks
- Demonstrate ways to cope with new situations using reality testing, problem solving, and positive affirmations within 4 to 8 weeks
- Identify realistic goals and start to develop desired skills/abilities that will increase self-esteem within 2 to 8 weeks
- Name two things child likes about self within 1 week
- Use social skills to develop rewarding peer relationships within 4 to 8 weeks

Interventions and Rationales

Intervention	Rationale
1. Give "unconditional positive regard" without reinforcing negative behaviors.	1. The client often sets up situations in which the behavior brings rejection and further confirms the lack of self-worth.

◆ NANDA accepted; ● In addition to NANDA.

2. Reinforce the client's self-worth with time and attention.

3. Help the client identify positive qualities and accomplishments.

4. Help the client identify behaviors needing changing and set realistic goals.

5. Use a behavior modification program that rewards the client for trying new behaviors and evaluates results.

2. Giving one-on-one time or attention in group activity confirms the client's self-worth.

3. An accurate appraisal of accomplishments can help dispel unrealistic expectations.

4. To change, the client needs goals and knowledge of new behaviors.

5. Rewarding the client's efforts will increase the positive behaviors and foster the development of self-esteem.

Altered Parenting

Inability of the primary caregiver to create an environment that promotes the optimum growth and development of the child

---

Related To (Etiology)

◆ Physical illness (impaired neurological development or dysfunction)
◆ Attention-deficit/hyperactivity disorder
◆ Lack of fit with that of parent/caregiver
◆ Lack of knowledge about parenting or the special needs of the child
◆ Role strain or overload (multiple stressors)
◆ Mental or physical illness
● Child's birth temperament
● Disturbance in attachment or bonding with the parent/caregiver

As Evidenced By (Assessment Findings/Diagnostic Cues)

◆ Behavioral disorder
◆ Poor cognitive development
◆ Cannot control child

◆ NANDA accepted; ● In addition to NANDA.

- Disturbed relationship between parent/caregiver and child (lack of trust, abuse, neglect, conflicts, inadequate role models, disorganized family system)
- Unrealistic expectations of self, or the child

Outcome Criteria

Parent/caregiver will:

- Have the resources to help client reach his or her age-related potential
- Learn the necessary parenting skills to deal with the client's problematic behavior(s)

Short-Term Goals

Parent/caregiver will:

- Participate in the client's therapeutic program within 1 to 2 weeks
- Increase knowledge of normal growth and development, the client's diagnosis, medications, and parenting skills needed within 2 to 6 weeks
- Set realistic, age-appropriate behavioral goals for client when at home within 4 weeks
- Learn at least four new skills that will help provide for client's biological and psychosocial needs when at home within 2 to 4 weeks
- Learn the skills necessary to facilitate the development of client's competencies and coping skills when at home within 4 to 6 weeks
- Develop a support system to assist them in parenting within 4 to 6 weeks
- Use available resources to advocate for the client's needs within 2 to 4 weeks

Interventions and Rationales

Intervention	Rationale
1. Explore the impact of the problematic behavior on the life of the family.	1. Helps nurse understand parent's/caregiver's situation. Feeling understood and supported can help foster an alliance.
2. Assess the parent/caregiver's level of knowledge of growth and development, and parenting skills.	2. Problem identification and analysis of learning needs is necessary before intervention begins.

◆ NANDA accepted; ● In addition to NANDA.

3. Assess the parent/caregiver's understanding of the diagnosis, treatment, and medications.

3. Knowledge will increase the parent/caregiver's participation, motivation, and satisfaction.

4. Help the parent/caregiver identify the client's biological and psychosocial needs.

4. Adequate parenting involves being able to identify client's actual-age appropriate needs.

5. Involve the parent in identifying a realistic plan for how these needs will be met when the client is at home.

5. Parents/caregivers have the opportunity to learn the skills necessary to meet the client's needs.

6. Work with the parent/caregiver to set behavioral goals; help set realistic ones for when the client is at home.

6. Mutually set goals provide for continuity and keep the client from using splitting or manipulation to sabotage treatment.

7. Teach behavior modification techniques; give parent/caregiver support in using them and evaluating effectiveness.

7. Education and follow-up support is the key to successful treatment program.

8. Assess the parent/caregiver's support system; use referrals to establish additional supports.

8. Self-help groups and special programs such as respite care can increase the parent/caregiver's ability to cope.

9. Give information on legal rights and available resources that can assist in advocating for child services.

9. Parent/caregiver frequently lacks information on how to secure services for the child.

◆ THERAPY AND PSYCHOPHARMCOLOGY FOR CHILDHOOD AND ADOLESCENT DISORDERS

Treatment of childhood and adolescent disorders requires a multimodal approach in most all instances. Close work with schools, the availability of remediation services, and the incorporation of behavior modification techniques should all be part of the intervention. Therapies including cognitive-behavioral therapies, social skills groups, family therapy, parent training in behavioral techniques, and individual therapy focused on esteem issues have all

Table 4–4 ♦ Psychopharmacology of Child and Adolescent Disorders and Symptoms

DISORDER AND/OR SYMPTOMS	TYPE OF DRUG	EXAMPLES AND COMMENTS
Pervasive developmental disorders	Antipsychotics SSRIs	Haloperidol (Haldol) can reduce irritability and labile affect.
Autistic disorder (AD)	Antipsychotics Propranolol SSRI	Inderal reduces rage outbursts, aggression, and severe anxiety. Clomipramine (Anafranil) may help treat anger and compulsive behavior.
Attention-deficit/hyperactivity disorder (ADHD)	Stimulants Antidepressants Alpha-adrenergic agonists	Methylphenidate (Ritalin) is most used; dextroamphetamine (Dexedrine), and pemoline (Cylert) are also used. Nortriptyline (Aventyl), Bupropion (Wellbutrin), Fluoxeline (Prozac) For example, Clonidine (Catapres) can be used for aggressiveness, impulsivity, and hyperactivity in ADHD clients.
Conduct disorders	Antipsychotics Stimulants Antidepressants Mood stabilizers Alpha-adrenergic agonists	Carbamazepine (Tegretol) Clonidine (Catapres) may help with impulsive and disordered behaviors.
Anxiety disorders • Panic and school phobia	Antidepressants (TCAs, MAOIs, SSRIs) Benzodiazepines	TCA: imipramine (Tofranil) commonly used. Alprazolam use is short term.

• OCD	Antidepressants (SSRIs) Atypical anxiolytic	Clomipramine (Anafranil) Buspirone (BuSpar) is used as adjunct treatment in refractory OCD.
• Separation anxiety disorder	Antidepressants (TCAs, SSRIs)	TCA: imipramine (Tofranil), protriptyline (Vivactil) SSRI: fluoxetine (Prozac)
• Social phobia	TCAs Antianxiety	Protriptyline (Vivactil) Buspirone (BuSpar)
• PTSD	Antianxiety Atypical antipsychotic	Buspirone (BuSpar) Resperidone (Risperdal) is being used to control the flashbacks and aggression in PTSD.
Anxiety symptoms • Insomnia	Antihistamines	Diphenhydramine (Benadryl)
Depressive symptoms	Major depression and dysthymia • SSRIs • TCAs • Atypical antidepressants	Venlafaxine, Nefazodone
	With: Sleep disorders Anxiety Bipolar depression	Trazdone Nefazodone Bupropion
Psychotic symptoms	Antipsychotics	Chlorpromazine (Thorazine), haloperidol (Haldol), thioridazine (Mellaril), trifluoperazine (Stelazine)

MAOI, monoamine oxidase inhibitor; SSRI, selective serotonin reuptake inhibitor; TCA, tricyclic antidepressant.
Data from Schatzberg et al. (1997); Dunner and Rosenbaum (1999); Dunner (1997).

been found to be useful. Skills training may focus on a variety of areas depending on the child's or adolescent's presenting symptoms. For example, some children need to learn basic ADLs, others have difficulty with their impulse control and frustration tolerance, and those with anxiety disorders may benefit from anxiety reduction skills. Many children and adolescents benefit from a variety of social skills (problem solving, decision making, initiating and maintaining contacts with peers) that will help them negotiate satisfying and productive relationships and friendships in the outside world. Many young people suffer from severe symptoms of depression, and although medication may be immediately useful, family and individual therapies should be made a pivotal part of the youngster's treatment. Rarely, if ever is medication alone treatment of choice.

However, there are many indications for the use of medications. Medications that target specific symptoms can make a decided difference in the family's ability to cope and their quality of life, and can enhance the child's or adolescent's optimal potential for growth. Table 4–4 identifies some child/adolescent disorders and medications used in the treatment of such disorders.

♦ NURSE AND PARENT/CAREGIVER RESOURCES—MENTAL DISORDERS OF CHILDHOOD AND ADOLESCENCE

Books for Parents

Barkley, R.A. (1995). Taking Charge of ADHD: The Complete Authoritative Guide for Parents. New York: Guilford Press.

Barkley, R.A., and Benton, C.M. (1998). Your Defiant Child: 8 Steps to Better Behavior. New York: Guilford Press.

Burt, S., and Perlis, L. (1998). Parents as Mentors. Rocklin, CA: Prima Publishing.

Gardner, R.A. (1997). Understanding Children. Northvale, NJ: Jason Aronson.

Greenspan, S.I., and Salmon, J. (1995). The Challenging Child: Understanding, Raising and Enjoying Five Different Types of Children. Reading, PA: Perseus Books.

Maurice, C., Green, G., and Luce, S. (1996). Behavioral Interventions for Your Children with Autism: A Manual for Parents and Professionals. Austin, TX: PRO-ED.

Powers, M.D. (ed.). (1993). A Parent's Guide to Autism. Rockville, MD: Woodbine House.

Schaefer, C.E. (1991). Teach Your Child to Behave. New York: Penguin.

Witkin, G. (1999). Kid Stress: Effective Strategies Parents Can Teach Kids for School, Family, Peers, the World and Everything. New York: Viking Penguin.

References for Nurses

Berg, B. (1986). The changing family game: Cognitive-behavioral interventions for children of divorce. In Schaefer, C.E., and Reid, S.E. (eds.), Game Play: Therapeutic Use of Childhood Games. New York: Wiley.

Cittone, R.A., and Madonna, J.M. (1997). Play Therapy with Sexually Abused Children. New York: Jason Aronson.

Greenspan, S.I., and Wieder, S. (1998). The Child with Special Needs: Encouraging Intellectual and Emotional Growth. Reading, PA: Perseus Books.

Kaduson, H. (1997). Play therapy for children with attention-deficit hyperactivity disorder. In Kaduson, H., Cangelosi, D., and Schaefer, C.E. (eds.), The Playing Cure: Individualized Play Therapy for Specific Childhood Problems. New York: Jason Aronson.

Kaduson, H., and Schaefer, C.E. (1997). 101 Favorite Play Therapy Techniques. New York: Jason Aronson.

King, N.J., and Ollendick, T.H. (1997). Treatment of childhood phobias. Journal of Child Psychology and Psychiatry 38:389–400.

Maurice, C., Green, G., and Luce, S. (1996). Behavioral Interventions for Your Children with Autism: A Manual for Parents and Professionals. Austin, TX: PRO-ED.

Pfefferbaum, B. (ed.). (1998). Stress in children. Child and Adolescent Psychiatric Clinics of North America 7(1).

Shelby, J.S. (1997) Rubble, disruption, and tears: Helping young survivors of natural disaster. In Kaduson, H., Cangelosi, D., and Schaefer, C.E. (eds.), The Playing Cure: Individualized Play Therapy for Specific Childhood Problems. New York: Jason Aronson.

Tait, D., and Depta, T. (1997). Play group therapy for bereaved children. In Webb, N.B. (ed.), Helping Bereaved Children. New York: Guilford Press.

Internet Sites

Autism Society of America Home Page
http://www.autism-society.org

Autism Resources
http://www.autism-resources.com

**Children and Adults with Attention
Deficit/Hyperactivity Disorder**
http://www.chadd.org

ADD Medical Treatment Center of Santa Clara Valley
http://www.addmtc.com

Oppositional Defiant Disorder
http://www.conductdisorders.com

Children and Anxiety (Anxiety-Panic Internet Resource)
http://www.algy.com/anxiety/children.html

Adolescent Depression (Internet Mental Health)
http://www.mentalhealth.com/magl/p51-dp01.html

**Mood Disorders in Children and Adolescents
(Mental Health Info Source)**
http://www.mhsource.com/advocacy/narsad/childmood.html

American Academy of Child and Adolescent Psychiatry
http://www.aacap.org

**Association of Child and Adolescent Psychiatric Nurses
(ACAPN)**
http://www.acapn.org

CHAPTER 5

Personality Disorders

C lients diagnosed as having personality disorders (PDs) have multiple needs that pose many challenges to nurses and other health care providers. PDs occur in about 10% of the population; however, they are often overdiagnosed in clients who are ethnically and culturally different from the health care practitioner (Kaplan and Sadock, 1996). Therefore, it is important that assessment be performed in the context of the client's national, cultural, spiritual, and ethnic background.

PDs are a major source of long-term disability and frequently occur in conjunction with other psychiatric disorders, or with general medical conditions. For example, both major depression and panic disorder have a high rate of comorbidity (co-occurrence) with PDs, estimated to occur in about 25% to 50% of clients. Comorbid PDs are likely to be found in clients with somatization, eating disorder, chronic pain, recurrent suicide attempts, and post-traumatic stress disorder (see Chapter 6) (Goldberg, 1995). People with a substance abuse problem may also have a comorbid PD, which can complicate the therapeutic working relationship and interfere with treatment.

PDs are made up of personality traits that are maladaptive, persistent, and inflexible. The intensity and manifestation of presenting problems may vary widely among clients with PDs depending upon diagnoses and individual characteristics. Some clients with PDs may have milder forms of disability, whereas other clients' symptoms may present as extreme, even psychotic. However, all of the PDs have four characteristics in common:

1. Inflexible and maladaptive responses to stress
2. Disability in working and loving
3. Ability to evoke interpersonal conflict in nurse as well as family and friends
4. Capacity to have an intense effect on others (this process is often unconscious and generally produces undesirable results)

Box 5–1 identifies the DSM-IV criteria for a person with a PD. The DSM IV organizes the 10 personality disorders into three clusters (Box 5–2).

Because each of the personality disorders have their own characteristics, personality traits, and effects on self and others, it is best to deal with them individually. The following sections (1) describe the defining characteristics, (2) identify some intervention guidelines, and (3) offer the most recent treatment modalities for each PD.

Some of the most problematic behaviors that nurses are confronted with in the health care setting are similar for many of the personality disorders. These behaviors in part include manipula-

---

❖   B O X   5 – 1   ❖

General Diagnostic Criteria for a Personality Disorder

1. An enduring pattern of inner experience and behavior that deviates markedly from the expectations of the individual's culture. This pattern is manifested in two (or more) of the following areas:
   • Cognition (i.e., ways of perceiving and interpreting self, other people, and events)
   • Affect (i.e., the range, intensity, lability, and appropriateness of emotional response)
   • Interpersonal functioning
   • Impulse control
2. The enduring pattern is inflexible and pervasive across a broad range of personal and social situations.
3. The enduring pattern leads to clinically significant distress or impairment in social, occupational, or other important areas of functioning.
4. The pattern is stable and of long duration and its onset can be traced back at least to adolescence or early adulthood.
5. The enduring pattern is not better accounted for as manifestation or consequence of another mental disorder.
6. The enduring pattern is not due to the direct physiological effects of a substance (e.g., a drug of abuse, a medication) or a general medical condition (e.g., head trauma).

Adapted from American Psychiatric Association. (1994). Diagnostic and Statistical Manual of Mental Disorders, 4th ed. Washington, DC: American Psychiatric Press, p. 633; reprinted with permission. Copyright 1994 American Psychiatric Association.

❖   B O X   5 – 2   ❖
Personality Disorder Clusters

Cluster A Disorders—Odd or Eccentric
Paranoid Personality Disorder
Schizoid Personality Disorder
Schizotypal Personality Disorder

Cluster B Disorders—Dramatic, Emotional, or Erratic
Antisocial Personality Disorder
Borderline Personality Disorder
Histrionic Personality Disorder
Narcissistic Personality Disorder

Cluster C Disorders—Anxious or Fearful
Dependent Personality Disorder
Obsessive-Compulsive Personality Disorder
Avoidant Personality Disorder

tion (see Chapter 17), self-mutilation, suicide (see Chapter 13), anger and hostility (see Chapter 14), low self-esteem, ineffective coping and/or impaired social interaction, and nonadherence to medication or treatment (see Chapter 18). Self-mutilation, low self-esteem, and impaired social interaction are covered in this chapter. The other common nursing diagnoses of clients with PD are covered in separate chapters. All of these behaviors are commonly seen in a host of disorders, and the guidelines for intervention are similar for all clients. Table 5–1 identifies other possible nursing diagnoses for a PD client that may warrant intervention.

Although people with PDs may be hospitalized briefly during a crisis, for the most part long-term treatment takes place in clinics and community settings.

◆ CLUSTER A DISORDERS—ODD OR ECCENTRIC

Cluster A disorders, often referred to as "odd" or "eccentric," comprise PDs that have been established to have some relationship to schizophrenia. Of the Cluster A disorders, schizotypal PD is most strongly related to schizophrenia. The following discussion gives defining characteristics, guidelines for care, and *treatments* for the Cluster A disorders.

Table 5–1 ◆ Potential Nursing Diagnoses—Personality Disorder

SYMPTOMS	NURSING DIAGNOSIS
Crisis, high levels of anxiety	**Ineffective Individual Coping**
	Anxiety
Anger and aggression; child, elder, or spouse abuse	**Risk for Violence Directed at Others**
	Ineffective Individual Coping
	Altered Parenting
	Ineffective Family Coping: Disabling
Withdrawal	**Social Isolation**
Paranoia	**Fear**
	Sensory/Perceptual Alteration
	Altered Thought Process
	Defensive Coping
Depression	**Hopelessness**
	Helplessness
	Risk for Violence: Self-Directed
	Self-Mutilation
	Self-Esteem/Chronic Low Self-Esteem
	Spiritual Distress
Difficulty in relationships, manipulation	**Ineffective Individual Coping**
	Impaired Social Interaction
	Defensive Coping
	Altered Family Processes
	Risk for Loneliness
Not keeping medical appointments, late for appointments, not following prescribed medical procedure/ medication	**Ineffective Management of Therapeutic Regimen**
	Nonadherence to Medications or Treatments (specify)

◆ OVERVIEW OF THE DSM-IV PERSONALITY DISORDERS

Paranoid Personality Disorder (PPD)

Defining Characteristics

1. Vigilant and suspicious of others' motives—believe people mean to exploit, harm, or deceive them in some manner
2. Bear grudges; are unforgiving of insults, injuries, or slights
3. Read hidden, demeaning, or threatening meanings into benign remarks or events
4. Have difficulty establishing close relationships; usually work alone
5. Perceived as cold and unemotional, and do not share their thoughts with others; lack a sense of humor

6. Very critical of others but have great deal of difficulty accepting criticism
7. Are prone to file suit

≡	NURSING GUIDELINES

1. Avoid being too "nice" or "friendly."
2. Give clear and straightforward explanations of tests and procedures beforehand.
3. Use simple clear language; avoid ambiguity.
4. Project a neutral but kind affect.
5. Warn about any changes, side effects of medications, and reasons for delay. Such interventions may help allay anxiety and minimize suspiciousness.
6. A written plan of treatment may help encourage co-operation.

Treatment

Paranoid clients will initially mistrust their therapist's motives and find it difficult to share personal information. For that reason, therapy is often not sought or sustained among these clients. However, when a person with PPD does enter therapy, initially supportive therapy may help the client experience trust and even begin to feel some amount of safety in an interpersonal relationship. If a therapeutic alliance can be achieved, cognitive and behavioral techniques may be useful to the client. The focus is on enhancing coping strategies and relieving stress and worry that are expressed as hypervigilance and social withdrawal (Zale et al., 1997). Severe symptoms of paranoia may be attenuated with careful use of antipsychotic medication.

Schizoid Personality Disorder

Defining Characteristics

1. Neither desire nor enjoy close relationships, even within their own family
2. Prefer to live apart from others, choose solitary activities, have little interest in sexual activity with others, and may describe themselves as "loners"
3. Show emotional coldness, detachment, or flattened affect
4. Occupation often involves little interpersonal contact

NURSING GUIDELINES
1. Avoid being too "nice" or "friendly."
2. Do not try to re-socialize these clients (Goldberg, 1995).
3. A thorough diagnostic assessment may be needed to identify symptoms or disorders that the client is reluctant to discuss.

Treatment

A schizoid individual is apt to seek treatment only in a crisis situation, and only then to seek relief from acute symptoms. In some cases, supportive psychotherapy with cognitive-behavioral techniques may help reinforce socially outgoing behaviors. Group therapy may be appropriate if the individual needs of each client are addressed. In some cases social skills training groups may be an effective intervention (Zale et al., 1997). Short-term use of psychopharmacology may be appropriate for treating anxiety or depression. Low-dose antipsychotic medication can target symptoms such as anger, hostility, paranoia, and ideas of reference if such symptoms are part of the clinical picture.

Schizotypal Personality Disorders

Defining Characteristics

1. Share many of the withdrawn, aloof, and socially distant characteristics listed for the schizoid PD client described above
2. Ideas of reference, odd beliefs, magical thinking, or unusual perceptual experiences, including bodily illusions, may be present.
3. Excessive and unrelieved social anxiety frequently associated with paranoid fears
4. Lack of close friends and confidants
5. Inappropriate or constricted affect
6. Behavior or appearance that is odd, eccentric, or peculiar
7. Some individuals diagnosed with schizotypal PD will go on to present with a full-blown schizophrenic illness.

NURSING GUIDELINES
1. Respect the client's need for social isolation.
2. Be aware of client's suspiciousness and employ appropriate interventions (see Chapter 9).
3. As with the schizoid client, careful diagnostic assessment may be needed to uncover any other medical or psychological symptoms that may need intervention (e.g., suicidal thoughts).

Treatment

As with the schizoid client, allowing distance and providing supportive measures may encourage the gradual development of a therapeutic alliance. Cognitive and behavioral measures may help clients gain basic social skills. Low-dose therapy with the newer atypical antipsychotics (risperidone [Risperdal], olanzapine [Zyperxa]) may be effective in allowing the schizotypal client to be more comfortable, less anxious, less prone to suspiciousness, and more organized in his or her thinking (Zale et al., 1997).

◆ **CLUSTER B DISORDERS—DRAMATIC, EMOTIONAL OR ERRATIC**

These four disorders appear to share dramatic, erratic, or flamboyant behavior as part of their presenting symptoms. As yet, no empirical evidence for this manner of clustering exists (Zale et al., 1997), but there does seem to be a high degree of overlap among these disorders. There is also a great deal of comorbidity with Axis I disorders such as substance abuse, mood, and anxiety disorders as well as other personality disorders (cluster A, B, or C) that are found on Axis II. It is often difficult for the clinician to know which disorder is primary and which should take precedence in treatment (Zale et al., 1997).

Antisocial Personality Disorder (ASPD)

Defining Characteristics

1. An extended history of antisocial behaviors (stealing, persistent lying, cruelty to animals or people, vandalism, substance abuse) usually beginning before the age of 15 and continuing into adulthood

2. Deceitfulness (use of aliases, conning others for personal profit or pleasure, repeated lying)
3. Consistent irresponsibility (failure to honor financial obligations, work responsibilities, family/parenting obligations)
4. Impassivity and repeated aggressiveness toward others
5. Total lack of remorse for physically or emotionally hurting or mistreating others or swindling or stealing from others
6. At times may present as charming, self-assured, and adept.
7. Interaction with others through **manipulation, aggressiveness,** and **exploitation,** totally lacking in empathy or concern for others
8. Substance abuse is the most frequent comorbid Axis I disorder.
9. There is a significant familial pattern to criminality in general and ASPD in particular (McGee and Linehan, 1997).

NURSING GUIDELINES

1. Try to prevent or reduce untoward effects of manipulation (flattery, seductiveness, instilling guilt).
   - Set clear and realistic limits on specific behavior.
   - All limits should be adhered to by all staff involved.
   - Carefully document objective physical signs of manipulation or aggression when managing clinical problems.
   - Document behaviors objectively (give times, dates, circumstances).
   - Provide clear boundaries and consequences.
2. Be aware that antisocial clients can instill guilt when they are not getting what they want. Guard against being manipulated through feeling guilty.
3. Treatment of substance abuse is best handled through a well-organized treatment *before* counseling and other forms of therapy are started.

Treatment

Unfortunately, there is no treatment of choice for ASPD. The most useful approach is to target specific problem behaviors that have been shown to be amenable to modification, combined with other therapies such as psychopharmacology and family therapy. Lithium carbonate, divalproex sodium (Depakote), and carbamazepine have effectively decreased violent behaviors in some individuals. The selective serotonin reuptake inhibitors (SSRIs) (e.g., fluoxetine) have been effective in decreasing the occurrence of aggressive behaviors in others (McGee and Linehan, 1997). Some positive results have been obtained through milieu programs (e.g., token economy systems and therapeutic communities).

Borderline Personality Disorder (BPD)

Defining Characteristics

1. Relationships with others are intense and unstable, and alternate between intense dependence and rejection.
2. Behaviors are often impulsive and self-damaging (e.g., spending, unsafe sex, substance abuse, reckless driving, binge eating).
3. Recurrent suicidal and/or self-mutilating behaviors are common, often in response to perceived threats of rejection, separation.
4. Chronic feelings of emptiness or boredom, and an absence of self-satisfaction.
5. Frantic efforts to avoid real or imagined abandonment.
6. Intense affect is manifested in outbursts of anger, hostility, depression, and/or anxiety.
7. Intense and primitive rage often complicates therapy and takes the form of extreme sarcasm, enduring bitterness, and angry outbursts at others.
8. Major defense is **splitting,** which often manifests in pitting one person or group against another (good guy vs. bad guy).
9. Splitting is only one form of **manipulation** that individuals with BPD use.
10. Rapid idealization-devaluation is a classic signal behavior suggestive of borderline psychopathology or some other primitive personality.
11. Transient quasi-psychotic symptoms may develop in the form of paranoid or dissociate symptoms during times of stress.

NURSING GUIDELINES

1. Set realistic goals, use clear action words.
2. Be aware of manipulative behaviors (flattery, seductiveness, guilt instilling).
3. Provide clear and consistent boundaries and limits.
4. Use clear and straightforward communication.
5. When behavioral problems emerge, calmly review the therapeutic goals and boundaries of treatment.
6. Avoid rejecting or rescuing.
7. Assess for suicidal and self-mutilating behaviors, especially during times of stress.

Treatment

There is no one treatment that has emerged as a guaranteed treatment for BPD. Although psychodynamically oriented therapy is commonly recommended for BPD, there are no randomized, controlled trials demonstrating the efficacy of any psychodynamic approach. Linehan has developed a behaviorally based testament that targets the highly dysfunctional behaviors seen in clients with BPD. Her treatment approach is called dialectical behavioral therapy, and has proved promising in a randomized, controlled study (McGee and Linehan, 1997). Therapy is often marked by a period of improvement with alternating periods of worsening. Short-term hospitalization is not uncommon during periods of suicidal or self-mutilating behaviors or severe depression. Long-term outpatient therapy, and at times carefully chosen group therapy if appropriate for the client, has shown improvement over time for many clients.

A combination of psychotherapy and medication appears to provide the best results for treatment of clients diagnosed with BPD. Medications can reduce anxiety, depression, and disruptive impulses. About 50% of people with BPD experience serious episodes of depression. Low-dose antipsychotics may prove useful for severely cognitively disturbed individuals. The newer antidepressants (SSRIs) have helped some BPD clients in dealing with their anger. The anticonvulsant carbamazepine has demonstrated some efficacy in decreasing the frequency and severity of behavioral dyscontrol episodes, suicidality, and temper outbursts (McGee and Linehan, 1997).

Clients with BPD pose great challenges for nurse clinicians, and supervision is advised to help with the inevitable strong countertransference issues.

Histrionic Personality Disorder (HPD)

Defining Characteristics

1. Consistently draw attention to themselves; very concerned about being attractive and use physical appearance to gain center stage.
2. Show excessive emotionality and attention-getting behavior (e.g., display sexually seductive, provocative, or self-dramatizing behaviors).
3. Intense emotional expressions are shallow, with rapid shifts from person to person or idea to idea.
4. Prone to describe more intimacy in a relationship than is there (e.g., show intense attention to a casual acquaintance).

5. Are suggestible, (easily influenced by others or circumstances).
6. Others experience them as smothering, destructive; unable to understand/insensitive to anyone else's experience.
7. Without instant gratification or admiration from others, clients can experience depression and become suicidal.

NURSING GUIDELINES
1. Understand seductive behavior as a response to distress.
2. Keep communication and interactions professional, despite temptation to collude with the client in a flirtatious and misleading manner.
3. Encourage and model the use of concrete and descriptive rather than vague and impressionistic language.
4. Teach and role model assertiveness.

Treatment

People with HPD use indirect means to get others to take care of them (physical attractiveness, charm, temper outbursts), and this can greatly complicate the therapeutic process. Therapeutic approaches used are psychoanalytic and cognitive-behavioral methods; however, research on the treatment of HPD is lacking. Most of the literature consists of case reports using various approaches (McGee and Linehan, 1997).

Narcissistic Personality Disorder (NPD)

Defining Characteristics

1. Exploit others to meet their own needs and desires.
2. Come across as arrogant and demonstrate a demeanor of "persistent entitlement."
3. Portray a demeanor of grandiosity, a need for admiration, and a lack of empathy for others (APA, 1994).
4. May begrudge others their success or possessions, feeling that they deserve the admiration and privileges more (APA, 1994).
5. Relationships are characterized by disruption (frequently provoke arguments) or control (consistently in power struggles).

	NURSING GUIDELINES

1. Remain neutral, avoid power struggles or becoming defensive in response to the client's disparaging remarks, no matter how provocative the situation may be.
2. Convey unassuming self-confidence.

Treatment

There have been no controlled trials of efficacy for any one therapeutic approach. The main approaches are supportive or insight-oriented psychotherapy. Milieu therapy may be useful for some NPD clients. Treatment difficulties lie in preserving the client's self-esteem in the face of psychiatric interventions (Kaplan and Sadock, 1996). Most of these clients do not seek treatment unless they seek treatment for an Axis I disorder and have comorbid NPD.

◆ CLUSTER C DISORDERS—ANXIOUS OR FEARFUL

These disorders have been clustered together because their common property is the experience of high levels of anxiety and the outward signs of fear. These personality types also show social inhibitions, mostly in the sexual sphere (e.g., shyness or awkwardness with potential sexual partners; impotence or frigidity). Many people with a Cluster C disorder have a fearful reluctance to express irritation or anger, even in an interpersonal encounter that justifies these feelings (Stone, 1997).

Inhibited clients tend to *internalize* blame for the frustrations in their lives even when they are not to blame for these frustrations. This willingness to accept responsibility for contributing to their own unhappiness can foster a good working relationship between clinician and client. Therefore, this can be a useful trait. Those who blame others for their problems (*externalize* blame outward), such as antisocial, paranoid, and sadistic people, pose great challenges in therapy and have a guarded prognosis (Stone, 1997).

Dependent Personality Disorder (DPD)

Defining Characteristics

1. May manifest an unusual degree of agreeableness or friendliness.

2. These qualities are meant to enhance the dependent person's ability to attach to another who can act as protector. Urgently seeks another relationship as a source of care and support when a close relationship ends.

3. Clinging is a common manifestation, but unfortunately this trait eventually alienates people and threatens to drive them away.

4. Often perfecting the techniques of clinging to others takes the place of outside interests, reading, cultivation of friends, or other sustaining activities.

5. Have difficulty making everyday decisions without excessive advice and support from others.

6. Go to excessive lengths to obtain nurture and support from others, even to the point of being mistreated or abused, or suffering extreme self-sacrifice.

7. Need others to assume responsibility for most major areas of life. When others do not take initiative or take responsibility for them, their needs go unmet.

8. Difficulty expressing disagreements with others for fear of loss of support or approval.

9. The DPD client is at risk for anxiety and mood disorders, and DPD can occur with BPD, avoidant personality disorder, and HPD.

10. Fear not getting enough care, and often insist on having everything done for them.

NURSING GUIDELINES

1. Identify and help address current stresses.
2. Try to satisfy client's needs at the same time as you set up limits in such a manner that the client does not feel punished and withdraw.
3. Strong countertransference often develops in clinicians because of the client's excessive clinging (demands of extra time, nighttime calls, crisis before vacations); therefore, supervision is well advised.
4. Teach and role model assertiveness.

Treatment

A variety of therapies are useful, and may all be appropriate during different phases while working on specific issues. Therapies include psychoanalytic psychotherapy, supportive therapy, cognitive-behavioral therapy, group therapy, and family therapy. Therapy is usually long term and is dependent upon the motivation of the client and how realistic the goals are (Stone, 1997).

Obsessive-Compulsive Personality Disorder (OCPD)

Defining Characteristics

1. Inflexible, rigid, and need to be in control
2. Perfectionists to a degree that interferes with completion of work; cannot delegate
3. Overemphasis on work to the exclusion of friendships and pleasurable leisure activities
4. Preoccupied with details to the extent that decision-making is impaired
5. Intimacy in relationships is superficial and rigidly controlled, even though clients with OCPD may feel deep and genuine affection for friends and family.
6. Highly critical of self and others in matters of morality, ethics, or values
7. The term *compulsive* refers to the behavioral aspects: preoccupation with lists, rules, schedules, and more. Other traits include indecisiveness, hoarding, and stinginess with money or time.
8. Clients with OCPD are often overwhelmed with a concern about loss of control (being too messy, sexy, or naughty), hence their need to overcontrol and dominate people and situations in their lives (Stone, 1997) .

NURSING GUIDELINES
1. Guard against engaging in power struggles with an OCPD client. Need for control is very high for these clients.
2. Intellectualization, rationalization, and reaction formation are the most common defense mechanisms clients with OCD use.

Treatment

Individual psychotherapy, supportive or insight-oriented therapy, and cognitive-behavioral therapy may all be useful depending on goals and the ego strengths of the client. Therapeutic issues usually include those of control, submission, and intellectualization. Some medications found to be useful for the obsessional component are clomipramine (tricyclic antidepressant [TCA]), fluoxetine (SSRI), and clonazepam (anxiolytic). Group therapy can also be a useful adjunct to therapy.

Avoidant Personality Disorder (APD)

Defining Characteristics

1. Pervasive pattern of social inhibition. Virtually all people with APD have social phobias.
2. Strong feelings of inadequacy. APD clients experience fear of rejection and/or criticism. These individuals are very reticent in social situations because of this fear.
3. Avoid occupational activities that involve significant interpersonal contact because of fears of criticism, disapproval, or rejection.
4. View themselves as socially inept, personally unappealing, or inferior to others.
5. APD clients may be inhibited and reluctant to involve themselves in new interpersonal situations or new activities.
6. Not uncommon for some clients with APD to have comorbid agoraphobia and obsessive-compulsive disorder as well as social phobia.

NURSING GUIDELINES

1. A friendly, gentle, reassuring approach is the best way to treat clients with APD.
2. Being pushed into social situations can cause extreme and severe anxiety for APD clients.

Treatment

Each client needs to be assessed individually. For example, if the client has been taught fearfulness and withdrawal by avoidant parents, treatment would differ from that for the client whose behavioral and cognitive traits stem from parental brutalization, incest, or sexual molestation in childhood (Stone, 1997). Because of the inherent social phobia, various forms of treatment can prove useful, such as cognitive therapy, densensitization, social skills training, and other cognitive-behavioral techniques. Group therapy has not proven advantageous over one-to-one supportive or exploratory psychotherapies. However, in the case of incest or other interpersonal trauma, special groups that include people with similar backgrounds are considered quite beneficial (Stone, 1997). Social anxiety may respond to a monoamine oxidase inhibitor (MAOI). Benzodiazepine anxiolytics may help to contain brief panic episodes. The lowering of the frightening anxiety can help clients engage more readily into therapy and can aid compliance when clients are very fearful and anxious.

◆ ASSESSING FOR A PERSONALITY DISORDER

History

In assessing for a PD, the client's history may reveal persistent traits held over long periods of time causing distress or impairment in functioning. Does the client:

Cluster A

1. Suspect others of exploiting or deceiving him or her? Bear grudges and not forget insults?
2. Detach self from social relationships? Not desire close relationships or being part of a family? Take pleasure in few, if any, activities?
3. Have a history of social and interpersonal deficits marked by acute discomfort? Have any cognitive or perceptual distortions?

Cluster B

4. Have a pervasive pattern of disregard for and violation of the rights of others? Act deceitful (repeated lying, use others for own needs)? Act consistently irresponsible toward others?
5. Have a pattern of unstable and chaotic personal relationships? Have a history of suicide attempts or self-mutilation? Have chronic feelings of emptiness, or show intense anger, intense anxiety, and dysphoria?
6. Have a pattern of excessive emotionality and attention-seeking behaviors (e.g., sexually seductive or provocative)? Have very self-dramatic, theatrical, and exaggerate expressions of emotion?
7. Act grandiose, need admiration, lack empathy for others? Have unreasonable expectations of favored treatment? Act interpersonally exploitive?

Cluster C

8. Persistently avoid social situations because of feelings of inadequacy and hypersensitivity to negative evaluation? View self as socially inept or inferior to others?
9. Have an excessive need to be taken care of, show clinging behaviors within relationships, have intense fear of separation?

Have difficulty making everyday decisions without excessive amount of advice and reassurance from others?

10. Have a preoccupation with neatness, perfectionism, and mental and interpersonal control? Show rigidity and stubbornness?

Presenting Symptoms

1. Client usually comes to the attention of the health care system through a crisis situation.

2. Antisocial clients most often come into the health care system through the courts by means of a court order.

3. Suicide attempts, self-mutilation, or substance abuse are common crises that bring people with PD into treatment.

Box 5–3 provides sample questions the nurse clinician/counselors may use to identify specific traits and personality characteristics.

❖   B O X   5 – 3   ❖

Sample Questions To Identify Personality Traits

The nurse uses a variety of therapeutic techniques to obtain the answers to the following questions. Use your discretion and decide which questions are appropriate to complete your assessment.

The following questions are NOT meant to be used in a checklist fashion. They should be woven into the assessment, using only a few of the questions for each diagnosis. Often the answer to one can eliminate certain diagnoses.

Obsessive-Compulsive Personality

1. Do you tend to drive yourself pretty hard, frequently feeling like you need to do just a little more? (yes)
2. Do you think that most people would view you as witty and light-hearted? (no)
3. Do you tend toward being perfectionist? (yes)
4. Do you tend to keep lists or sometimes feel a need to keep checking things, like is the door locked? (yes)

Dependent Personality

1. Is it sort of hard for you to argue with your spouse, because you're worried that he or she will really get mad at you and start to dislike you? (yes)
2. When you wake up in the morning, do you need to plan your day around the activities of your husband or wife? (yes)

Continued

3. Do you enjoy making most decisions in your house or would you prefer that others make most important decisions? (prefers others to make decision)
4. When you were younger, did you often dream of finding someone who would take care of you and guide you? (yes)

Avoidant Personality

1. Throughout most of your life, have you found yourself being worried that people won't like you? (yes)
2. Do you often find yourself sort of feeling inadequate and not up to new challenges and tasks? (yes)
3. Do you tend to be very careful about selecting friends, perhaps only having one or two close friends in your whole life? (yes)
4. Have you often felt hurt by others, so that you are pretty wary of opening yourself to other people? (yes)

Schizoid Personality

1. Do you tend to really enjoy being around people, or do you much prefer being alone? (much prefers being alone)
2. Do you care a lot about what people think about you as a person? (tends not to care)
3. Are you a real emotional person? (no, feels strongly that he or she is not emotional)
4. During the course of your life, have you had only about one or two friends? (yes)

Antisocial Personality

1. If you felt like the situation really warranted it, do you think that you would find it pretty easy to lie? (yes)
2. Have you ever been arrested or pulled over by the police? (yes)
3. Over the years have you found yourself able to take care of yourself in a physical fight? (yes)
4. Do you sometimes find yourself resenting people who give you orders? (yes)

Histrionic Personality

1. Do people of the opposite sex frequently find you attractive? (answered with an unabashed "yes")
2. Do you frequently find yourself being the center of attention, even if you don't want to be? (yes)
3. Do you view yourself as being a powerfully emotional person? (yes)
4. Do you think that you'd make a reasonably good actor or actress? (yes)

Continued

Narcissistic Personality

1. Do you find that, when you get really down to it, most people aren't quite up to your standards? (yes)
2. If people give you a hard time, do you tend to put them in their place quickly? (yes)
3. If someone criticizes you, do you find yourself getting angry pretty quickly? (yes)
4. Do you think that, compared with other people, you are a very special person? (answered with a self-assured "yes")

Borderline Personality

1. Do you frequently feel let down by people? (yes)
2. If a friend or family member hurts you, do you sometimes feel like hurting yourself, perhaps by cutting at yourself and burning yourself? (yes)
3. Do you find that other people cause you to feel angry a couple of times per week? (yes)
4. Do you think that your friends would view you as sort of moody? (yes)
5. Does anxiety make you want to self-mutilate? (yes)

Schizotypal Personality

1. Do you tend to stay by yourself, even though you would like to be with others? (yes)
2. Do you sometimes feel like other people are watching you or have some sort of special interest in you? (yes)
3. Have you ever felt like you had some special powers like ESP or some sort of magical influence over others? (yes)
4. Do you feel that people often want to reject you or that they find you odd? (yes)

Paranoid Personality

1. Do you find that people often have a tendency to be disloyal or dishonest? (yes)
2. Is it fairly easy for you to get jealous, especially if someone is making eyes at your spouse? (yes)
3. Do you tend to keep things to yourself just to make sure the wrong people don't get the right information? (yes)
4. Do you feel that other people take advantage of you? (yes)

Adapted from Roberts, J.K.A. (1984). Differential Diagnoses in Neuropsychiatry. Chichester: John Wiley & Sons Limited, p. 26 and Shea, S.C. (1998). Psychiatric Interviewing: The Art of Understanding. Philadelphia: W.B. Saunders, pp. 420–422; with permission.

ASSESSMENT ALERTS
1. Assessment about personality functioning needs to be viewed within the person's ethnic, cultural, and social background.
2. PDs are often exacerbated following the loss of significant supporting people or in a disruptive social situation.
3. A change in personality in middle adulthood or later signals the need for a thorough medical work-up or assessment for unrecognized substance abuse disorder.
4. Be cognizant that social stereotypes can muddy a clinician's judgment in that a particular diagnosis may be over- or underdiagnosed (e.g., for males or females because of sexual bias; because of social class or immigrant status).

◆ NURSING DIAGNOSES WITH INTERVENTIONS

The data the nurse clinician collects provide information about the client's presenting problem or behaviors, emotional state, precipitating situations, and maladaptive coping behaviors. Clients with PDs present with any number of problematic behaviors. These behaviors may or may not be pathological or maladaptive. Behaviors that are repetitive or rigid, or those that present an obstacle to meaningful relationships or functioning, are considered behaviors that will be focused on during management of care. Many of the dysfunctional thought processes and behaviors have been described in the individual presentation of these disorders.

Short-term goals usually center on the client's safety and comfort, and are pertinent to the client's physical and mental well-being. Often the first goals for the management of an *acute crisis* are to evaluate the need for medication and to identify appropriate verbal interventions to decrease the client's immediate emotional stress (Profiri, 1998). **Keep in mind that clients have varied degrees of cognitive functioning and disabilities. What may be a short-term goal for one is likely a long-term goal for another client.** The goals cited here and in other chapters are helpful guidelines, but often the clinician is the one to best estimate client strengths, capabilities, supports, and current level of functioning when setting specific time limits on goals. (For more on this topic, see Chapter 1.)

Outcome criteria are targeted for the long term, and center on skill attainment. It is important to keep goals realistic. Changing lifelong patterns of behaviors that are inflexible and persistent takes a great deal of time, as well as engagement by the client. Outcome criteria usually include the following areas (Profiri, 1998).

- Linking consequences to both functional and dysfunctional behaviors
- Learning and mastering skills that facilitate functional behaviors
- Practicing the substitution of functional alternatives during crisis
- Ongoing management of anger, anxiety, shame, and happiness
- Creating a lifestyle that prevents regressing (e.g., **HALT**: never getting too **H**ungry, too **A**ngry, too **L**onely, or too **T**ired)
- Nursing crisis intervention strategies

These clients often act very impulsively. The nurse will be called upon to intervene in many acting-out behaviors, often marked by impulsivity, such as self-mutilation and/or suicide attempts, anger and hostility toward the nurse clinician, extreme paranoia and blaming others for problems, manipulation and splitting, and intense anxiety, to name but a few. Acting-out behaviors are often most intense during the initial phases of therapy. Dealing with clients when they are acting out, especially during crises, takes persistence, patience, and learned skill on the part of the clinician. Some of the more common behavioral defenses PD clients employ require rigorous interventions. Because it is impossible to deal with all the problem areas of the 10 personality disorders, we will identify common behaviors for which all nurses are encouraged to develop skills. Common phenomena related to PD clients are (1) manipulation, (2) self-mutilation/suicide attempts, (3) intense low self-esteem, (4) intense anxiety, (5) anger and physical fighting, (6) projecting identification and projecting blame to others, and (7) impulsivity. PD clients are often very demanding of health care personnel and others.

Among the common phenomena and nursing diagnoses three are presented here: **Risk for Self-Mutilation (scratching, burning, cutting), Chronic Low Self-Esteem, and Impaired Social Interaction.** Nursing interventions for minimizing and preventing **manipulation** are presented in Chapter 17. **Suicide** is covered in Chapter 13. Intense **anger and hostility** are addressed in Chapter 14.

People with PDs have great difficulty getting along with others and often elicit intense negative feelings from others. The following behaviors are found in a variety of combinations: demanding, angry, fault finding, suspicious, insensitive to the needs of others, manipulative, clinging, at times withdrawn, and often intensely lonely. Therefore, their relationships with others are often chaotic and unsatisfying for all concerned. **Impaired Social Interaction (Defensive Coping/Avoidance Coping, Ineffective Individual Coping)** is one of the key nursing diagnoses for people with PD and is always present, most often in response to intense feelings of powerlessness. Table 5–1 identifies other possible nursing diagnoses.

Many people with PDs leave therapy after a crisis is over and things have settled down somewhat. Therefore, nonadherence to therapy or medication is common. **Non-adherence to medications or treatment** is addressed in Chapter 18.

Keep in mind, however, each client is uniquely individual, so, although many of the phenomena are shared among several of the PDs, the manifestations of these behaviors can take many forms. The difficulty PD clients have in their interpersonal relationships is carried over to the health care setting, and poses challenges for nurses, physicians, and actually all health care personnel.

Supervision and case discussion are usually extremely useful in guarding against getting caught up in countertransferential power struggles and nontherapeutic encounters that threaten any therapeutic alliance.

Whatever nursing diagnoses you choose, keep in mind that nursing diagnoses need to be uniquely crafted to the specific individual, the presenting symptoms, the individual circumstances, and the personal manifestation of these symptoms. This is especially true for people with PDs.

	OVERALL GUIDELINES FOR NURSING INTERVENTION
	1. Understand that creating a therapeutic alliance with clients with PD is going to be difficult. A history of interrupted therapeutic alliances, in addition to the client's suspiciousness, aloofness, secretive style, and hostility, can be a setup for failure.
	2. Giving PD clients some choices (e.g., time they wish to set up appointments) may enhance compliance, because these clients often require a sense of control.
	3. A feeling of being threatened and vulnerable may lead to blaming or verbally attacking others.
	4. Clients with PD are hypersensitive to criticism, so one of the most effective methods of teaching new behaviors is to build upon their own existing skills.

Continued

5. Setting limits is an important part of the work with PD clients. It is important for nurses to take time setting clear boundaries (nurse's responsibilities and client's responsibility) and repeat the limits frequently when working with PD clients.

Risk for Self-Mutilation

A state in which an individual is at high risk to perform an act upon the self to injure, not kill, which produces tissue damage and tension relief

Related To (Etiology)

- ◆ High-risk populations (BPD, psychotic states)
- ◆ History of self-injury
- ◆ History of physical, emotional, or sexual abuse
- ◆ Feelings of depression, rejection, self-hatred, separation anxiety, guilt, and depersonalization
- ◆ Emotionally disturbed or battered children
- ◆ Mentally retarded and autistic children
- ● Ineffective coping skills
- ● Desperate need for attention
- ● Inability to verbally express feelings verbally
- ● Impulsive behavior

As Evidenced By (Assessment Findings/Diagnostic Cure)

- ● Signs of old scars on wrists and other parts of the body (cigarette burns, superficial knife/razor marks)
- ● Fresh superficial slashes on wrists or other parts of the body
- ● Statements as to self-mutilation behaviors
- ● Intense rage focused inward

Outcome Criteria

Client will:

- • Be free of self-inflicted injury
- • Participate in therapeutic regimen
- • Demonstrate new coping skills for when tension mounts and impulse returns

---

◆ NANDA accepted; ● In addition to NANDA.

Short-Term Goals

Client will:

- Respond to external limits
- Sign a "no-harm" contract that identifies steps he or she will take when urges return (date)
- Express feelings related to stress and tension instead of acting-out behaviors (date)
- Discuss alternative ways client can meet demands of current situation (date)

Interventions and Rationales

Intervention	Rationale

1. Assess client's history of self-mutilation:
  a. Types of mutilating behaviors
  b. Frequency of behaviors
  c. Stressors preceding behavior
	1. Identify patterns and identifying circumstances surrounding self-injury helps nurse plan interventions and teaching strategies to fit the individual.

2. Identify feelings experienced before and around the act of self-mutilation.	2. Feelings are a guideline for future intervention (e.g., rage at feeling left out or abandoned).

3. Explore with client what these feelings may mean.	3. Self-mutilation might also be
	  a. a way to gain control over others,
	  b. a way to feel alive through pain, and/or
	  c. an expression of guilt or self-hate.

4. Secure a written or verbal no-harm contract with the client. Identify specific steps (e.g., persons to call upon when prompted to self-mutilate).	4. Client is encouraged to take responsibility for healthier behavior. Talking to others and learning alternative coping skills can reduce frequency and severity until such behavior ceases.
5. Use a matter-of-fact approach when self-mutilation occurs. Avoid criticizing or giving sympathy.	5. A neutral approach prevents blaming, which increases anxiety, giving special attention that encourages acting out.

Intervention	**Rationale**
6. After treatment of the wound, discuss what happened right before, and the thoughts and feelings that the client had immediately before self-mutilating.	6. Identify dynamics for both client and clinician. Allows for identifying less harmful responses to help relieve intense tensions.

7. Work out a plan identifying alternatives to self-mutilating behaviors.
  a. Anticipate certain situations that may lead to increased stress (e.g., tension or rage).
  b. Identify actions that may modify the intensity of such situations.
  c. Identify two or three people the client can contact to discuss and examine intense feelings (rage, self-hate) when they arise.
	7. Plan is periodically reviewed and evaluated. Offers a chance to deal with feelings and struggles that arise.

8. Set and maintain limits on acceptable behavior and make clear client's responsibilities. If client is hospitalized at the time, be clear regarding the unit rules.	8. Clear and nonpunitive limit setting is essential for decreasing negative behaviors.
9. Be consistent in maintaining and enforcing the limits, using a nonpunitive approach.	9. Consistency can establish a sense security.

Chronic Low Self-Esteem

Longstanding negative self-evaluation/feelings about self or self-capabilities

Related To (Etiology)

- Childhood physical/sexual/psychological abuse and/or neglect
- Avoidant and dependent patterns
- Lack of integrated self-view persistent, with splitting as a defense
- Shame and guilt
- Substance abuse
- Lack of realistic ego boundaries
- Dysfunctional family of origin

As Evidenced By (Assessment Findings/Diagnostic Cues)

- ◆ Longstanding or chronic self-negating verbalizations; expressions of shame/guilt
- ◆ Evaluates self as unable to deal with events
- ◆ Rationalizes away/rejects positive feedback and exaggerates negative feedback about self
- ◆ Hesitant to try new things/situations
- ◆ Overly conforming, dependent on others' opinions, indecisive
- ◆ Excessively seeks reassurance
- ◆ Expresses longstanding shame/guilt

Outcome Criteria

Client will:

- Demonstrate ability to reframe and dispute cognitive distortions (date)
- State a willingness to work on realistic future goals (date)
- Identify one new skill he or she has learned to help meet personal goals

Short-Term Goals

Client will:

- Identify three strengths in work/school life by (date)
- Identify two cognitive distortions that affect self-image
- Reframe and dispute one cognitive distortion with nurse
- Set one realistic goal with nurse that he or she wishes to pursue
- Identify one skill he or she will work on to meet future goals by (date)

◆ NANDA accepted; ● In addition to NANDA.

Interventions and Rationales

Intervention	Rationale
1. Maintain a neutral, calm, and respectful manner, although with some clients this is easier said than done.	1. Helps client see himself or herself as respected as a person even when behavior may not be appropriate.
2. Keep in mind PD clients may defend against feeling of low-self esteem through blaming, projection, anger, passivity, and demanding behaviors.	2. Many behaviors seen in PD clients cover a fragile sense of self. Often these behaviors are the crux to clients interpersonal difficulties in all their relationships.

3. Assess with clients their self-perception. Target different areas of the client's life.
  a. Strengths and weaknesses in performance at work /school/daily life tasks
  b. Strengths and weaknesses as to physical appearance, sexuality, personality
	3. Identify with client *realistic* areas of strength and weakness. Client and nurse can then work on the realities of the self-appraisal, and target those areas of assessment that do not appear accurate.

4. Review with the client the types of cognitive distortions that affect self-esteem (e.g., self-blame, mind reading, overgeneralization, selective inattention, all-or-none thinking).	4. These are the most common cognitive distortions people use. Identifying them is the first step to correcting distortions that forms one's self-view.
5. Work with client to recognize cognitive distortions. Encourage client to keep a log.	5. Cognitive distortions are automatic. Keeping a log helps make automatic, unconscious thinking clear.
6. Teach client to reframe and dispute cognitive distortions. Disputes need to be strong, specific, and nonjudgmental.	6. Practice and belief in the disputes over time help clients gain a more realistic appraisal of events, the world, and themselves.

7. Discourage client from dwelling on and "reliving" past mistakes.

7. ***The past cannot be changed.*** Dwelling on past mistakes prevents the client from appraising the present and planning for the future.

8. Discourage client from making repetitive self-blaming and negative remarks.

8. Unacceptable behavior does not make the client a bad person, it means that the client made some poor choices in the past.

9. Focus questions in a positive and active light; helps client refocus on the present and look to the future. For example: **"What could you do differently now?"** *or* **"What have you learned from that experience?"**

9. Allows client to look at past behaviors differently, and gives the client a sense that he or she has choices in the future.

10. Give the client honest and genuine feedback regarding your observations as to his or her strengths, and areas that could use additional skills.

10. Feedback helps give clients a more accurate view of self, strengths, areas to work on, as well as a sense that someone is trying to understand them.

11. Do not flatter or be dishonest in your appraisals.

11. Dishonesty and insincerity undermine trust and negatively affect any therapeutic alliance.

12. Set goals realistically, and re-negotiate goals frequently. Remember that client's negative self-view and distrust of the world took years to develop.

12. Unrealistic goals can set up hopelessness in clients and frustration in nurse clinicians. Clients may blame the nurse for not "helping them," and nurses may blame the client for not "getting better."

Intervention	**Rationale**
13. Discuss with client his or her plans for the future. Work with client to set realistic short-term goals. Identify skills to be learned to help client reach his or her goals.	13. Looking toward the future minimizes dwelling on the past and negative self-rumination. When realistic short-term goals are met, client can gain a sense of accomplishment, direction, and purpose in life. Accomplishing goals can bolster a sense of control and enhance self-perception.

Impaired Social Interaction

The state in which an individual participates in an insufficient or excessive quantity or ineffective quality of social exchange

---

Related To (Etiology)

- ◆ Unacceptable social behavior or values
- ◆ Immature interests
- ● Biochemical changes in the brain
- ● Genetic factors
- ● Disruptive or abusive early family background

As Evidenced By (Assessment Findings/Diagnostic Cues)

- ◆ Observed use of unsuccessful social interaction behaviors
- ◆ Dysfunctional interaction with peers, family, and /or others
- ● Alienating others through angry, clinging, demeaning, and/or manipulative behavior or ridicule toward others
- ● Destructive behavior toward self or others

Outcome Criteria

Client will:

- • Demonstrate an ability to use constructive criticism
- • Demonstrate newly acquired social skills in social situations
- • Identify and problem solve with counselor factors that interfere with social interaction

---

◆ NANDA accepted; ● In addition to NANDA.

- Demonstrate a willingness to participate in follow-up therapy
- Demonstrate a reduction in clinging, splitting, manipulation, and other distancing behaviors

Short-Term Goals

Client will:

- Begin to demonstrate a reduction in manipulative behaviors as evidenced by nurse/staff
- Begin to demonstrate an increase in nonviolent behaviors as evidenced by reported outbursts
- Identify two personal behaviors that are responsible for relationship difficulties within 2 weeks
- Verbalize decreased suspicion and increased security
- Identify one specific area that requires change
- Identify and express feelings as they occur with nurse
- State he or she is willing to continue in follow-up therapy
- Keep follow-up appointments

Interventions and Rationales

Intervention	Rationale
1. In a respectful, neutral manner, explain expected client behaviors, limits, and responsibilities during sessions with nurse clinician. Clearly state rules and regulations of institution, and the consequences when these rules are not adhered to.	1. From the beginning, clients needs to have explicit guidelines and boundaries for expected behaviors on their part, as well what client can expect from the nurse. Clients needs to be fully aware that they will be held responsible for their behaviors.

2. Set limits on any manipulative behaviors:
  a. Arguing or begging
  b. Flattery or seductiveness
  c. Instilling guilt, clinging
  d. Constantly seeking attention
  e. Pitting one person, staff, group against another
  f. Frequently disregarding the rules
	2. From the beginning, limits need to be clear. It will be necessary to refer to these limits frequently, because it is to be expected that the client will test these limits repeatedly.

Intervention	**Rationale**
g. Constant engagement in power struggles	
h. Angry, demanding behaviors	
3. Intervene in manipulative behavior.	3. Clients will test limits, and, once they understand that the limits are solid, this understanding can motivate them to work on other ways to get their needs met. Hopefully, this will be done with the nurse clinician through problem-solving alternative behaviors and learning new effective communication skills.
a. All limits should be adhered to by all staff involved.	
b. Carefully document objective physical signs in managing clinical problems.	
c. Document behaviors objectively (give times, dates, circumstances).	
d. Provide clear boundaries and consequences.	
e. Enforce the consequences.	
4. Expand limits by making clear expectation for clients in a number of settings.	4. When time is taken in initial meetings to clarify expectations, confrontations and power struggles with clients can be minimized and even avoided.
5. Collaborate with the client, as well as the multidisciplinary team, to establish a reward system for compliance with clearly defined expectations (Krupnick and Wade, 1993).	5. Tangible reinforcement for meeting expectations can strengthen the client's positive behaviors (Krupnick and Wade, 1993).
6. Monitor own thoughts and feelings constantly regarding your response to the PD client. Supervision is strongly recommended for new and seasoned clinicians alike when working with PD clients.	6. Strong and intense countertransference reactions to PD clients are bound to occur. When the nurse is enmeshed in his or her own strong reactions toward the client (either positive or negative), nurse effectiveness suffers and the therapeutic alliance may be threatened.

7. Problem solve and role play with client acceptable social skills as ways to get needs met effectively and appropriately.

7. Over time, alternative ways of experiencing interpersonal relationships may emerge. Take one small skill that client is willing to work on, break it down into small parts, and work on it with client.

8. Assess need for and encourage skills training workshop.

8. Skills training workshops offer the client ways to increase social skills through role play and interactions with others who are learning similar skills. This often acts as a motivating factor where positive feedback and helpful suggestions are readily available.

9. Understand that PD clients in particular will be resistant to change and that this is symptomatic of PDs. This is particularly true in the beginning phases of therapy.

9. Responding to client's resistance and seeming lack of change in a neutral manner is part of the foundation for setting up some trust. In other words, the nurse does not have a vested interest in the client "getting better." The nurse remains focused on the client's needs and issues in any event.

◆ PSYCHOPHARMACOLOGY FOR PERSONALITY DISORDERS

There are no medications for treating PDs per se. There are, however, medications that can target some of the symptoms clients' experience, and, prescribed on an individual basis, can be very helpful for many clients as an adjunct in their therapy. Counseling/psychotherapy is probably the best primary approach to care, but psychopharmacology can be an important part of the therapeutic regimen in decreasing a client's anxiety, paranoia, aggressiveness, or other symptoms. Specific medications that are often used for a particular PD are mentioned in the earlier discussions of each of the PDs. Medications can facilitate a client's comfort, and make people with PDs more amenable to therapy.

Inherent in the diagnosis of PDs are longstanding traits that interfere with a person's social, occupational, and/or intimate relationships and functioning, and usually the person's sense of well-being as well. Therefore, as mentioned earlier, changing or modifying dysfunctional traits may take a long time.

◆ NURSE, CLIENT, AND FAMILY RESOURCES—PERSONALITY DISORDERS

Association

National Alliance for the Mentally Ill (NAMI)
200 North Glebe Road, Suite 1015
Arlington, VA 22203-3754
1-800-950-6264

Internet Sites

StrongeR—Destroying the Myth of Self Harm
Recovery information for those who self-mutilate
http://victorian.fortunecity.com/rembrant/441

Borderline Personality Disorder Sanctuary
Recovery information for people with BPD
http://www.navicom.com/~patty/

Self-Injury Page
Self-mutilation
http://www.palace.net/~llama/psych/injury.html

BPD Central
Borderline personality disorder web site
http://www.bpdcentral/index.html
http://www.bpdcentral.com

Borderline Personality Disorder Page
http://mentalhelp.net/disorders

Internet Mental Health
For a good overview of all the personality disorders
http://www.mentalhealth.com

Avoidant Personality Disorder Home Page
http://www.geocities.com/hotsprings/3764

CHAPTER 6

Anxiety and Anxiety Disorders

◆ ANXIETY

Anxiety is a normal response to threatening situations. Anxiety can be a positive motivating factor in our lives. For example, the anxiety a student experiences before taking a test gives the student help with awareness and sharpens focus. Anxiety *does* become a problem when it:

- Interferes with adaptive behavior
- Causes physical symptoms
- Becomes intolerable to the individual

Anxiety is conceptualized on four levels, mild (+), moderate (++), severe (+++), and panic (++++). When working with people who are anxious, it is helpful to distinguish between these levels of anxiety, primarily because the interventions are different for mild to moderate levels of anxiety versus severe to panic levels of anxiety. Following a discussion of the various anxiety disorders and nursing assessment of symptoms seen in anxiety disorders, nursing interventions are presented that are effective for clients with moderate levels of anxiety, and for clients with severe to panic levels of anxiety. The rest of the chapter is devoted to targeting common problem areas (nursing diagnoses) and identifying useful nursing actions for these problem areas.

◆ ANXIETY DISORDERS

Anxiety disorders are a group of disorders that have as their primary symptom anxiety levels that are so high that they interfere with personal, occupational, or social functioning. Anxiety disorders produce symptoms that range from mild to severe, and they tend to be persistent and often disabling. These disorders have a lifetime prevalence of 10% to 30% in the general population, and they are the most prevalent of all psychiatric disorders. Physicians and nurses, however, need to be alerted to the fact that anxiety may not be caused by the client's psychosocial condition. Anxiety can be a symptom of a physical disease, medical problem, or substance use problem. **Therefore, medical causes and drug-induced anxiety must be ruled out before a diagnosis of anxiety disorder can be made.**

People who have anxiety disorders are usually treated in the community setting. Rarely is hospitalization needed unless the client is suicidal or the symptoms are severely out of control (e.g., client is employing self-mutilating behaviors). The best treatment for anxiety disorders is often a combination of medication and therapy (cognitive/behavioral). The final section of this chapter discusses medications and therapies that seem to prove most effective for each of the anxiety disorders. Anxiety disorders include panic disorder (with or without agoraphobia), phobias, obsessive-compulsive disorder (OCD), generalized anxiety disorder (GAD), and stress disorders.

Panic Disorder (with or without Agoraphobia)

A diagnosis of panic disorder is made in the presence or history of recurrent, unexpected panic attacks that do not have an underlying medical or chemical etiology. A **panic attack** involves extreme apprehension or fear, usually associated with feelings of impending doom or terror. During an attack, normal functioning is suspended, the peripheral field of vision is severely limited, and misinterpretations of reality may occur. Individuals experiencing panic attacks often have the terrifying belief they are having a heart attack. These signs and symptoms can be mistaken for a heart attack by hospital personnel because the symptoms of a panic attack can be similar to those of a myocardial infarction (shortness of breath, chest pain, feelings of impending doom). (See Box 6–1 for the signs and symptoms of a panic attack.) Panic attacks can also be present in other anxiety disorders, including social phobia, simple phobia, and post-traumatic stress disorders (PTSD). (Box 6–2 presents the DSM-IV diagnostic criteria for panic disorder.

Agoraphobia is frequently seen with panic disorder. Individuals who are agoraphobic avoid places or situations from which escape might be difficult or embarrassing, or where help might not be available if a panic attack occurred. Agoraphobia is a phobia and is discussed further under phobias. About 67% of panic clients lose or quit their jobs because they can no longer tolerate traveling to

---

❖   B O X   6 – 1   ❖

Signs and Symptoms of a Panic Attack

Panic attack is defined as a discrete period of intense fear or discomfort, starting abruptly and reaching a peak within 10 minutes.
 1. Palpitations, tachycardia
 2. Sweating
 3. Shaking or trembling
 4. Choking
 5. Chest pain/discomfort
 6. Nausea, abdominal distress
 7. Dizziness, faintness
 8. Feeling unreal or detached from oneself
 9. Fear of "going crazy"
10. Fear of dying
11. Paresthesias
12. Chills or hot flashes

Adapted from American Psychiatric Association. (1994). Diagnostic and Statistical Manual of Mental Disorders, 4th ed. Washington, DC: American Psychiatric Press, p. 395; reprinted with permission. Copyright 1994 American Psychiatric Association.

❖   B O X   6 – 2   ❖

Diagnostic Criteria for Panic Disorder

1. Both A and B
   a. Recurrent episodes of panic attacks
   b. At least one of the attacks has been followed by 1 month (or more) of the following:
      • Persistent concern of having additional attacks
      • Worry about consequences ("going crazy," having a heart attack, losing control)
      • Significant change in behavior
2. Absence of Agoraphobia = **Panic disorder without agoraphobia**
3. Presence of Agoraphobia = **Panic disorder with agoraphobia**

Adapted from American Psychiatric Association. (1994). Diagnostic and Statistical Manual of Mental Disorders, 4th ed. Washington, DC: American Psychiatric Press, pp. 402–403; reprinted with permission. Copyright 1994 American Psychiatric Association.

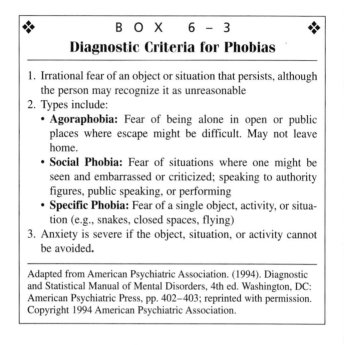

❖   B O X   6 – 3   ❖
Diagnostic Criteria for Phobias

1. Irrational fear of an object or situation that persists, although the person may recognize it as unreasonable
2. Types include:
   • **Agoraphobia:** Fear of being alone in open or public places where escape might be difficult. May not leave home.
   • **Social Phobia:** Fear of situations where one might be seen and embarrassed or criticized; speaking to authority figures, public speaking, or performing
   • **Specific Phobia:** Fear of a single object, activity, or situation (e.g., snakes, closed spaces, flying)
3. Anxiety is severe if the object, situation, or activity cannot be avoided.

Adapted from American Psychiatric Association. (1994). Diagnostic and Statistical Manual of Mental Disorders, 4th ed. Washington, DC: American Psychiatric Press, pp. 402–403; reprinted with permission. Copyright 1994 American Psychiatric Association.

their place of business. Approximately 20% of people with panic disorder attempt suicide (Weissman et al., 1989).

Phobias

Phobias are irrational fears of an object or situation that persist although the person may recognize them as unreasonable. There are three categories of phobias; agoraphobia, social phobia, and specific phobia. (See Box 6–3 for DSM-IV criteria for phobias.)

Obsessive-Compulsive Disorder

A person with OCD has either *obsessions* (intrusive thoughts, impulses, or images) that break into their conscious awareness and are perceived as senseless and intrusive, *compulsions* (repetitive behaviors or mental acts that the person feels driven to perform in order to reduce distress or prevent a dreaded event or situation), or both. Common compulsions involve touching, counting, cleaning, and arranging things. People with OCD often present in a physician's office with a complaint of compulsive hand washing, compulsive cleanliness, or alopecia resulting from pulling out their hair (trichotillomania). Box 6–4 presents the DSM-IV diagnostic criteria for OCD.

> ❖ **B O X 6 – 4** ❖
> ## Diagnostic Criteria for Obsessive-Compulsive Disorder (OCD)
>
> ---
>
> 1. Either obsessions or compulsions
>   a. Preoccupation with persistent intrusive thoughts, impulses, or images (**obsession**), *or*
>   b. Repetitive behaviors or mental acts that the person feels driven to perform in order to reduce distress or prevent a dreaded event or situation (**compulsion**)
> 2. Person knows the obsessions/compulsions are excessive and unreasonable.
> 3. The obsession/compulsion can cause increased distress and is time consuming.
>
> ---
>
> Adapted from American Psychiatric Association. (1994). Diagnostic and Statistical Manual of Mental Disorders, 4th ed. Washington, DC: American Psychiatric Press, pp. 422–423; reprinted with permission. Copyright 1994 American Psychiatric Association.

Generalized Anxiety Disorder

People are diagnosed with GAD when they have chronic and excessive anxiety or worry most of the time over a 6-month period of time. Other symptoms include restlessness, fatigue, difficulty concentrating, irritability, muscle tension, and sleep problems. The symptoms cause the individual to have significant distress, and these individuals tend to have impairment in their social and occupational functioning. Box 6–5 presents the DSM-IV diagnostic criteria for GAD.

Stress Disorders

Two other disorders that are included in the anxiety disorders are **Post-traumatic Stress Disorder** (PTSD) and **Acute Stress Disorder** (ASD). Both of these disorders follow exposure to an extremely traumatic event, usually outside of the range of normal experiences (e.g., natural disasters, crime-related events, prisoner of war, diagnosis of a life-threatening disease, rape). They also share similar symptoms:

1. Re-experiencing the symptoms through dreams or images
2. Reliving the event through flashbacks, illusions, hallucinations

---

❖   **B O X   6 – 5**   ❖
Diagnostic Criteria for
Generalized Anxiety Disorder (GAD)

---

1. Excessive anxiety or worry more days than not over 6 months
2. Cannot control the worrying
3. Anxiety and worry associated with three or more of the following symptoms:
   - Restlessness, keyed-up
   - Easily fatigued
   - Difficulty concentrating, mind goes blank
   - Irritability
   - Muscle tension
   - Sleep disturbance
4. Anxiety or worry or physical symptoms cause significant impairment in social, occupational, or other areas of important functioning.

Adapted from American Psychiatric Association. (1994). Diagnostic and Statistical Manual of Mental Disorders, 4th ed. Washington, DC: American Psychiatric Press, pp. 435–436; reprinted with permission. Copyright 1994 American Psychiatric Association.

---

3. Marked symptoms of anxiety
   a. Difficulty falling/staying asleep
   b. Irritability/outbursts of anger
   c. Difficulty concentrating
4. Avoidance of stimuli associated with the trauma that could arouse memory of the trauma

The main difference is one of time. ASD lasts from 2 days to 4 weeks, and occurs within 4 weeks of the traumatic event. PTSD lasts for *more* than 1 month and may last for years. Boxes 6–6 and 6–7 present for DSM-IV diagnostic criteria for these two stress responses.

◆ ASSESSING FOR ANXIETY DISORDERS
History

1. Does the client have a history of an anxiety disorder (e.g., phobia, OCD, PTSD, panic attacks)?
2. Does the client have another psychological disorder (e.g., depression, substance abuse, sleep disorder, eating disorder)?
3. Is the client experiencing a loss or change (loss of job, move, death, retirement, illness, pregnancy)?

❖   B O X   6 – 6   ❖

Diagnostic Criteria for
Post-traumatic Stress Disorder (PTSD)

---

1. The person experienced, witnessed, or was confronted with an event that involved actual or threatened death to self or others, responding in fear, helplessness, or horror.
2. The event is persistently re-experienced:
   • Distressing dreams or images
   • Reliving the event through flashbacks, illusions, hallucinations
3. Persistent avoidance of stimuli associated with trauma:
   • Avoidance of thoughts, feelings, conversations
   • Avoidance of people, places, activities
   • Inability to recall aspects of trauma
   • Decreased interest in usual activities
   • Feelings of detachment, estrangement from others
   • Restriction in feelings (love, enthusiasm, joy)
   • Sense of shortened feelings
4. Persistent symptoms of increased arousal (two or more):
   • Difficulty falling/staying asleep
   • Irritability/outbursts of anger
   • Difficulty concentrating
5. **Duration more than 1 month**
   • *Acute*: Duration less than 3 months
   • *Chronic*: Duration 3 months or more
   • *Delayed*: If onset of symptoms is at least 6 months after stress

---

Adapted from American Psychiatric Association. (1994). Diagnostic and Statistical Manual of Mental Disorders, 4th ed. Washington, DC: American Psychiatric Press, pp. 427–429; reprinted by permission. Copyright 1994 American Psychiatric Association.

---

4. Is anxiety secondary to certain medical conditions (hyperthyroidism, multiple sclerosis)? **Medical or chemical conditions (diseases, conditions, substances) need to be ruled out.**

Presenting Symptoms

1. Might state they feel like they are going to die or have a sense of impending doom
2. Narrowing of perceptions, difficulty concentrating, problem-solving inefficient
3. Increased vital signs (blood pressure, pulse, respirations), increased muscle tension, sweat glands activated, pupils dilated

---

❖   B O X   6 – 7   ❖
Diagnostic Criteria for
Acute Stress Disorder (ASD)

---

1. The person experienced, witnessed, or was confronted with an event that involved actual or threatened death to self or others, responding in fear, helplessness, or horror.
2. Three or more of the following dissociative symptoms:
   • Sense of numbing, detachment, or absence of emotional response
   • Reduced awareness of surroundings (e.g., "in a daze")
   • Derealization
   • Depersonalization
   • Amnesia for an important aspect of the trauma
3. The event is persistently re-experienced by:
   • Distressing dreams or images
   • Reliving the event through flashbacks, illusions, hallucinations
4. Marked avoidance of stimuli that arouse memory of trauma (thoughts, feelings, people, places, activities, conversations)
5. Marked symptoms of anxiety:
   • Difficulty falling/staying asleep
   • Irritability/outbursts of anger
   • Difficulty concentrating
6. Causes impairment in social, occupational, and other functioning, or impairs ability to complete some memory tasks.
7. **Lasts from 2 days to 4 weeks, and occurs within 4 weeks of the traumatic event.**

Adapted from American Psychiatric Association. (1994). Diagnostic and Statistical Manual of Mental Disorders, 4th ed. Washington, DC: American Psychiatric Press, pp. 431–432; reprinted with permission. Copyright 1994 American Psychiatric Association.

---

4. Palpitations, urinary urgency/frequency, nausea, tightening of throat, unsteady voice
5. Complaints of fatigue, difficulty sleeping, irritability, disorganization

Sample Questions

The nurse uses a variety of therapeutic techniques to obtain the answers to the following questions. Use your discretion and decide which questions are appropriate to complete your assessment.

1. "What are you concerned about or afraid might happen?"
2. "Describe how you see your future."
3. "When you get frightened, what happens to you?"
4. "Do you have times of great fear or anxiety attacks? When? What triggers them? How long do they last?"
5. "Are there any distressing memories of a traumatic event that keep coming back to you? Please share them with me."
6. "Are there situations or places you avoid because they really upset you?"
7. "Are there behaviors or habits that you feel compelled to repeat?"
8. "Are there certain thoughts that go through your mind over and over?"

Preliminary Screening Guide for Assessing Anxiety Symptoms

There are a number of tools that help the health care worker assess for anxiety symptoms. The Hamilton Rating Scale For Anxiety (Table 6–1) helps the clinician to identify a client's level of anxiety. Box 6–8 presents a simple screening guide that can be done quickly, and can elicit specific anxiety symptoms that the client might not offer without being asked. Any positive answers alert the nurse clinician that more detailed assessment is needed.

ASSESSMENT ALERTS
1. A sound physical and neurological exam helps to determine if the anxiety is primary or secondary to another psychiatric disorder, medical condition, or substance.
2. Assess for potential for self-harm, because it is known that people suffering from high levels of intractable anxiety may become desperate and attempt suicide.
3. Many people with anxiety disorder greatly benefit from cognitive and behavioral techniques, as well as certain medications. Assess client's community for appropriate clinics, groups, and counselors who offer these techniques. Table 6–2 on page 146 identifies which approaches and medications seem to be the most effective for each of the anxiety disorders.

◆ NURSING DIAGNOSES WITH INTERVENTIONS

Several nursing diagnoses target symptoms for people with high levels of anxiety and anxiety disorders. The nursing diagnosis

Table 6–1 ◆ Hamilton Rating Scale for Anxiety

Max Hamilton designed this scale to help clinicians gather information about anxiety states. The symptom inventory provides scaled information that classifies anxiety behaviors and assists the clinician in targeting behaviors and achieving outcome measures. Provide a rating for each indicator based on the following scale:

0 = None	3 = Disabling
1 = Mild	4 = Severe, Grossly Disabling
2 = Moderate	

ITEM	SYMPTOMS	RATING
Anxious mood	Worries, anticipation of the worst, fearful anticipation, irritability	_____
Tension	Feelings of tension, fatigability, startle response, moved to tears easily, trembling, feelings of restlessness, inability to relax	_____
Fear	Of dark, strangers, of being left alone, of animals, of traffic, of crowds	_____
Insomnia	Difficulty in falling asleep, broken sleep, unsatisfying sleep and fatigue on waking, dreams, nightmares, night terrors	_____
Intellectual (cognitive)	Difficulty in concentration, poor memory	_____
Depressed mood	Loss of interest, lack of pleasure in hobbies, depression, early waking, diurnal swings	_____
Somatic (sensory)	Tinnitus, blurring of vision, hot and cold flushes, feelings of weakness, prickling sensation	_____
Somatic (muscular)	Pains and aches, twitchings, stiffness, myoclonic jerks, grinding of teeth, unsteady voice, increased muscular tone	_____
Cardiovascular symptoms	Tachycardia, palpitations, pain in chest, throbbing of vessels, fainting feelings, missing beat	_____
Respiratory symptoms	Pressure of constriction in chest, choking feelings, sighing, dyspnea	_____
Gastrointestinal symptoms	Difficulty in swallowing, wind, abdominal pain, burning sensations, abdominal fullness, nausea, vomiting, borborygmi, looseness of bowels, loss of weight, constipation	_____

(Continued)

Genitourinary symptoms	Frequency of micturition, urgency of micturition, amenorrhea, menorrhagia, development of frigidity, premature ejaculation, loss of libido, impotence	_____
Autonomic symptoms	Dry mouth, flushing, pallor, tendency to sweat, giddiness, tension headache, raising of hair	_____
Behavior at interview	Fidgeting, restlessness or pacing, tremor of hands, furrowed brow, strained face, sighing or rapid respiration, facial pallor, swallowing, belching, brisk tendon jerks, dilated pupils, exophthalmos	_____

Adapted from Hamilton, M. (1959). The assessment of anxiety states by rating. British Journal of Medical Psychology; reprinted with permission. © The British Psychological Society.

Anxiety is most often used. When using the nursing diagnosis of Anxiety, the nurse needs to clarify the level of anxiety because different levels of anxiety call for different intervention strategies. For example, the diagnosis should be stated **Anxiety—Moderate Level**, or **Anxiety—Severe–Panic Level**.

Ineffective Individual Coping is another frequently used diagnosis because high levels of anxiety lead to interference in ability to work, disruptions in relationships, and changes in ability to interact satisfactorily with others. For example, people with phobias often develop avoidance behaviors, and people with obsessions and compulsions make it difficult for others to relate to them other than under rigid circumstances.

People with anxiety disorders often have **Altered Thought Processes**. Individuals with OCD are preoccupied with their obsessive thoughts, and people with panic disorder are filled with fear and terror during anxiety attacks when their ability to problem solve, use sound judgment, or understand directions is totally impaired. Individuals with PTSD and ASD suffer from intrusive thoughts and memories that increase levels of anxiety so that their ability to function and think clearly is greatly hampered for brief periods of time.

The nursing diagnoses Anxiety—Moderate, Anxiety—Severe-Panic, Ineffective Individual Coping, and Altered Thought Processes are presented here with suggested nursing interventions for each diagnosis.

OVERALL GUIDELINES FOR NURSING INTERVENTION

1. Identify community resources that can offer client the development of skills that have been proven to be highly effective for people with a variety of anxiety disorders:
   - Cognitive restructuring
   - Relaxation training
   - Modeling techniques
   - Systematic desensitization/graduated exposure
   - Flooding (implosion therapy)
   - Behavior therapy
2. Identify community support groups for people with specific anxiety disorders.
3. Assess need for interventions for families and significant others (support groups, family therapy, and help with issues that may be leading to relationship stress and turmoil).
4. When medications are used in conjunction with therapy, clients and their significant others will need thorough teaching. Written information and instructions are given to client/family/partner.

Anxiety

Increased to extreme level of arousal with selective attention or scattered focus associated with expectation of a threat (unfocused) to the self or significant relationships

---

Related To (Etiology)

- ◆ Perceived threat to self-concept, health status, socioeconomic status, role function, interaction patterns or environment
- ◆ Perceived threat of death
- ◆ Unconscious conflict
- ◆ Unmet needs
- ● Exposure to phobic object or situation
- ● Cessation of ritualistic behavior
- ● Traumatic experience
- ● Fear of panic attack
- ● Intrusive unwanted thoughts
- ● Flashbacks

◆ NANDA accepted; ● In addition to NANDA.

❖   B O X   6 – 8   ❖

Preliminary Screening for Assessing Anxiety Symptoms

1. Do you ever experience a sudden, unexplained attack of intense fear, anxiety, or panic for no apparent reason?
2. Have you been afraid of not being able to get help or not being able to escape in certain situations, like being on a bridge, in a crowded store, or in similar situations?
3. Do you find it difficult to control your worrying?
4. Do you spend more time than is necessary doing things over and over again, such as washing your hands, checking things, or counting things?
5. Do you either avoid or feel very uncomfortable in situations involving people, such as parties, weddings, dating, dances, or other social events?
6. Have you ever had an extremely frightening, traumatic, or horrible experience like being a victim of a crime, seriously injured in a car accident, sexually assaulted, or seeing someone injured or killed?

From National Mental Illness Screening Project. (1999). National Anxiety Disorders Screening Day page: Sample test for anxiety disorder screening. http://www.nmisp.org; reprinted with permission. © 1999.

As Evidenced By (Assessment Findings/Diagnostic Cure)

◆ Autonomic signs and symptoms (tachycardia, rapid breathing, palpitations, muscle tension, diaphoresis)
◆ Narrowing focus of attention
◆ Perceptual focus shattered
◆ Restlessness to purposeless activity to immobilization
◆ Feelings of dread, apprehension, nervousness, or concern
● Increase in symptoms (compulsions, phobias, obsessions, nightmares/flashbacks)
● Inability to complete tasks

Outcome Criteria

Client will:

• Demonstrate three anxiety reducing skills that work for him or her by (date)

◆ NANDA accepted; ● In addition to NANDA.

Table 6–2 ◆ Accepted Treatment for Selected Anxiety Disorders

DISORDER	PHARMACOTHERAPY*	THERAPEUTIC MODALITY	COMMENTS
Panic disorder	**Antidepressants** a. TCAs (imipramine) b. SSRIs c. MAOIs (2nd line because of dietary restrictions)	Cognitive-behavioral therapy (CBT) Behavioral Relaxation	Current CBT emphasizes: a. Information on anxiety and the panic cycle b. Symptom management (relaxation-breathing) c. Cognitive restructuring d. Systematic desensitization e. In vivo exposure aimed at elementary avoidance behavior
	Benzodiazepines (short-term) a. Alprazolam (Xanax) b. Lorazepam (Ativan) c. Clonazepam (Klonopin)	Breathing techniques	Systematic desensitization Deep muscle relaxation Rebreathing techniques Self-hypnosis Biofeedback
Agoraphobia	a. Treatment of panic attacks (above) if present b. Phenelzine (Nardil) an MAOI, may have antiagoraphobic effects	Behavioral Cognitive therapy Insight-oriented psychotherapy	Recognition of irrational beliefs Stopping irrational thoughts Replacing irrational thoughts with new thoughts or activities Especially for agoraphobia without history of panic disorder

Generalized anxiety disorder	a. Benzodiazepines—short-term only b. Buspirone c. TCAs, especially imipramine d. SSRIs (paroxetine [Paxil])	Cognitive therapy Behavioral therapy
Post-traumatic stress disorder	a. MAOIs (especially phenelzine) may diminish nightmares and flashbacks b. TCAs (imipramine and amitriptyline) and SSRIs for depressive symptoms	Psychotherapy Family therapy Vocational rehabilitation Group therapy Relaxation techniques	More than one treatment modality should be used[†] a. Establish support b. Focus on abreaction, survivor guilt or shame, anger, and helplessness.
Obsessive-compulsive disorder	a. SSRIs (fluvoxamine [Luvox] and fluoxetine [Prozac]) b. Clomipramine (Anafranil) (TCA)	Behavioral therapy	Effective and necessary in addition to serotonergic medications. Exposure in vivo plus response prevention are the crucial essential factors.

Data from Billings, C.K. (1993). An update on panic disorder, agoraphobia and social phobia. Workshop sponsored by U.S. Psychiatric & Mental Health Congress, New Orleans, December 3, 1993; Menninger, W.W. (1995). Coping with anxiety: Integrated approaches to treatment. Bulletin of the Menninger Clinic 59(2): A4–A26.
*MAOI, monoamine oxidase inhibitor; SSRI, selective serotonin reuptake inhibitor; TCA, tricyclic antidepressant.
[†]The sooner treatment begins, the more successful recovery is likely to be.

- State that he or she feels comfortable and physical symptoms of anxiety are absent
- Problem solve without assistance
- Identify negative "self-talk" and reframe thoughts successfully
- Demonstrate ability to reframe problems in solvable terms by (date)
- Demonstrate ability to get needs met using assertive communication skills

Short-Term Goals

- Client will demonstrate skills at reframing anxiety-provoking situations (date).
- Client will demonstrate one relaxation technique that works well for him or her (date).
- Client will role play with the nurse two behavioral techniques that help reduce feelings of anxiety to tolerable levels by (date).
- Client's anxiety level will go from severe (+++) to moderate (++) within 2 hours on (date).
- Client will role play with nurse *assertive* communication skills.

Interventions and Rationales

ANXIETY

Intervention	Rationale

1. Provide a safe, calm environment:
  a. Decrease environmental stimuli.
  b. Listen to and reassure client that he or she can feel more in control.
	1. When people feel fearful and vulnerable, being heard in an atmosphere of calm helps to foster a sense of connectedness with someone and control over what will happen.

2. Encourage client to talk about feelings and concerns.	2. When concerns are stated out loud, problems can be discussed and feelings of isolation decreased.
3. Reframe the problem in a way that is solvable. Provide a new perspective and correct distorted perceptions.	3. Correcting distortions increases the possibility of finding workable solutions to a realistically defined problem.
4. Identify thoughts or feelings prior to the onset of anxiety: "What were you doing/	4. Identify triggers for escalating anxiety, and a chance to understand why these

thinking right before you started to feel anxious?"

5. Identify any "self-talk" clients may use at this time (e.g., "I'll never be able to do this right." *or* "This means I'll never succeed in anything").

6. Teach relaxation techniques (deep breathing exercises, meditation, progressive muscle relaxation).

7. Refer client and significant others to support groups, self-help programs, or advocacy groups when appropriate.

8. Administer medications or obtain an order for medications when appropriate.

triggers are so frightening to the client.

5. Identify what thoughts trigger anxious feelings. Then cognitive skills can be used to help client to reframe his or her thinking so that problems can be solved.

6. When clients learn to lower levels of anxiety, their ability to assess a situation and utilize their own problem-solving skills are improved.

7. Clients with specific problems are known to greatly benefit from being around others who are grappling with similar issues. Provides the client with information and support and lowers feelings of isolation in stressful and difficult situations.

8. Use least restrictive interventions to decrease anxiety.

Ineffective Individual Coping

Impairment of adaptive behaviors and abilities of a person in meeting life's demands and roles

---

Related To (Etiology)

● Severe to panic levels of anxiety—panic attack, GAD
● Excessive negative beliefs about self—GAD, OCD, other
● Hypervigilance after a traumatic event—PTSD, ASD
● Presence of obsessions and compulsions associated with fear of contamination—OCD, phobia
● Avoidance behavior associated with phobia (list phobia)—phobia

---

◆ NANDA accepted; ● In addition to NANDA.

As Evidenced By (Assessment Findings/Diagnostic Cues)

◆ Verbalization of inability to cope or inability to ask for help
◆ Inability to problem solve
◆ Expression of anxiety
● Disturbance in vocational and social functioning related to (phobias, obsessions, compulsions, panic attacks, post-trauma symptoms)
● Panic attacks, severe obsessive acts, disturbing thoughts, disabling phobia(s), post-trauma symptoms

Outcome Criteria

Clients will:

• Function at previous level of independence without interference from phobias, compulsions, obsessions, post-trauma event, panic attacks, disabling anxiety.
• Verbalize ability to cope effectively with anxiety using two new stress-reducing skills.
• Demonstrate new coping skills (cognitive, behavioral, relaxation techniques, insight) that allay anxiety symptoms, such as visualization, deep breathing, and thought stopping techniques.

Short-Term Goals

Client will:

• Demonstrate knowledge of breathing techniques and relaxation skills by end of first/second session with nurse
• Describe the different therapies that are effective in treating their particular anxiety disorder (cognitive, behavioral, group) (see Table 6–2)
• Demonstrate one new anxiety reduction technique that works best for him or her within 2 weeks
• Accurately describe the desired effects, side effects, and toxic effects of any medication he or she might be given as an adjunct to therapy within 2 days

Interventions and Rationales

Intervention	Rationale
1. Monitor and reinforce client's use of positive coping skills and healthy defense mechanisms.	1. Identifies what does and does not work for client. Nurse uses client's strengths to build upon.

◆ NANDA accepted; ● In addition to NANDA.

2. Teach new coping skills to substitute for ineffective ones.

2. Gives client options.

3. At client level of understanding, explain the *"fight-or-flight"* response and the *relaxation response* of the autonomic nervous system. Address how breathing and relaxation techniques can be used to elicit the *relaxation response.*

3. Understanding the physiologic aspects of anxiety, and how people have some degree of control over their physiologic responses, gives people hope and a sense of control in their lives.

4. When the client's level of anxiety is mild to moderate, teach client proper *breathing techniques* and breathe with the client. (See Box 6–9 for client instructions for abdominal breathing.)

4. Breathing techniques can prevent anxiety from escalating. Doing exer-*cises with client helps* foster compliance.

5. When the client's level of anxiety is mild to moderate, teach client *relaxation techniques* (such as imaging, visualization [Box 6–10]).

5. Help the client gain some control over switching the parasympathetic nervous system from the "fight-or-flight" response to the relaxation response.

❖   B O X   6 – 9   ❖
Teaching Abdominal Breathing

Instruct the client to:
1. Place one hand on your abdomen beneath your rib cage.
2. Inhale slowly and deeply through your nose, sending air as far down into your lungs as you can. Your hand should rise.
3. After taking the full breath, pause for a moment, then exhale slowly and fully.
4. As you exhale, allow your whole body to go limp.
5. Count each breath up to 10 by saying the appropriate number after each exhalation.
6. Doing two or three "sets" of 10 abdominal breaths will produce a state of considerable relaxation.

From Varcarolis, E. (1998). Foundations of Psychiatric Mental Health Nursing, 3rd ed. Philadelphia: W.B. Saunders Company, p. 472; reprinted with permission.

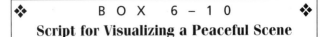

❖   B O X   6 – 1 0   ❖
Script for Visualizing a Peaceful Scene

Imagine releasing all the tension in your body . . . letting it go.

Now, with every breath you take, feel your body drifting down deeper and deeper into relaxation . . . floating down . . . deeper and deeper.

Imagine your peaceful scene. You're sitting beside a clear, blue mountain stream. You are barefoot, and you feel the sun-warmed rock under your feet. You hear the sound of the stream tumbling over the rocks. The sound is hypnotic, and you relax more and more. You see the tall pine trees on the opposite shore bending in the gentle breeze. Breathe the clean, pine-scented air, each breath moving you deeper and deeper into relaxation. The sun warms your face.

You are very comfortable. There is nothing to disturb you. You experience a feeling of well-being.

You can return to this peaceful scene by taking time to relax. The positive feelings can grow stronger and stronger each time you choose to relax.

You can return to your activities now, feeling relaxed and refreshed.

Intervention	Rationale
6. Identify for client which therapies have been highly effective with individuals who have the same disorder (cognitive, behavioral) (see Table 6–2).	6. Not only do cognitive and behavioral approaches work to decrease clients' anxiety and improve quality of life, they also foster chemical changes in the brain that lessen the brain's response to anxiety.
7. Use a cognitive approach.	7. Helps the client recognize that thoughts and beliefs can cause anxiety.
8. Teach client proven behavioral techniques. Client can become desensitized to a feared object or situation over time.	8. Cognitive and behavioral techniques are extremely effective interventions for treating anxiety disorders. Once they are learned, clients can draw upon these skills for the rest of their lives.

9. Keep focus on manageable problems; define them simply and concretely.

9. Concrete, well-defined problems lend themselves to intervention.

10. Provide behavioral rehearsals (role play) for anticipated stressful situations.

10. Predetermination of previous effective or new coping strategies, along with practice, increases potential for success.

11. Some clients respond well to biofeedback and feel more comfortable with physiologic manipulations than one-to one therapy.

11. Biofeedback is extremely useful for decreasing anxiety levels. Some clients may feel less "shame" in getting help.

12. Many anxiety disorders respond to medications along with therapy (e.g., SSRIs for OCD, buspirone [Buspar] for GAD). Therefore, medication teaching is extremely important, especially with the anxiolytics.

12. Clients need to know what the medications can and cannot do. They need to know that "more is not better," the side effects and toxic effects, and what to do if an untoward reaction occurs. This information should always be given to clients in writing after instructions with the nurse clinician.

Altered Thought Processes

A state in which an individual experiences a disruption in cognitive operations and activities

Related To (Etiology)

◆ Severe levels of anxiety
● Distorted perceptions
● Intrusive obsessional thoughts
● Anticipatory anxiety

As Evidenced By (Assessment Findings/Diagnostic Cues)

◆ Hypervigilance
◆ Distractibility

◆ NANDA accepted; ● In addition to NANDA.

◆ Inaccurate interpretation of the environment
● Flashbacks
● Intrusive obsessional thinking

Outcome Criteria

Client will:

• Recognize when anxiety begins to escalate and link anxiety to precipitating thoughts or feelings
• Demonstrate techniques that can distract and distance self from thoughts and feelings that are anxiety producing
• Reframe automatic thoughts and self-judgments that lead to increase in anxiety and lowering of self-worth

Short-Term Goals

Client will:

• Identify two thoughts or feelings that precede increases in anxiety and will discuss with the nurse within 1 week or (date)
• Share daily journal with counselor/nurse regarding thoughts, feelings preceding anxiety (date)
• Rate the anxiety on a scale from 1 to 10, then re-rate anxiety after using breathing, relaxation, cognitive, behavioral, or other anxiety-reducing skills
• Demonstrate one cognitive or behavioral technique after 1 week (date)

Interventions and Rationales

Intervention	Rationale
1. Explore with client the thoughts that lead up to client's anxious feelings and relief behaviors.	1. Recognition of precipitating thoughts or feelings leading to anxiety behaviors may give clues to how to arrest escalating anxiety.
2. Link client's relief behaviors to thoughts and feelings.	2. Client becomes aware of how anxiety can be the result of thoughts, and people can have some control over their thoughts and thus their anxiety levels, with practice.

◆ NANDA accepted; ● In addition to NANDA.

3. Teach cognitive principles:
   a. Anxiety is the result of dysfunctional appraisal of a situation.
   b. Anxiety is the result of automatic thinking.

3. Again, introduces the concept to clients that they can have some control over their thoughts and feelings, and instills some hope and stimulates compliance to try new ways of thinking.

4. Teach some brief cognitive techniques that the client can try out right away (see Box 6–11).

4. Increases self-awareness while distancing self from own anxiety. In a sense, helps distract client from feelings of anxiety, and allows him or her to be more of an observer.

5. Teach client behavioral techniques that can interrupt intrusive unwanted thoughts (see Box 6–12).

5. Can help distract client and interrupt escalating anxiety. During this time, alternative coping skills can be employed.

6. Role play and rehearse with client alternative coping strategies that can be used in threatening

6. Gives client chance to be proactive, giving client a choice of alternatives instead of client employ-

---

❖   B O X   6 – 1 1   ❖
Brief Cognitive Techniques

1. Instruct client to refer to self by first name and comment on own anxiety or thoughts (e.g., "Mary's heart is beating fast"; "Ted thinks everyone is looking at him now").
2. Work with the client to recognize his or her automatic thinking, and how certain words can trigger anxiety (e.g., *should, never, always*). Help client use words that are more objective and neutral; for example:
   • **Change:** "I should have gone to college."
     to: "I would have benefited from going to college, and if I still wish to go, I still can."
   • **Change:** "I always use poor judgment when it comes to money; I'll never get it right!"
     to: "Although I have made mistakes regarding money in the past, it would be useful for me to get some advice and check out my ideas more thoroughly in the future."

❖   B O X   6 – 1 2   ❖
                Brief Behavioral Techniques
───

- Have client wear a rubber band around his or her wrist. When intrusive repetitive thoughts start to occur (as in OCD), have client snap the rubber band hard on his or her wrist.
- When client is experiencing intrusive painful memories, clap your hands loudly in front of client, then teach client and family to do the same thing.

Intervention	**Rationale**
or anxiety-provoking situations.	ing usual unsatisfactory automatic reactions.
7. Encourage client to keep a daily journal of thoughts, situations that seem to precede anxiety, and coping strategies used.	7. Allows client to monitor "triggers" and evaluate useful coping strategies over time.
8. Teach client to *rate* his or her anxiety levels on a scale from 1 to 10, where 1 is the least and 10 the highest. Have client document situations and anxiety levels in the journal.	8. Allows client to evaluate effectiveness of coping strategies and monitor decrease in anxiety levels over time.
9. Review journal with client and identify which strategies worked and which did not work. Review with client progress made and give credit for the client's hard work.	9. Helps client see what seems to be working and what does not and encourages compliance when going through phases of feeling discouraged.
10. Teach client to recognize triggers of anxiety.	10. Gives client opportunity to use alternative responses and skills.
11. Refer client to support groups in the community in which people are dealing with similar issues.	11. Groups can foster a sense of belonging and diminish feelings of isolation and alienation. Positive feedback from others helps foster compliance and enhances self-esteem.

| 12. | Review with client and significant others stress reduction techniques (see Box 6–13). Encourage client and family members to practice relaxation techniques; give handout and references. | 12. | Everyone around the client may be tense. Sometimes simple steps make big differences in people's lives. |
| 13. | Refer family members and significant others to appropriate resources in the community. Resources might include family therapy, couples counseling, financial counseling, support groups, or classes in meditation and other relaxation techniques. | 13. | Family and others close to the client may need a great deal of support. They may benefit from learning new coping strategies that can lessen conflicts and stress on the whole family unit. |

◆ PSYCHOPHARMACOLOGY FOR ANXIETY DISORDERS

At one time, the predominant treatment for the anxiety disorders was antianxiety medications, or anxiolytics, as they are presently referred to. The benzodiazepines were often the treatment of choice and still are used for severe anxiety. However, today there are a number of groups of medications that can be used effectively with clients with anxiety disorders. Each group seems to be helpful for specific disorders. For example, the TCAs (e.g., *imipramine*) seem to be effective in targeting **panic attacks**. The MAOI antidepressants seem to have **antiagoraphobic** effects. Although the benzodiazepines are useful in **GAD**, they are best used for a short time because they can become addicting. Benzodiazepines may also cause "rebound anxiety" when they are stopped. Clinicians may switch to *buspirone*, which is not addicting nor does the client develop a tolerance for the drug. The downside is that it can take a long time for buspirone to work (3 weeks or much longer for some). The client can be maintained with buspirone for a long time. The SSRI antidepressants (e.g., fluvoxamine [Luvox], fluoxetine [Prozac]) have been found to be very effective for people with **OCD**.

Table 6–2 gives a good example of effective drugs for each of the anxiety disorders. Note that it is best when these drugs are

---

❖ B O X   6 – 1 3 ❖
Selected Stress Reduction Techniques

Relaxation Techniques

1. Induce a relaxation state more physiologically refreshing than sleep
2. Neutralize stress energy, producing a calming effect

Reframing

1. Changes the way we look and feel about things
2. There are many ways to interpret the same reality (seeing the glass as half full rather than half empty).
3. Reassess situation. Most situations we can learn from. Ask:
   • "What positive came out of the situation/experience?"
   • "What did you learn in this situation?"
   • "What would you do differently next time?"
4. Getting inside another person's shoes can help dissipate tension and help step outside ourselves. We might even feel some compassion toward the person.
   • "What might be going on with your (spouse, boss, teacher, friend) that they (said, did) that?"
   • "Are they having problems? Feeling insecure? Under pressure?"

Sleep

1. Chronically stressed people are often fatigued.
2. Go to sleep 30 to 60 minutes earlier each night for a few weeks.
3. If still fatigued, try going to bed another 30 minutes earlier.
4. Sleeping later in the morning is not helpful and can throw off body rhythms.

Exercise (Aerobic)

1. Exercise can dissipate chronic and acute stress.
2. Recommended at least for 30 minutes, three times a week.

Lower/Cut Out Caffeine Intake

1. Such a simple thing can lead to more energy, and fewer muscle aches, and help people feel more relaxed.
2. Wean off coffee, tea, colas, and chocolate drinks.

---

given as an adjunct to therapy. Drugs are not a cure. Therapy gives clients options on how to assess situations and how to deal with situations in ways that are appropriate and effective, and, in doing so, enhances the client's quality of life. Drugs cannot do that. Therefore, review Table 6–2 for the most effective medication and most effective therapies for each of the anxiety disorders.

♦   B O X   6 – 1 4   ♦
Client Teaching for Antianxiety Medications

CAUTION CLIENT:

1. Not to increase dose or frequency of ingestion without prior approval of therapist. **Benzodiazepines can become addicting.**

2. These medications reduce ability to handle mechanical equipment such as cars, saws, and machinery.

3. Avoid alcoholic beverages or take other antianxiety drugs because there is potential for dangerous central nervous system depression.

4. Avoid beverages that contain caffeine because it decreases the desired effects of the drug.

5. If pregnant, notify your physician right away. Benzodiazepines can increase the risk of congenital anomalies.

6. Do not breast-feed infants. Benzodiazepines are excreted in the milk and can have serious adverse effects on the infant.

7. Abrupt stoppage of benzodiazepines after 3 to 4 months of daily use may cause withdrawal symptoms. Drugs need to be tapered down.

8. Report symptoms of sore throat, fever, malaise, easy bruising, unusual bleeding, or motor restlessness immediately to your physician. Possible signs of agranulocytosis or thrombocytopenia; both need immediate attention.

9. If client is a heavy drinker, has a seizure disorder, plans to become pregnant, or takes other illicit drugs, have him or her discuss this with the nurse clinician or physician before taking these medications.

10. Lower doses are preferrred for elderly clients.

♦ NURSE, CLIENT, AND FAMILY RESOURCES—ANXIETY DISORDER

Associations

Anxiety Disorder Association of America
11900 Parklawn Drive, Suite 100
Rockville, MD 20852
1-301-231-9350
http://www.adaa.org/

Obsessive-Compulsive Foundation, Inc.
PO Box 70
Milford, CT 06460-0070
1-203-878-5669
http://www.ocfoundation.org

Internet Sites

Panic/Anxiety Disorders Guide
http://www.panicdisorder.about.com

Anxiety Panic Internet Resource
http://www.algy.com/anxiety/index.shtml

David Baldwin's Trauma Information Page
Site focuses on emotional trauma and traumatic stress, including PTSD
http://www.trauma-pages.com/

National Center for PSD
http://www.dartmouth.edu/dms/ptsd/

Anxiety Disorders Page
http://mentalhelp.net

Obsessive-Compulsive Disorder Home Page
http://www.fairlite.com/ocd/

CHAPTER 7

Mood Disorders

DEPRESSIVE DISORDERS

Mood refers to an emotion that dominates a person's mental life. Happiness and unhappiness are appropriate responses to life events. When sadness, grief, or elation is extremely intense and the mood unduly prolonged, a mood disorder results. Depressive symptoms often coexist in people with alcohol or substance abuse problems. Depressive symptoms are common in people who have other psychiatric disorders or behaviors (anorexia nervosa, borderline disorders, phobias, and schizophrenia), or people who have been physically or mentally abused (post-trauma behaviors). Depression may also be a critical symptom of many medical disorders or conditions (hepatitis, mononucleosis, multiple sclerosis, dementia, cancer, diabetes, chronic pain). Depression may also be directly related to the intake of many commonly prescribed medications (antihypertensive medications, steroids, hormones, digitalis, stimulants). Therefore, mood disorders can be caused by a medical condition, psychoactive drugs, and medications, as well as a host of psychiatric conditions. **Risk for suicide is an essential component of a thorough assessment regardless of the cause of depression.**

Primary mood disorders are of two types, *depressive disorders* and *bipolar disorders*. This chapter, covering the depressive disorders, is followed by a chapter on bipolar disorders.

◆ DEPRESSIVE DISORDERS
Major Depressive Disorder

In major depressive disorder, a severely depressed mood, usually recurrent, causes clinically significant distress or impairment in social, occupational, or other important areas of the person's life. The depressed mood can be distinguished from the person's usual functioning and may occur suddenly or gradually. Major depression is considered to be a "severe biologically-based mental illness" as determined by medical science in conjunction with the DSM-IV (National Alliance for the Mentally Ill [NAMI], 1999).

Major depression may be characterized by certain features. For example:

- Psychotic features—*delusions or hallucinations*
- Seasonal affective disorder (SAD)—*most prominent during certain seasons (e.g., winter or summer).* SAD is more prevalent in climates with longer periods of darkness in a 24-hour cycle.
- Catatonic features—*for example, peculiarities of voluntary movement, motor immobility, purposeless motor activity, echolalia or echopraxia*
- Melancholic features—*severe symptoms, loss of feelings of pleasure, worse in morning, early morning awakening, significant weight loss, excessive feelings of guilt*
- Postpartum onset—*within 4 weeks of delivery*

Box 7–1 presents the DSM-IV diagnostic criteria for major depressive disorder.

Dysthymic Disorder

Dysthymic disorder (dysthymia) is characterized by less severe, usually chronic depressive symptoms that have been present for at least 2 years (1 year for children or adolescents). Although dysthymia is not as severe as a major depression, the symptoms may cause significant distress or impairment in major areas of the person's life.

See Box 7–2 for a summary of the DSM-IV diagnostic criteria for dysthymia.

♦ ASSESSING FOR DEPRESSION

History

Does client have a(n):

1. Past history or family history of a mood disorder?
2. Substance abuse/alcohol problem?
3. Personality disorder (e.g., borderline) or eating disorder?
4. Recent bereavement (loss)?
5. Acute or chronic medical condition?

❖   B O X   7 – 1   ❖
Diagnostic Criteria for Major Depressive Disorder

1. Represents a change in previous functions.
2. Symptoms cause clinically significant distress or impair social, occupational, or other important areas of functioning.
3. **Five or more** of the following occur nearly every day for most waking hours over the same 2-week period:
   - Depressed mood
   - Anhedonia
   - Significant weight loss or gain (more than 5% of body weight in 1 month)
   - Insomnia or hypersomnia
   - Increased or decreased motor activity
   - Anergia (fatigue or loss of energy)
   - Feelings of worthlessness or inappropriate guilt (may be delusional)
   - Decreased concentration or indecisiveness
   - Recurrent thoughts of death or suicidal ideation (with or without pain)

Adapted from American Psychiatric Association. (1994). Diagnostic and Statistical Manual of Mental Disorders, 4th ed. Washington, DC: American Psychiatric Press, p. 327; reprinted by permission. Copyright 1994 American Psychiatric Association.

Presenting Symptoms

1. Depressed mood (or irritability in children or adolescents)
2. Diminished interest in or pleasure in most all activities
3. Alterations in eating, sleeping, activity level (fatigue), and libido
4. Feelings of worthlessness or guilt
5. Difficulty with concentration, memory, and making decisions
6. Recurrent thoughts of death and/or self-harm

Sample Questions

The nurse uses a variety of therapeutic techniques to obtain the answers to the following questions. Use your discretion and decide which questions are appropriate to complete your assessment.

1. "How is your general health? Has it changed recently?"
2. "How is your sleep/elimination/sex drive/appetite? Have they changed recently?"

❖ BOX 7 – 2 ❖
Diagnostic Criteria for Dysthymia

1. Occurs over a 2-year period (1 year for children and adolescents), presence of depressed mood.
2. Symptoms cause clinically significant distress in social, occupational, and other important areas of functioning.
3. Presence of two or more of the following:
   - Decreased or increased appetite
   - Insomnia or hypersomnia
   - Anergia or chronic fatigue
   - Anhedonia
   - Decreased self-esteem
   - Poor concentration or difficulty making decisions
   - Perceived inability to cope with routine responsibilities
   - Feelings of hopelessness and despair
   - Pessimistic about the future, brooding over the past, or feeling sorry for self
   - Recurrent thoughts of death or suicide

Adapted from American Psychiatric Association. (1994). Diagnostic and Statistical Manual of Mental Disorders, 4th ed. Washington, DC: American Psychiatric Press, p. 349; reprinted by permission. Copyright 1994 American Psychiatric Association.

3. "When you get sad or down, how long does it last?"
4. "Do you find yourself avoiding people?" Give an example.
5. "Do you go out less than you used to?" Give an example.
6. "Are you hard on yourself? Have you been harder on yourself lately?" Give an example.
7. "What do you see for yourself in the future?"
8. "When people get depressed, they sometimes think of dying. Have you had thoughts like that?"
9. "Have you thought of hurting yourself?"

Assessment Guide

There are a number of useful assessment guides available. Table 7–1 presents sample items from the **Beck Depression Inventory.**

◆ NURSING DIAGNOSES WITH INTERVENTIONS

There are a number of areas in a person's life that can be severely affected by depression. **Risk of harm to self** is the number one pri-

Table 7–1 ◆ Sample Items from the Beck Depression Inventory

Name _____ Date _____

The questionnaire provides groups of statements. Clients are asked to read all statements in the group and to circle the number that best describes their feelings. The following are two samples.

1. 0 I get as much satisfaction out of things as I used to.
    1 I don't enjoy things the way I used to.
    2 I don't get real satisfaction out of anything anymore.
    3 I am dissatisfied or bored with everything.
2. 0 I have not lost interest in other people.
    1 I am less interested in other people than I used to be.
    2 I have lost most of my interest in other people.
    3 I have lost all of my interest in other people.

From Beck Depression Inventory. Copyright © 1987, 1993 by Aaron T. Beck. Adapted and reproduced by permission of the publisher, The Psychological Corporation. All rights reserved. "Beck Depression Inventory" and "BDI" are registered trademarks of The Psychological Corporation.

ASSESSMENT ALERTS

1. A thorough physical and neurological exam helps to determine if the depression is primary or secondary to another disorder. Depression is a mood that can be secondary to a host of medical or other psychiatric disorders, as well as drugs/medications. Essentially, the nurse evaluates if:
   • The client is psychotic
   • The client has taken drugs or alcohol
   • Medical conditions are present
2. Always evaluate the client's risk of harm to self or others. Overt hostility is highly correlated with suicide. (**See Chapter 13 for assessment of and interventions for dealing with suicidal ideation and suicide attempts.**)

---

ority for assessment and intervention. **Chapter 13 deals with assessment and nursing interventions for people who are suicidal.** Risk for suicide is a concern with people who have a variety of psychiatric disorders (schizophrenia, bipolar disorder, substance abuse, borderline personality disorder) as well as medical disorders and syndromes.

Depression drastically affects a person's life and often affects cognitive ability. Poor concentration, lack of judgment and difficulties with memory can all affect cognitive abilities (**Altered**

Thought Processes). Feelings of self-worth plummet (**Self-Esteem Disturbance**), and ability to gain strength from their usual religious activities dwindles (**Spiritual Distress**). **Feelings of hopelessness** are common. Most noticeably, the ability to interact and gain solace from others is markedly reduced (**Impaired Social Interactions**).

The vegetative signs of depression can lead to physical complications such as lack of sleep (**Sleep Pattern Disturbance**), change in eating patterns (**Altered Nutrition**), and change in elimination (most often **Constipation**, although diarrhea may also occur in agitated clients). Therefore, **Self-Care Deficit** is often an obvious occurrence.

Table 7–2 identifies some potential nursing diagnoses for depressed clients.

The following list of overall nursing interventions will guide the nurse's care. Specific nursing interventions targeted to meet selected client problems (nursing diagnoses) are given below.

Related To (Etiology)

- Severe anxiety or depressed mood
- Biochemical/neurophysical imbalances
- Overwhelming life circumstances
- Persistent feelings of extreme anxiety, guilt, or fear
- Biological/medical factors
- Prolonged grief reaction

As Evidenced By (Assessment Findings/Diagnostic Cues)

- ◆ Memory deficit/problems
- ◆ Inaccurate interpretation of the environment
- ◆ Hypovigilance
- Impaired perception, judgment, decision making
- Impaired attention span/easily distracted
- Impaired ability to grasp ideas or order thoughts
- Negative ruminations
- Impaired insight
- Decreased problem-solving abilities

Outcome Criteria

- Client will give examples showing that short-term memory and concentration have improved to usual levels.

◆ NANDA accepted; ● In addition to NANDA.

Table 7–2 ◆ Potential Nursing Diagnoses for Depressive Disorders

SIGNS AND SYMPTOMS	POTENTIAL NURSING DIAGNOSES
Previous suicidal attempts, putting affairs in order, giving away prized possessions, suicidal ideation (has plan, ability to carry it out), makes overt or covert statements regarding killing self, feelings of worthlessness, hopelessness, helplessness	**Risk for Violence: Self-Directed** **Risk for Self-Mutilation**
Lack of judgment, memory difficulty, concentration poor, inaccurate interpretation of environment, negative ruminations, cognitive distortions	**Altered Thought Processes**
Difficulty with simple tasks, inability to function at previous level, poor problem solving, poor cognitive functioning, verbalizations of inability to cope	**Ineffective Individual Coping** **Altered Family Processes** **Risk for Altered Parent/Infant/ Child Attachment** **Altered Role Performance**
Difficulty making decisions, poor concentration, inability to take action	**Decisional Conflict**
Feelings of helplessness, hopelessness, powerlessness	**Helplessness** **Hopelessness** **Powerlessness**
Questions meaning of life, own existence, unable to participate in usual religious practices, conflict over spiritual beliefs, anger toward spiritual deity or religious representatives	**Spritual Distress**
Feelings of worthlessness, poor self-image, negative sense of self, self-negating verbalizations, feels like a failure, expressions of shame or guilt, hypersensitive to slights or criticism	**Self-Esteem Disturbance** **Chronic Low Self-Esteem** **Situational Low Self-Esteem**
Withdrawn, noncommunicative, speaks only in monosyllables, shies away from contact with others	**Impaired Social Interaction** **Social Isolation** **Risk for Loneliness**
Vegetative signs of depression: Changes in sleep, eating, grooming and hygiene, elimination, sexual patterns	**Self-Care Deficit (bathing/hygiene, dressing/ grooming)** **Altered Nutrition** **Sleep Pattern Disturbance** **Constipation** **Sexual Dysfunction**

OVERALL GUIDELINES FOR NURSING INTERVENTIONS

1. Convey caring, empathy, and potential for change by spending time with the client, even in silence, anticipating client's needs.
2. **The instillation of hope is a key tool for recovery.**
3. Enhance the person's sense of self by highlighting past accomplishments and strengths.
4. Whether in the hospital or in the community:
   - Assess needs for self-care and offer support when appropriate.
   - Monitor and intervene to help maintain adequate nutrition, hydration, and elimination.
   - Monitor and intervene to help provide adequate balance of rest, sleep, and activity.
   - Monitor and record increases/decreases in symptoms, what nursing interventions are effective.
   - Involve the client's support system and find supports for the client and family members in the community appropriate to their needs.
5. The dysfunctional attitude or learned helplessness and hopelessness seen with depressed people requires cognitive therapy or other psychotherapeutic interventions to counter.
6. **Continuously assess for the possibility of suicidal thoughts and ideation throughout the client's course of recovery.** (Refer to Chapter 13 for suicide assessment and interventions.)
7. Primary depression is a disease and responds well to psychopharmacology and electro-convulsive therapy (ECT). Be sure clients and those closely involved with them both understand the nature of the disease and have written information about the specific medications the client is taking. **Psychoeducation and a support system are essential.**
8. Assess family's and significant others' need for teaching, counseling, self-help groups, knowledge of community resources.

Altered Thought Processes

A state in which an individual experiences a disruption in cognitive operations and activities

- Client will demonstrate an increased ability to make appropriate decisions when planning with nurse.
- Client can identify negative thoughts and rationally counter them and/or reframe them in a positive manner.
- Client will show improved mood as demonstrated by the Beck Depression Inventory.

Short-Term Goals

Client will:

- Remember to keep appointments, attend activities, and attend to grooming with minimal reminders from others within 1 to 3 weeks
- Identify two goals he or she wants to achieve from treatment, with aid of nursing intervention, within 1 to 2 days
- Discuss with nurse two irrational thoughts about self and others by the end of the first day
- Reframe three irrational thoughts with nurse by (date)

Interventions and Rationales

Intervention	Rationale
1. Identify client's previous level of cognitive functioning (from client, family, friends, previous medical records).	1. Establishing a baseline of ability allows for evaluation of client's progress.
2. Help the client to postpone important major life decision making.	2. Making rational major life decisions requires optimal psychophysiological functioning.
3. Minimize client's responsibilities while severely depressed.	3. Decreases feelings of pressure and anxiety and minimizes feelings of guilt.
4. Use simple, concrete words.	4. Slowed thinking and difficulty concentrating impair comprehension.
5. Allow client plenty of time to think and frame responses.	5. Slowed thinking necessitates time to formulate a response.

Intervention	**Rationale**
6. Help client and significant others structure an environment that can help re-establish set schedules and predictable routines during severe depression.	6. A routine that is fairly repetitive and nondemanding is easier to both follow and remember.
7. Allow more time than usual for client to finish usual activities of daily living (ADL), for example, dressing, eating.	7. Usual tasks may take long periods of time; demands that the client hurry only increase anxiety and slow down ability to think clearly.
8. Work with client to recognize negative thinking and thoughts. Teach client to reframe and/or refute negative thoughts.	8. Negative ruminations add to feelings of hopelessness and are part of a depressed person's faulty thought processes. Intervening in this process aids in healthier and more useful outlook.

Chronic Low Self-Esteem

Longstanding negative self-evaluation/feelings about self or self-capabilities

---

Related To (Etiology)

- Biochemical/neurophysicological imbalances
- Impaired cognitive self-appraisal
- Unrealistic expectations of self
- Shame and guilt
- Repeated past failures

As Evidenced By (Assessment Findings/Diagnostic Cues)

- ◆ Negative feedback about self
- ◆ Self-negating verbalizations
- Repeated expressions of worthlessness

◆ NANDA accepted; ● In addition to NANDA.

- Inability to recognize own achievements
- Negative view of abilities
- ◆ Rejection of positive feedback

Outcome Criteria

Client will:

- Give an accurate and nonjudgmental account of four positive qualities as well as identify two areas he or she wishes to improve
- Demonstrate the ability to modify unrealistic self-expectations
- Report decreased feelings of shame, guilt, and self-hate by using a scale of 1 to 10 (1 lowest, 10 highest)

Short-Term Goals

Client will:

- Identify one or two strengths by the end of the day
- Identify two unrealistic self-expectations and reformulate more realistic life goals with nurse by the end of the day
- Keep a daily log and identify on a scale of 1 to 10 (1 lowest, 10 highest) feelings of shame, guilt, self-hate
- Identify three judgmental terms (e.g., "I am lazy") client uses to describe self and identify objective terms to replace them (e.g., "I do not feel motivated to") by (date)

Interventions and Rationales

Intervention	Rationale
1. Work with the client to identify cognitive distortions that encourage negative self-appraisal. For example:	1. Cognitive distortions reinforce negative, inaccurate perception of self and the world.
a. Overgeneralizations	a. Taking one fact or event and making a general rule out of it ("He always"; "I never").
b. Self-blame	b. Consistent self-blame for everything perceived as negative.
c. Mind reading	c. Assuming others don't like you, etc., without any real evidence that assumptions are correct.
d. Discounting positive attributes	

Intervention

Rationale

> d. Focusing on negative qualities.

2. Teach visualization techniques that help client replace negative self-images with more positive thoughts and images.

2. Promotes a healthier and more realistic self-image by helping the client choose more positive actions and thoughts.

3. Work with client on areas that he or she would like to improve using problem-solving skills. Evaluate need for more teaching in this area.

3. Feelings of low self-esteem can interfere with usual problem-solving abilities.

4. Evaluate client's need for assertiveness training tools in order to pursue things he or she wants or needs in life. Arrange for training through community-based programs, personal counseling, literature, etc.

4. People with low self-esteem often feel unworthy and have difficulty asking appropriately for what they need and want.

5. Role model assertiveness.

5. Example client can follow.

6. Encourage participation in a support/therapy group where others are experiencing similar thoughts, feelings, and situations.

6. Decrease feelings of isolation and provide an atmosphere where positive feedback and a more realistic appraisal of self is available.

Spiritual Distress

A disruption in the life principle that pervades a person's entire being and that integrates and transcends biological and psychosocial nature

---

Related To (Etiology)

◆ Separation from religious/cultural ties
◆ Beliefs and values challenged as a result of severe suffering, loss, moral dilemmas, etc.

◆ NANDA accepted; ● In addition to NANDA.

- Death of a significant other
- Lack of purpose and meaning in life
- Serious illness
- Overwhelming life changes
- Overwhelming loss

As Evidenced By (Assessment Findings/Diagnostic Cues)

- ◆ Questions meaning of own existence
- ◆ Expresses concern with meaning of life/death or belief systems
- ◆ Unable to participate in usual religious practices
- Recognition of one's mortality
- Searching for a spiritual source of strength
- Expresses intense feelings of guilt
- Expresses hopelessness and helplessness

Outcome Criteria

Clients will:

- State that they gain comfort from previous spiritual practices
- State that they feel their life is meaningful

Short-Term Goals

Client will:

- Talk to nurse or spiritual leader about spiritual conflicts and concerns within 3 days
- Discuss with nurse two things that gave his or her life meaning in the past within 3 days
- Keep a journal tracking thoughts and feelings for 1 week

Interventions and Rationales

Intervention	Rationale
1. Assess what spiritual practices have offered comfort and meaning to the client's life when not ill.	1. Evaluates neglected areas in the person's life that, if reactivated, might add comfort and meaning during a painful depression.
2. Discuss with the client what has given meaning and com-	2. When depressed, clients often struggle for meaning

---

◆ NANDA accepted; ● In addition to NANDA.

Intervention	**Rationale**
fort to the person in the past.	in life and reasons to go on when feeling hopeless and despondent.
3. Encourage client to write in a journal every day expressing daily thoughts and reflections.	3. Helps some to identify significant personal issues and one's thoughts and feelings surrounding spiritual issues. Journal writing is an excellent way to explore deeper meanings of life.
4. If client is unable to write, have client use a tape recorder.	4. Often speaking aloud helps a person clarify thinking and explore issues.
5. Provide information on referrals, when needed, for religious or spiritual information (e.g., readings, programs, tapes, community resources).	5. When hospitalized, spiritual tapes and readings may be useful; when the client is in the community, client may express other needs.
6. Suggest spiritual leader in or affiliated with the facility to contact client.	6. Spiritual leaders in an institution or community are familiar with spiritual distress and may offer comfort to client.

Impaired Social Interaction

The state in which an individual participates in an insufficient or excessive quantity or ineffective quality of social exchange

Related To (Etiology)

◆ Self-concept disturbance (negative view of self)
◆ Absence of available significant others/peers (support system deficit)
◆ Altered thought processes
● Fear of rejection
● Feelings of worthlessness
● Anergia (lack of energy and motivation)

◆ NANDA accepted; ● In addition to NANDA.

As Evidenced By (Assessment Findings/Diagnostic Cues)

◆ Family reports change of style or patterns of interaction.
◆ Verbalized or observed discomfort in social situations (e.g., inability to receive or communicate a satisfying sense of belonging, caring, interest, or shared history).
◆ Dysfunctional interaction with peers, family, and/or others.
● Remains secluded, lacks eye contact, avoids contact with others.

Outcome Criteria

Clients will:

• State and demonstrate resumption of sustaining relationships with friends and family members
• State that they enjoy interacting with others in activities and one-to-one interactions to the extent they did before becoming depressed

Short-Term Goals

Client will:

• Participate in one activity by the end of each day
• Discuss three alternative actions to take when feeling the need to withdraw by (date)
• Identify two personal behaviors that might discourage others from seeking contact by (date)
• Eventually voluntarily attend individual/group therapeutic meetings within a therapeutic milieu (hospital or community) (date)

Interventions and Rationales

Intervention	Rationale
1. While client is most severely depressed, involve the client in one-to-one activity.	1. Maximizes the potential for interactions while minimizing anxiety levels.
2. Engage the client in activities involving gross motor activity that call for limited concentration (e.g., taking a walk)	2. Physical activities can help relieve tensions and may help to elevate mood.

◆ NANDA accepted; ● In addition to NANDA.

Intervention	**Rationale**
3. Initially, provide activities that require very little concentration (playing simple card games, looking through a magazine, drawing).	3. Concentration and memory are poor in depressed people. Activities that have no "right or wrong" or "winners or losers" minimize opportunities for the client to put himself or herself down.
4. Eventually increase the client's contacts with others (first one other, then two others, etc.).	4. Contact with others distracts the client from self-preoccupation.
5. Eventually involve the client in group activities (e.g., dance therapy, art therapy, group discussions).	5. Socialization decreases feelings of isolation. Genuine regard for others can increase self-worth.
6. Refer the client as well as the family to self-help groups in the community.	6. Both client and family may gain tremendous support and insight from people sharing their experiences.

Self-Care Deficit (Specify Level)

Inability to complete feeding, bathing, toileting, dressing, and grooming of self

---

Related To (Etiology)

◆ Perceptual or cognitive impairment
◆ Decreased or lack of motivation (anergia)
◆ Severe anxiety
● Severe preoccupation

Outcome Criteria

Client will:

• Gradually return to weight consistent for height and age or baseline before illness

---

◆ NANDA accepted; ● In addition to NANDA.

- Sleep between 6 and 8 hours per night
- Maintain adequate hygiene and be appropriately groomed and dressed (shave/makeup, clothes clean and neat)
- Experience normal elimination

Short-Term Goals

- Client will gain 1 pound a week with encouragement from family, significant others, and/or staff if significant weight loss exists.
- Client will sleep between 4 and 6 hours with aid of medication and/or nursing measures.
- Client will groom and dress appropriately with help from nursing staff and/or family.
- Client's elimination pattern will become more normal with aid of foods high in roughage, increased fluids, and exercise daily (also with aid of medications).

Interventions and Rationales

ALTERED NUTRITION

Intervention	**Rationale**
1. Encourage small, high-calorie and high-protein snacks and fluids frequently throughout the day and evening if weight loss exists.	1. Minimize weight loss, dehydration, and constipation.
2. Encourage eating with others.	2. Increase socialization, decrease focus on food.
3. Serve foods or drinks the client likes.	3. Clients are more likely to eat the foods they like.
4. Weigh the client weekly and observe the client's eating patterns.	4. Give the information needed for revising the intervention.

SLEEP PATTERN DISTURBANCE

Intervention	**Rationale**
1. Provide rest periods after activities.	1. Fatigue can intensify feelings of depression.
2. Encourage the client to get up and dress and to stay out of bed during the day.	2. Minimizing sleep during the day increases the likelihood of sleep at night.

Intervention	**Rationale**
3. Encourage relaxation measures in the evening (e.g., backrub, tepid bath, or warm milk).	3. These measures induce relaxation and sleep.
4. Reduce environmental and physical stimulants in the evening—provide decaffeinated coffee, soft lights, soft music, and quiet activities.	4. Decreasing caffeine and epinephrine levels increases the possibility of sleep.
5. Teach relaxation exercises (see Chapter 6).	5. Besides deeply relaxing the body, relaxation exercises often lead to sleep.

SELF-BATHING HYGIENE DEFICIT

Intervention	**Rationale**
1. Encourage the use of toothbrush, washcloth, soap, makeup, shaving equipment, and so forth.	1. Being clean and well groomed can temporarily raise self-esteem.
2. Give step-by-step reminders, such as "Wash the right side of your face, now the left . . . ."	2. Slowed thinking and difficulty concentrating make organizing simple tasks difficult.

CONSTIPATION

Intervention	**Rationale**
1. Monitor intake and output, especially bowel movements.	1. Many depressed clients are constipated. If this condition is not checked, fecal impaction can occur.
2. Offer foods high in fiber and provide periods of exercise.	2. Roughage and exercise stimulate peristalsis and help evacuation of fecal material.
3. Encourage the intake of nonalcoholic/non-caffeinated fluids, 6 to 8 glasses/day.	3. Fluids help prevent constipation.
4. Evaluate the need for laxatives and enemas.	4. These prevent the occurrence of fecal impaction.

♦ PSYCHOPHARMACOLOGY FOR DEPRESSION

Depression is a recurring disorder. About 75% to 95% of people with a primary depression have multiple episodes. However, the discovery of effective antidepressants has resulted in depression being one of the most "treatable" disorders (Zajecka, 1995). Keller (1995) noted that:

- 65% to 75% of depressed clients "respond" to antidepressant treatment.
- 25% to 35% of clients with a major depression fail to respond meaningfully to presently available treatment.

However, waiting too long to start treatment leads to (Greden, 1995):

- Greater morbidity
- Greater disability
- Greater expense
- Greater resistance to treatment and increased potential for relapse

All depressed individuals need to be evaluated for suicide risk, whether they are in the hospital or the community. When a depressed person is hospitalized, staff members need to check to make sure that all medications are swallowed (not placed in the cheek or under the tongue). If a client is being treated in an outpatient setting, only a week's supply should be given to a severely depressed person to minimize client overdosing.

Antidepressant drugs can improve poor self-concept, degree of withdrawal, vegetative signs of depression, and activity level.

Basic Assumptions Guiding Nursing Care with Medications

1. Primary depression is a disease and responds well to psychopharmacology. Be sure client and family both understand the nature of the disease and have written information about the specific medications the client is taking. **Client and family teaching is vital.**
2. Clients and significant others need a sound understanding of the side effects and toxic effects of all of their medications, and need to know what to do and whom to call if severe or toxic side effects occur. **This information should be writ-**

Continued

> ten down in the client's own language. Names and tele-
> phone numbers of whom to call in an emergency need to
> be written down and given to the client as well.
>
> 3. Combined psychopharmacotherapy and psychotherapy has
>   been found to be more effective in the treatment of major
>   depression and the delay of return of symptoms than either
>   treatment alone (Slaby, 1994).
> 4. Successful management of a depressive episode entails ad-
>   herence to medication provided over the course of months
>   and sometimes years.
> 5. To prevent relapse, clients should take antidepressants con-
>   tinuously for 1 year after the symptoms have subsided.

The major types of antidepressant drugs are the:

- Selective serotonin reuptake inhibitors (**SSRIs**)
- Selective serotonin/norepinephrine reuptake inhibitors (**SSNRIs**)
- Tricyclic antidepressants (**TCAs**)
- Monoamine oxidase inhibitors (**MAOIs**)
- Atypical—bupropion (Wellbutrin), trazodone (Desyrel)

There are guidelines that physicians and advanced clinical practice
nurses use in identifying which medications may be most useful
for which clients. Table 7–3 identifies some of these guidelines.
Table 7–4 gives an overview of the initial and maximum adult
dosages for the commonly prescribed antidepressant medications.

Selective Serotonin Reuptake Inhibitors

SSRIs and the SSNRIs are recommended as first-line therapy in
all depressions except severe inpatient depression (in which ECT
may be the first choice) or melancholic depression, or mild outpatient depression (Maxman and Ward, 1995). The SSRIs block
the reuptake of serotonin in the brain, permitting serotonin to act
for an extended period of time at the synaptic binding sites in
the brain.

SSRI antidepressant drugs have a lower incidence of anticholinergic side effects (dry mouth, blurred vision, urinary retention),
less cardiotoxicity, and faster onset than the TCAs. For most
clients, the SSRIs are better tolerated than the TCAs. The SSRIs
are also being used successfully with many individuals who have
anxiety disorders and eating disorders.

Table 7–3 ◆ Special Problems and Medications of Choice

PROBLEM	DRUGS OF CHOICE
1. High suicide risk	1. Trazodone, fluoxetine, sertraline, paroxetine, bupropion, venlafaxine
2. Concurrent depression and panic attacks	2. Phenelzine, imipramine, fluoxetine, paroxetine
3. Chronic pain with or without depression	3. Amitriptyline, doxepin
4. Weight gain on other antidepressants	4. Fluoxetine, bupropion, sertraline, paroxetine
5. Sensitivity to anticholinergic side effects	5. Trazodone, fluoxetine, phenelzine, tranylcypromine, bupropion, sertraline, paroxetine
6. Orthostatic hypotension	6. Nortriptyline, bupropion, sertraline
7. Sexual dysfunction	7. Bupropion, nefazodone

From Preston, J., and Johnson, J. (1998). Clinical Psychopharmacology Made Ridiculously Simple. Miami: MedMaster; reprinted with permission.
Note: Most antidepressants are quite toxic when taken in an overdose. Extreme caution should be taken in prescribing to high-risk suicidal patients. Of the existing antidepressants, trazodone appears to have the lowest degree of cardiotoxicity.

The main complaints (side effects) of individuals taking these drugs is that the drugs may cause sleeping difficulties, loss of appetite, and sexual dysfunction (primarily anorgasmia, erectile dysfunction) in selected individuals.

One rare toxic effect of these drugs is central serotonin syndrome. Table 7–5 identifies the main side and toxic effects of the SSRIs.

Client and family teaching is extremely important for all medications. Medication information, side effects, and cautions should always be written down and given to the client. Discussion and teaching with the nurse should always be done, and questions should be elicited and clarifications made. (For a guide to client and family teaching with the SSRIs, see Box 7–3.)

Tricyclic Antidepressants

TCAs benefit about 65% to 80% of people with nondelusional depressive disorders. It may take up to 10 to 14 days before these agents start to work. The full effect may take from 4 to 8 weeks to be seen. As with all drugs, side effects and toxic effects are present. Presently, the **SSRIs** are considered the drugs of choice.

Table 7-4 ◆ Adult Dosages for Antidepressants

GENERIC NAME	TRADE NAME	INITIAL DOSE*† (mg/day)	DOSE AFTER 4–8 WEEKS* (mg/day)	MAXIMUM DOSE‡ (mg/day)
Selective Serotonin Reuptake Inhibitors (SSRIs)				
Fluoxetine	Prozac	20	20–40	80
Fluvoxamine	Luvox	50–100	50–300	300
Paroxetine	Paxil	20	20–50	50
Sertraline‡	Zoloft	50	50–200	200
Selective Serotonin/Norepinephrine Reuptake Inhibitors (SSNRIs)				
Venlafaxine	Effexor	50	75–225	375
Nefazodone	Serzone	200	300–600	600
Atypical Antidepressants				
Amoxapine	Asendin	50–150	200–300	400
Bupropion	Wellbutrin	200	300	450
Maprotiline	Ludiomil	50–150	100–150	225
Trazodone	Desyrel	150	150–200	400

Tricyclic Antidepressants (TCAs)

Amitriptyline	Elavil, Endep	50–150	100–200	300
Desipramine	Norpramin, Pertofrane	50–150	75–200	300
Doxepin	Adapin, Sinequan	50–150	100–200	300
Imipramine	Tofranil	50–150	100–200	300
Nortriptyline	Aventyl, Pamelor	25–100	75–150	150
Protriptyline	Vivactil	10–40	15–40	60
Trimipramine	Surmontil	50–150	75–250	250
Monoamine Oxidase Inhibitors (MAOIs)				
Isocarboxazid	Marplan	20–30	20–30	30
Phenelzine	Nardil	45–75	45–75	75
Tranylcypromine	Parnate	20–30	20–30	30

Data from Lehne, R.A., et al. (1998).

*Doses listed are total daily doses. Depending on the drug and the patient, the total dose may be given in a single dose or in divided doses.

†Initial doses are employed for 4 to 8 weeks, the time required for most symptoms to respond. The smaller dose within the range listed is used initially. Dosage is gradually increased as required.

‡Doses higher than these may be needed for some people with severe depression.

**Table 7–5 ◆ Side Effects and Toxic Effects of
Selective Serotonin Reuptake Inhibitors**

Note: *Do not administer SSRIs to patients who are taking MAOIs. The
drug interaction can result in serious or fatal reactions.*

SIDE EFFECTS	COMMENTS
1. Rash or allergic reaction	1. Discontinue drug; ask physician about treatment with antihistamines or steroids.
2. Anxiety, nervousness, insomnia	2. Discontinue the drug. Giving the drug in AM may help decrease insomnia.
3. Anorexia, weight loss, nausea	3. Particularly common in underweight, depressed clients. If significant weight loss occurs, ask physician about changing to a different drug.
4. Tremors, sweating, dizziness, lightheadedness	4. Most of the effects listed in 4, 5, and 6 are transient and disappear when drug is discontinued.
5. Drowsiness and fatigue	5. SSRIs can affect cognitive motor ability.
6. Decreased or altered libido/ erectile dysfunction	6. If change in libido or ability to perform becomes a problem for client, ask doctor about changing the drug.
7. Weight gain	7. Weight gain is a reason for nonadherence to medication in some women. Needs to be addressed.
8. Nonadherence to drug	8. Approximately 33% of clients experience sexual dysfunction.

SEROTONERGIC SYNDROME: TOXIC EFFECTS

1. Hyperactivity/restlessness
2. Tachycardia $\longrightarrow$ cardiovascular shock
3. Fever $\longrightarrow$ hyperpyrexia
4. Elevated blood pressure
5. Altered mental states (delirium)
6. Irrationality, mood swings, hostility
7. Seizures $\longrightarrow$ status epilepticus
8. Myoclonus, incoordination, tonic rigidity
9. Abdominal pain, diarrhea, bloating
10. Apnea $\longrightarrow$ death

From Varcarolis, E. (1998). Clinical Companion for Foundations of Psychiatric
Mental Health Nursing, 3rd ed. Philadelphia: W.B. Saunders Company, pp. 11–12;
reprinted with permission.

People taking TCAs can have adverse reactions to numerous other medications. For example, use of a MAOI along with a TCA is contraindicated.

Clients and families need to be aware of the side effects and toxic effects of the medications as well as other relevant informa-

---

❖   **B O X   7 – 3**   ❖
Client and Family Teaching: SSRIs

- SSRIs may cause sexual dysfunction or lack of sex drive. Inform nurse or physician.
- SSRIs may cause insomnia, anxiety, and nervousness. Inform nurse or physician.
- SSRIs may interact with other medications. Be sure physician knows other medications client is taking (digoxin, warfarin). SSRIs should not be taken within 14 days of the last dose of an MAOI.
- Do not take any over-the-counter drugs without first notifying the physician.
- Common side effects include fatigue, nausea, diarrhea, dry mouth, dizziness, tremor, fatigue, and sexual dysfunction or lack of sex drive.
- Because of the potential for drowsiness and dizziness, client should not drive or operate machinery until these side effects are ruled out.
- Avoid alcohol.
- Client should have liver and renal function tests performed and blood counts checked periodically.
- Do not discontinue medication abruptly. If side effects become bothersome, client should ask physician about changing to a different drug, but be aware that the medication will have to be phased out over a period of time.

Report any of the following symptoms to physician immediately:
- Rash or hives
- Rapid heart beat
- Sore throat
- Difficulty urinating
- Fever, malaise
- Anorexia/weight loss
- Unusual bleeding
- Initiation of hyperactive behavior
- Severe headache

From Varcarolis, E. (1998). *Clinical Companion for Foundations of Psychiatric Mental Health Nursing*, 3rd ed. Philadelphia: W.B. Saunders Company, pp. 12–13; reprinted with permission.

❖   B O X   7 – 4   ❖

Teaching Clients and Their Families About Tricyclic Antidepressants

1. Tell the client and the client's family that mood elevation may take from 7 to 28 days. It may take up to 6–8 weeks for the full effect to take place and for major depression symptoms to subside.
2. Have the family reinforce this frequently to the depressed family member because depressed people have trouble remembering and respond to ongoing reassurance.
3. Reassure the client that drowsiness, dizziness, and hypotension usually subside after the first few weeks.
4. When the client starts taking tricyclic antidepressants (TCAs), caution the client to be careful working around machines, driving cars, and crossing streets because of possible altered reflexes, drowsiness, and/or dizziness.
5. Alcohol can block the effects of antidepressants. Tell the client to refrain from drinking.
6. If possible, the client should take the full dose at bedtime to reduce the experience of side effects during the day.
7. If the client forgets the bedtime dose (or the once-a-day dose), the client should take the dose within 3 hours; otherwise, the client should wait for the next day. The client should *not* double the dose.
8. Suddenly stopping TCAs can cause nausea, altered heartbeat, nightmares, and cold sweats in 2 to 4 days. The client should call the doctor or take one dose of TCA until the physician can be contacted.

From Varcarolis, E. (1998). Foundations of Mental Health Nursing, 3rd ed. Philadelphia: W.B. Saunders Company, p. 572; reprinted with permission.

tion. This information should be written down and given to the family and client once teaching is complete. (See Box 7–4 for a guide to client and family teaching with the TCAs.)

Monoamine Oxidase Inhibitors

These drugs are usually *not* first-line drugs because of their serious side effects. A serious side effect of these drugs is that they interact with foods containing tyramine, a natural product of bacterial fermentation found in many cheeses, some wines, and chopped liver as well as certain medications, including sympathomimetic amines. The interaction results in a hypertensive crisis that may cause a stroke or even death.

Because these drugs have the danger of hypertensive crisis, they are usually contraindicated for people who are debilitated, elderly, or hypertensive; those who have cardiac or cerebrovascular disease; those who have severe renal and hepatic disease; and those unwilling or unable to adhere to dietary restrictions.

Client teaching is as important with these drugs as all others, perhaps even more so because of the danger of hypertensive crisis with tyramine-containing foods and with medications. Clients and their families need to know these foods and drugs, and be taught to read food labels very carefully, because some of these tyramine-containing foods may be present as an ingredient. Clients should also be told that, before they take *any* over-the-counter medication, they should first check with their physician. See Box 7–5.

❖ **B O X 7 – 5** ❖

Teaching Clients and Their Families About Monoamine Oxidase Inhibitors

- Tell the client and the client's family to avoid certain foods and all medications (especially cold remedies) unless prescribed by and discussed with the client's doctor. Give client and family a list of "forbidden foods" and drugs.
- Give the client a wallet card describing the monoamine oxidase inhibitor (MAOI) regimen (Parke-Davis will supply them if contacted at 1-800-223-6432).
- Instruct the client to avoid Chinese restaurants (sherry, brewer's yeast, and other products may be used).
- Tell the client to go to the emergency room right away if he or she develops a severe headache.
- Ideally, blood pressure should be monitored during the first 6 weeks of treatment (for both hypotensive and hypertensive effects).
- After stopping the MAOI, the client should maintain dietary and drug restrictions for 14 days.

From Varcarolis, E. (1998). Foundations of Mental Health Nursing, 3rd ed. Philadelphia: W.B. Saunders Company, p. 577; reprinted with permission.

◆ ELECTROCONVULSIVE THERAPY

ECT is indicated when antidepressant drugs have no effect. ECT is particularly effective in clients with major depression, especially when psychotic symptoms are present (delusions of guilt, somatic delusions, or delusions of infidelity). Clients who have depression with marked psychomotor retardation also respond well. A course of ECT for a depressed client is 6 to 12 treatments given two or three times per week.

◆ NURSE AND CLIENT RESOURCES — DEPRESSIVE DISORDERS

Associations

National Alliance for the Mentally Ill (NAMI)
200 North Glebe Road, Suite 1015
Arlington, VA 22203-3754
1-800-950-NAMI

Depressed Anonymous: Recovery from Depression
DSS, Inc.
P.O. Box 17471
Louisville, KY 40217
(502) 569–1989

National Foundation for Depressive Illness
P.O. Box 2257
New York, NY 10016
1-800-248-4344

National Organization for Seasonal Affective Disorders (NOSAD)
P.O. Box 40133
Washington, DC 20016

National Depressive & Manic-Depressive Association
730 N. Franklin, #501
Chicago, IL 60610
(312) 642-0049
http://www.ndmda.org

Internet Sites

Depression.com
Great general source
http://www.depression.com

NIMH—Depression/Awareness, Recognition, and Treatment
http://www.nimh.nih.gov/depression/index.html

Depression Resources List
http://www.execpc.com/~corbeau/

Internet Mental Health
Great resource for everything
http://www.mentalhealth.com

What You Should Know About Women and Depression
http://www.apa.org/pubinfo/depress.html

Pharmaceutical Information Network
Drug FAQS: Antidepressants
http://pharminfo.com/drugfaq/antidep_faq.html

Online Depression Screening Test
Short (10-question) assessment
http://www.med.nyu.edu/psych/screens/depres.html

# CHAPTER 8

Mood Disorders

BIPOLAR DISORDERS

Bipolar disorders are mood disorders that include one or more manic or hypomanic episodes (elevated, expansive, or irritable mood) and usually one or more depressive episodes. Bipolar disorders are essentially related to biochemical imbalances in the brain, and the disease is thought to be genetically transferred. Medication adherence is key if nursing and counseling interventions are to be effective.

An acute or severe manic phase usually warrants hospitalization. A person experiencing hypomania, on the other hand, rarely needs hospitalization unless there is a danger to self or others.

Bipolar disorders consist of two different categories of disorders: (1) **cyclothymia** and (2) **bipolar disorder (bipolar I and bipolar II)**. The symptoms seen in bipolar disorder (I and II) are more serious than those in cyclothymia.

◆ CYCLOTHYMIA

Cyclothymia is a chronic mood disturbance of at least 2 years' duration. Cyclothymia is the recurrent experience of some of the symptoms of *hypomania* alternating with *dysthymic depression*. People with cyclothymia **do not** have severe impairment in their social or occupational functioning, nor do they experience psychotic symptoms such as delusions.

◆ BIPOLAR DISORDER (BIPOLAR I AND BIPOLAR II) (APA, 1994)

The manic episode in bipolar I may begin suddenly and last a few days to months. There can be impairments in reality testing, and, when severe, these impairments may take the form of grandiose or

persecutory *delusions*. Considerable impairment in social, occupational, and interpersonal functioning exists. Hospitalization is often
required to protect the person from the consequences of poor judgment and hyperactivity. Bipolar disorder is classified as severe biologically based mental illness by medical science in conjunction
with the DSM-IV.

Bipolar I consists of one or more episodes of *major depression*
plus one or more periods of clear-cut *mania*.

Bipolar II consists of one or more periods of *major depression*
plus periods of *hypomania*.

The distinction between hypomania and mania is made clear for
diagnostic purposes in the DSM-IV, and is presented in Box 8–1.

Bipolar disorder can be grouped into three phases:

1. **Acute Phase**—Hospitalization is most always indicated for a
   client in the acute manic or severe manic phase of bipolar disorder (particularly bipolar I). Hospitalization protects client from
   harm (cardiac collapse, financial loss) and allows for medication
   stabilization.
2. **Continuation Phase**—usually lasts for 4 to 9 months, and the
   goal during this phase is to prevent relapse.
3. **Maintenance Treatment Phase**—aimed at preventing the recurrence of an episode of bipolar illness.

Many of the interventions in this chapter address the client in the
acute phase, because that is the phase that requires the most immediate and complex nursing care.

◆ ASSESSING FOR MANIA

History

1. Past history or family history of bipolar illness?
2. Has client had periods of elated or depressed moods in the past?
3. Is client on any mood-altering drugs? What are they?
4. Have all other medical or mental disorders been ruled out?

Presenting Symptoms

1. Periods of hyperactivity (paces, restless, speeded up)
2. Overconfident, exaggerated view of own abilities
3. Decreased need for sleep, no acknowledgment of fatigue
4. Poor social judgment, engaging in reckless and self-destructive
   activities (foolish business ventures, sexual indiscretions, buying sprees)
5. Rapid-fire speech, pressured speech, loud, garrulous, rhyming
   punning

❖   B O X   8 – 1   ❖
Diagnostic Criteria for Manic Symptoms

1. A distinct period of abnormality and persistently elevated, expansive, or irritable mood for at least:
   • 4 days for hypomania
   • 1 week for mania
2. During the period of mood disturbance, **at least three (or more)** of the following symptoms have persisted (four if the mood is only irritable) and have been present to a significant degree:
   • Inflated self-esteem or grandiosity
   • Decreased need for sleep (e.g., the person feels rested after only 3 hours of sleep)
   • Increased talkativeness or pressure to keep talking
   • Flight of ideas or subjective experience that thoughts are racing
   • Distractibility (i.e., the person's attention is too easily drawn to unimportant or irrelevant external stimuli)
   • Increase in goal-directed activity (either socially, at work or school, or sexually) or psychomotor agitation
   • Excessive involvement in pleasurable activities that have a high potential for painful consequences (e.g., the person engages in unrestrained buying sprees, sexual indiscretions, or foolish business investments)

Hypomania

1. The episode is associated with an unequivocal change in functioning that is uncharacteristic of the person when not symptomatic.
2. Absence of marked impairment in social or occupational functioning
3. Delusions are never present.
4. Hospitalization is not indicated.

Mania

1. Severe enough to cause marked impairment in occupational activities, usual social activities, or relationships
   or
2. Hospitalization is needed to protect client and others from irresponsible or aggressive behavior
   or
3. There are psychotic features (e.g., grandiose and/or paranoid delusions)

6. Brief attention span, easily distractible, flights of ideas, loosened associations, delusions
7. Expansive, irritable, or paranoid behaviors
8. Impatient, uncooperative, abusive, obscene, manipulative

Sample Questions

The nurse uses a variety of therapeutic techniques to obtain answers to the following questions. Use your discretion and decide which questions are appropriate to complete your assessment.

1. "Was there ever a time when you . . .
   a. ". . . talked too much and couldn't stop?"
   b. ". . . started things you couldn't finish?"
   c. ". . . were too happy without any reason?"
   d. ". . . did without sleep or much food for a day or two?"
   e. ". . . spent money recklessly/spent money you didn't have/ made extravagant gifts? Describe this to me."
2. "Have you ever found yourself pacing or moving and couldn't stop?"
3. "Was there ever a time you couldn't stop your mind racing? Couldn't concentrate? Describe such a time."

Assessment Guidelines

See Box 8–2 for a self-assessment test. Clients may want to take this test frequently to monitor symptoms.

 B O X   8 – 2 ❖
Mania Questionnaire

Use this questionnaire to help determine if you need to see a mental health professional for diagnosis and treatment of mania or manic-depression or bipolar disorder.

Instructions: You might reproduce this scale and use it on a weekly basis to track your moods. It also might be used to show your doctor how your symptoms have changed from one visit to the next. Changes of five or more points are significant. This scale is not designed to make a diagnosis of mania or take the place of a professional diagnosis. If you suspect you are manic, please consult with a mental health professional as soon as possible.

Continued

The 18 items below refer to how you have felt and behaved DURING THE PAST WEEK. For each item, indicate the extent to which it is true by circling the appropriate number next to the item.

Key:

0 = Not at all	**3 = Moderately**
1 = A little	**4 = Quite a lot**
2 = Somewhat	**5 = Very much**

1. My mind has never been sharper.   0 1 2 3 4 5
2. I need less sleep than usual.   0 1 2 3 4 5
3. I have so many plans and new ideas that it is hard for me to work.   0 1 2 3 4 5
4. I feel a pressure to talk and talk.   0 1 2 3 4 5
5. I have been particularly happy.   0 1 2 3 4 5
6. I have been more active than usual.   0 1 2 3 4 5
7. I talk so fast that people have a hard time keeping up with me.   0 1 2 3 4 5
8. I have more new ideas than I can handle.   0 1 2 3 4 5
9. I have been irritable.   0 1 2 3 4 5
10. It's easy for me to think of jokes and funny stories.   0 1 2 3 4 5
11. I have been feeling like "the life of the party."   0 1 2 3 4 5
12. I have been full of energy.   0 1 2 3 4 5
13. I have been thinking about sex.   0 1 2 3 4 5
14. I have been feeling particularly playful.   0 1 2 3 4 5
15. I have special plans for the world.   0 1 2 3 4 5
16. I have been spending too much money.   0 1 2 3 4 5
17. My attention keeps jumping from one idea to another.   0 1 2 3 4 5
18. I find it hard to slow down and stay in one place.   0 1 2 3 4 5

	ASSESSMENT ALERTS

1. Assess if danger to self or others:
   - Manic clients can exhaust themselves to the point of death.
   - Client may not eat or sleep for days at a time.
   - Poor impulse control may result in harm to others or self.
   - Uncontrolled spending
2. Clients may give away all of their money or possessions, so might need controls to protect them from bankruptcy.
3. Assess for need for hospitalization to safeguard and stabilize client.
4. Assess medical status. A thorough medical exam helps to determine if mania is primary (a mood disorder—bipolar/cyclothymia) or secondary to another condition. Mania can be:
   - Secondary to a general medical condition
   - Substance induced (use or abuse of drug, medication, or toxin exposure)
5. Assess the client's and family's understanding of bipolar disorder, knowledge of medications, support groups, and organizations that provide information on bipolar disorder.

◆ NURSING DIAGNOSES WITH INTERVENTIONS

During an acutely or extremely manic episode, hospitalization is recommended to prevent physical exhaustion and initiate and stabilize medication. The primary consideration is the prevention of exhaustion and death from cardiac collapse. Because of the client's poor judgment, excessive and constant motor activity, probably dehydration, and difficulty evaluating reality, the client is at risk for injury (**Risk for Injury**).

Aggression is a common feature in mania. At times, intrusive and taunting behaviors can induce others to strike out against these clients. Conversely, when in a manic state, a client may evidence inability to control behavior, and destructive, hostile, and aggressive behaviors (rage reaction) may occur and pose danger to the well-being of others and/or property (**Risk for Violence Directed at Self or Others**).

Grandiosity and poor judgment can result in giving away money and possessions indiscriminately, bankruptcy, and neglect of family. Clients may get involved in making foolish business deals or

Table 8–1 ◆ Potential Nursing Diagnosis—Bipolar Disorder

SIGNS AND SYMPTOMS	NURSING DIAGNOSIS
Excessive and constant motor activity Poor judgment Lack of rest and sleep Poor nutritional intake (Excessive/ relentless mix of above behaviors can lead to cardiac collapse.)	**Risk for Injury**
Loud, profane, hostile, combative, aggressive, demanding	**Risk for Violence: Directed at Self or Others**
Intrusive and taunting behaviors Inability to control behavior Rage reaction	**Ineffective Individual Coping**
Manipulative, angry, or hostile verbal and physical behaviors	**Defensive Coping** **Ineffective Individual Coping**
Impulsive speech and actions Can be destructive of property or lash out at others in a rage reaction.	
Racing thoughts, grandiosity, poor judgment	**Altered Thought Processes** **Ineffective Individual Coping**
Gives away valuables, neglect of family, impulsive major life changes (divorce, career changes)	**Altered Family Processes** **Caregiver Role Strain**
Continuous pressured speech jumping from topic to topic (**flights of ideas**)	**Impaired Verbal Communi- cation**
Constant motor activity, going from one person or event to another	**Impaired Social Interaction**
May annoy or taunt others; speech loud and crass. Provocative behaviors	
Too distracted, agitated, and dis- organized to eat, groom, bathe, dress self	**Altered Nutrition, Less than Body Requirements**
	Fluid Volume Deficit
Too frantic and hyperactive to sleep; sleep deprivation can lead to exhaustion and death	**Self-Care Deficit: (Bathing/ Hygiene, Dressing/ Grooming)**
	Sleep Pattern Disturbance

make impulsive major life changes (e.g., divorce, marriage, or career changes). Getting involved in impossible schemes, shady legal deals, and questionable business ventures may also be part of the picture. Because of the client's grandiose thinking and extremely poor judgment, **Altered Thought Processes** are present. The behaviors that stem from the client's faulty thinking usually result in **Ineffective Individual Coping**.

Clients when manic can be extremely manipulative, fault finding, and adept at exploiting other's vulnerabilities. They constantly push limits. Often the motivation for this manipulation is an attempt to gain a sense of control, when in fact the person is totally unable to control any aspect of his or her life: thoughts, feelings, and particularly behaviors. Therefore, **Defensive Coping** may be evidenced by the client's manipulative, angry, and hostile verbal behaviors.

The families of people with bipolar disorder often experience terrific disruptions in their lives, and may be in crises when their family member is in acute and severe mania. Infidelity and divorce is common, family savings may be wiped out and debt accumulated, relationships within the family unit may be strained beyond endurance, and friendships may be ruined. **Altered Family Processes** must always be assessed and information and referrals for support provided.

The client in the acute or extreme manic state may have numerous unmet physical needs. The manic client is too busy to eat, sleep, or be appropriately groomed or dressed and may be constipated. Therefore, **Fluid Volume Deficit, Altered Nutrition, Sleep Pattern Disturbance, Constipation, Dressing/Grooming Self-Care Deficit, and Bathing Hygiene Self-Care Deficit** are all areas that need to be carefully assessed. When the client is severely manic, the nurse could target interventions for all of the above using **Total Self-Care Deficits** (eating, sleeping, dressing/grooming, bathing/hygiene, bowel functioning).

See Table 8–1 for a list of potential nursing diagnoses.

GUIDELINES FOR NURSING INTERVENTION
1. Use a firm and calm approach.
2. Use short, concise explanations or statements.
3. Remain neutral, avoid power struggles.
4. Provide a consistent and structured environment.
5. Firmly redirect energy into appropriate and constructive channels.
6. Decrease environmental stimuli whenever possible.
7. Provide structured solitary activities; tasks that take minimal concentration are best. Avoid groups and stimulating activities until client can tolerate that level of activity.
8. Spend one-on-one time with the client if psychotic or anxious.
9. Provide frequent rest periods.

Continued

10. Provide high-calorie fluids and finger foods frequently throughout the day.
11. On a daily basis, monitor client's:
    - Sleep pattern
    - Food intake
    - Elimination (constipation often a problem)
12. Teach client and family about illness and be sure client has written information regarding his or her medications.
13. Ascertain that client and family have information on supportive services in their community for further information and support.

The following sections identify primary nursing diagnoses for use with a manic client, particularly in the acute and severely manic phases of the illness. Included are specific nursing interventions that are appropriate for meeting outcome criteria for each diagnosis.

Risk for Injury

A state in which the individual is at risk of injury as a result of environmental conditions interacting with the individual's adaptive and defensive resources

Related To (Etiology)

◆ Cognitive, affective, and psychomotor factors
● Biochemical/neurological imbalances
● Extreme hyperactivity/physical agitation
● Rage reaction
● Dehydration and exhaustion

As Evidenced By (Assessment Findings/Diagnostic Cues)

● Impaired judgment (reality testing, risk behavior)
● Excessive and constant motor activity—unable to rest for even short periods
● Lack of fluid ingestion
● Abrasions, bruises, cuts from running/falling into objects

◆ NANDA accepted; ● In addition to NANDA.

Outcome Criteria

Client will:

- Be free of injury:
  - Cardiac status stable
  - Well hydrated
  - Skin free of abrasions and scrapes
- Be free of excessive physical agitation and purposeless motor activity
- Take short voluntary rest periods during the day

Short-Term Goals

- The client's cardiac status will remain stable while in the hospital.
- While acutely manic, client will drink 8 oz of fluid every hour throughout the day.
- Client will spend time with the nurse in a quiet environment three to four times a day between 7 AM and 11 PM with the aid of nursing guidance.
- Client will remain free from falls and abrasions every day while in the hospital.
- Client will be free of dangerous levels of hyperactive motor behavior with the aid of medications and nursing interventions within 24 hours.

Interventions and Rationales

Intervention	Rationale
1. Maintain low level of stimuli in client's environment (e.g., away from bright lights, loud noises, and people).	1. Helps decrease escalation of anxiety.
2. Provide structured solitary activities with nurse or aide.	2. Structure provides security and focus.
3. Provide frequent high-calorie fluids.	3. Prevents serious dehydration.
4. Provide frequent rest periods.	4. Prevents exhaustion.
5. Redirect violent behavior.	5. Physical exercise can decrease tension and provide focus.
6. Acute mania may warrant the use of phenothiazines and seclusion to minimize physical harm.	6. Exhaustion and death can result from dehydration, lack of sleep, and constant physical activity.

Intervention	Rationale
7. Observe for signs of lithium toxicity.	7. There is a small margin of safety between therapeutic and toxic doses.
8. Protect client from giving away money and possessions. Hold valuables in hospital safe until rational judgment returns.	8. Client's "generosity" is a manic defense that is consistent with irrational, grandiose thinking.

Risk for Violence: Self-Directed or Directed at Others

The state in which an individual exhibits behaviors that can be physically, emotionally, and/or sexually harmful to self or others

---

Related To (Etiology)

- ◆ Psychotic symptomatology
- ◆ Rage reaction
- ◆ Impulsivity
- ◆ Manic excitement
- ● Biochemical/neurological imbalances

As Evidenced By (Assessment Findings/Diagnostic Cues)

- ◆ Verbal threats against others
- ◆ Verbal threats against self (suicidal threats/attempts, hitting or injuring self, banging head against wall)
- ◆ Provocative behaviors (e.g., argumentative)
- ● Loud, threatening, profane speech
- ● Poor impulse control
- ● Agitated behaviors (e.g., slamming doors, prowling hallways, increased muscle tension, knocking things over)

Outcome Criteria

Client will:

- • Display nonviolent behaviors toward self and others
- • Refrain from verbal threats and loud profane language toward others

---

◆ NANDA accepted; ● In addition to NANDA.

Short-Term Goals

Client will:

- Display nonviolent behavior toward others in the hospital, with the aid of medications and nursing interventions
- Refrain from provoking others to physical harm, with the aid of seclusion or nursing interventions
- Respond to external controls (medications, seclusion, nursing interventions) when potential or actual loss of control occurs

Interventions and Rationales

Intervention	Rationale
1. Use a calm and firm approach.	1. Provides structure and control for a client who is out of control.
2. Use short and concise explanations or statements.	2. Short attention span limits comprehension to small bits of information.
3. Maintain a consistent approach, employ consistent expectations, and provide a structured environment.	3. Clear and consistent limits and expectations minimize potential for client's manipulation of staff.
4. Remain neutral: avoid power struggles and value judgments.	4. Client can use inconsistencies and value judgments as justification for arguing and escalating mania.
5. Decrease environmental stimuli (keep away from loud music/noises, people, and bright lights).	5. Helps decrease escalation of anxiety and manic symptoms.
6. Assess client's behavior frequently (every 15 minutes) for signs of increased agitation and hyperactivity.	6. Early detection and intervention of escalating mania may help prevent harm to self or others, and decrease need for seclusion.
7. Redirect agitation and potentially violent behaviors with physical outlets in area of low stimulation (e.g., punching bag).	7. Can help to relieve pent-up hostility and relieve muscle tension.
8. Alert staff if potential for seclusion appears imminent.	8. If nursing interventions (quiet environment and

Intervention	**Rationale**
Usual priority of interventions would be: a. Firmly setting limits b. Chemical restraints (tranquilizers) c. Seclusion	firm limit setting) and chemical restraints (tranquilizers—e.g., haloperidol [Haldol]) have not helped dampen escalating manic behaviors, then seclusion may be warranted. **See Chapter 14 for guidelines on secluding an individual.**
9. Chart in nurse's notes behaviors, interventions, what seemed to escalate agitation, what helped to calm agitation, when as-needed (PRN) medications were given and their effect, and what proved most helpful.	9. Staff will begin to recognize potential signals for escalating manic behaviors and have a guideline for what might work best for the individual client.

Ineffective Individual Coping

Inability to form a valid appraisal of stressors, inadequate choice of practical responses, and/or inability to use available resources

---

Related To (Etiology)

◆ Disturbance in tension release
◆ Inadequate level of perception of control
● Ineffective problem-solving strategies/skills
● Biochemical/neurological changes in the brain

As Evidenced By (Assessment Findings/Diagnostic Cues)

◆ Inability to ask for help
◆ Inability to meet basic needs
◆ Inability to problem-solve
◆ Destructive behavior toward self or others
◆ Change in usual communication patterns
● Presence of delusions (grandeur, persecution)

◆ NANDA accepted; ● In addition to NANDA.

- Using extremely poor judgment in business and financial negotiations
- Giving away valuables and financial savings indiscriminately,
  often to strangers

Outcome Criteria

Client will:

- Report an absence of delusions, racing thoughts, and irresponsible actions as a result of medication adherence and environmental structures
- Be protected from making any major life decisions (legal, business, marital) during an acute or severe manic phase
- Demonstrate an absence of destructive behavior toward self or
  others
- Cease use of manipulation to get needs met and control others
- Return to precrisis level of functioning after acute/severe manic
  phase is past

Short-Term Goals

Client will:

- Seek competent medical assistance and legal protection when
  signing any legal documents regarding personal or financial matters during manic phase of illness
- Retain valuables or other possessions while in the hospital
- Respond to external controls (medication, seclusion, nursing interventions) when potential or actual loss of control occurs
- Respond to limit-setting techniques with aid of medication during acute and severe manic phase

Interventions and Rationales

Interventions	**Rationale**
1. Administer an antimanic medication and PRN tranquilizers, as ordered, and evaluate for efficacy, side and toxic effects.	1. Bipolar disorder is caused by biochemical/neurological imbalances in the brain. Appropriate antimanic medications allow psychosocial and nursing interventions to be effective.

◆ NANDA accepted; ● In addition to NANDA.

Interventions	**Rationale**
2. Observe for destructive behavior toward self or others. Intervene in the early phases of escalation of manic behavior. Intervene using **Risk for Violence** above and **Chapter 14 (Anger and Aggression)** as a guide for interventions.	2. Hostile verbal behaviors, poor impulse control, provocative behaviors, and violent acting out against others or property are some of the symptoms of this disease and seen in extreme and/or acute mania. Early detection and intervention can prevent harm to client or others in the environment.
3. Have valuables, credit cards, and large sums of money sent home with family or put in hospital safe until client is discharged.	3. During manic episodes, people give away valuables and money indiscriminately to strangers, often leaving themselves broke and in debt.
4. Maintain a firm, calm, and neutral approach at all times. **Avoid:** a. Getting involved in power struggles b. Arguing with the client c. Joking or "clever" repartee in response to client's "cheerful and humorous" mood	4. a–c. These behaviors by staff can have the effect of escalating environmental stimulation and consequently manic activity. Once the manic client is out of control, seclusion may be required, which can be traumatic to the manic individual as well as the staff and other clients.
5. Provide hospital legal service when and if client is involved in making or signing important legal documents during an acute manic phase.	5. Judgment and reality testing are both impaired during acute mania. Clients may need legal advice and protection against making important decision that are not in their best interest.
6. Assess and recognize early signs of manipulative behavior and intervene appropriately. For example: a. Taunting staff by pointing out faults or oversights. b. Pitting one staff member	6. Setting limits is an important step in the intervention of bipolar clients, especially when intervening in manipulative behaviors. Staff agreement on limits set and consistency is impera-

against another ("You are much more understanding than Nurse X . . . do you know what he did?") or pitting one group against another (evening vs. day shift).

c. Aggressively demanding behaviors that can trigger exasperation and frustration in staff

tive if the limits are to be carried out effectively. **(Refer to Chapter 17, Manipulation.)**

Impaired Social Interaction

The state in which an individual participates in an insufficient or excessive quantity or ineffective quality of social exchange

Related To (Etiology)

◆ Altered thought processes
● Biochemical imbalances
● Excessive hyperactivity and agitation

As Evidenced By (Assessment Findings/Diagnostic Cues)

◆ Observed use of unsuccessful social interaction behaviors
◆ Dysfunctional interaction with peers, family, and/or others
◆ Family reports change of style or patterns of interaction
● Intrusive and manipulative behaviors antagonizing others
● Loud, obscene, or threatening verbal behavior
● Poor attention span and difficulty focusing on one thing at a time
● Increase of manic behaviors around a highly stimulating environment (groups of people, loud music)

Outcome Criteria

• Client will initiate and maintain goal-directed and mutually satisfying activities/verbal exchanges with others.
• Client and family will state that there is an increase in stability and meaningfulness in social interactions.
• Client will put feelings into words instead of actions when experiencing anxiety or loss of control.

◆ NANDA accepted; ● In addition to NANDA.

Short-Term Goals

Client will:

- Focus on one activity requiring a short attention span for 5 minutes three times a day with nursing assistance by (date)
- Find one or two solitary activity(s) that can help relieve tensions and minimize escalation of anxiety with aid of nurse or occupational/activity therapist by (date)
- Sit through a short, small group meeting free from disruptive outbursts by (date)

Interventions and Rationales

Intervention	Rationale
1. When possible, provide an environment with minimal stimuli (e.g., quiet, soft music, dim lighting).	1. Reduction in stimuli lessens distractibility.
2. Solitary activities requiring short attention spans with mild physical exertion are best initially (e.g., writing, painting [finger painting, murals], woodworking, or walks with staff).	2. Solitary activities minimize stimuli; mild physical activities release tension constructively.
3. When less manic, client may join one or two other clients in quiet, nonstimulating activities (e.g., board games, drawing, cards). *Avoid competitive games.*	3. As mania subsides, involvement in activities that provide a focus and social contact becomes more appropriate. Competitive games can stimulate aggression and can increase psychomotor activity.

Total Self-Care Deficit

Inability to complete feeding, bathing, toileting, dressing, and grooming of self

---

Related To (Etiology)

- ◆ Perceptual or cognitive impairment
- ◆ Severe anxiety

◆ NANDA accepted; ● In addition to NANDA.

- Manic excitement
- Racing thoughts and poor attention span
- Inability to concentrate on one thing at a time

As Evidenced By (Assessment Findings/Diagnostic Cues)

◆ Observation or valid report of inability to eat, bathe, toilet, dress, and/or groom self independently

Outcome Criteria

- Client's weight will be within normal limits for age and height.
- Client will sleep 6 to 8 hours per night.
- Client will dress and groom self in appropriate manner consistent with precrisis level of dress and grooming.
- Client's bowel habits will be within normal limits.

Short-Term Goals

Client will:

- Eat one half to one third of each meal plus one snack between meals with aid of nursing intervention by (date)
- Sleep 6 hours out of 24 with aid of medication and nursing measures within 3 days
- Wear appropriate attire each day while in hospital
- Bathe at least every other day while in hospital
- Have normal bowel movements within 2 days with the aid of high-fiber foods, fluids, and, if needed, medication

Interventions and Rationales

ALTERED NUTRITION

Intervention	Rationale
1. Monitor intake, output, and vital signs.	1. Ensures adequate fluid and caloric intake; minimizes dehydration and cardiac collapse.
2. Encourage frequent high-calorie protein drinks and finger foods (e.g., sandwiches, fruit, milkshakes).	2. Constant fluid and calorie replacement are needed. Client may be too active to sit at meals. Finger foods allow "eating on the run."
3. Frequently remind the client to eat: *Tom, finish your milkshake. Sally, eat this banana.*	3. The manic client is unaware of bodily needs and is easily distracted. Needs supervision to eat.

◆ NANDA accepted; ● In addition to NANDA.

SLEEP PATTERN DISTURBANCE

Intervention	**Rationale**
1. Encourage frequent rest periods during the day.	1. Lack of sleep can lead to exhaustion and death.
2. Keep client in areas of low stimulation.	2. Promotes relaxation and minimizes manic behavior.
3. At night, encourage warm baths, soothing music, and medication when indicated. Avoid giving the client caffeine.	3. Promotes relaxation, rest, and sleep.

SELF-DRESSING/GROOMING DEFICIT

Intervention	**Rationale**
1. If warranted, supervise choice of clothes, minimize flamboyant and bizarre dress, sexually suggestive dress such as bikini tops and bottoms.	1. Lessens the potential for inappropriate attention, which can increase level of mania, or ridicule, which lowers self-esteem and increases the need for manic defense. Assists client in maintaining dignity.
2. Give simple step-by-step reminders for hygiene and dress. *Here is your razor. Shave the left side . . . now the right side. Here is your tooth brush. Put the toothpaste on the brush.*	2. Distractibility and poor concentration are countered by simple, concrete instructions.

CONSTIPATION

Intervention	**Rationale**
1. Monitor bowel habits; offer fluids and food that is high in fiber. Evaluate the need for laxative. Encourage client to go to the bathroom.	1. Prevents fecal impaction resulting from dehydration and decreased peristalsis.

Altered Family Processes

A change in family relationships and/or functioning

Related To (Etiology)

◆ Shift in health status of family member
◆ Situational crisis or transition (illness . . . manic episode of one member)
◆ Family role shift
● Erratic and out-of-control behavior of one family member with the potential for dangerous behavior affecting all family members (violence, leaving family in debt, risky behaviors in relationships and business, flagrant infidelities, unprotected promiscuous sex)
● Nonadherence to antimanic and other medications

As Evidenced By (Assessment Findings/Diagnostic Cues)

◆ Changes in effectiveness in completing assigned tasks
◆ Changes in participation in problem solving
◆ Changes in participation in decision making
◆ Changes in communication patterns
● Inability to deal with traumatic or crisis experiences constructively
● Deficient knowledge regarding disorder, need for medication adherence, and available support systems for both family members and client
● Family in crisis

Outcome Criteria

Family members/significant others:

• State that they find needed support and information in a support group(s)
• Can identify the signs of increase manic behavior in their family member
• State what they will do (whom to call, where to go) when client's mood begins to escalate to dangerous levels
• Demonstrate an understanding of what a bipolar disorder is, the medications, need for adherence to medication and treatment

Short-Term Goals

Family members/significant others will:

• Discuss with nurse/counselor three areas of family life that are most disruptive and seek alternative options with aid of nursing/counseling interventions by (date)

◆ NANDA accepted; ● In addition to NANDA.

- State and have in writing the names and telephone numbers of at least two bipolar support groups by (date)
- State that they have gained support from at least one support group on how to work with family member when he or she is manic by (date)
- State their understanding for the need for medication adherence, and be able to identify three signs that indicate possible need for intervention when their family member's mood escalates by (date)
- Briefly discuss and have in writing the names and addresses of two bipolar organizations, two Internet site addresses, and medication information regarding bipolar disorder by (date)

Interventions and Rationales

Intervention

1. During the first or second day of hospitalization, spend time with family identifying their needs during this time, for example:
   a. Need for information about the disease
   b. Need for information about lithium or other antimanic medications (e.g., need for adherence, side effects, toxic effects)
   c. Knowledge about bipolar support groups in the family's community and how they can help families going through crises

Rationale

1. This is a disease that can devastate and may destroy some families. During an acute manic attack, families experience a great deal of disruption and confusion when their family member begins to act bizarre, out of control, and at times aggressive. Families need to understand about the disease, what can and cannot be done to help control the disease, and where to go for help for their individual issues.

◆ PSYCHOPHARMACOLOGY FOR BIPOLAR DISORDER

Lithium

Lithium or other antimanic medication (particularly valproate [Depakote]) is an essential part of treatment. Lithium is particularly effective in reducing (Maxmen and Ward, 1995):

- Elation
- Flights of ideas

- Irritability and manipulativeness
- Anxiety

To a lesser extent, lithium controls:

- Insomnia
- Psychomotor agitation
- Threatening or assaultive behavior
- Distractibility

Lithium can calm manic clients, prevent or modify future manic episodes, and protect against future depressive episodes. Lithium must reach therapeutic levels in the client's blood to be effective. This usually takes from 7 to 14 days to be effective. Therefore, when a client is first brought to the hospital, he or she may be started on antipsychotic medications to help decrease psychomotor activity and aggressive behaviors, and prevent exhaustion, coronary collapse, and death.

As lithium reaches therapeutic levels, the antipsychotics are usually discontinued. A narrow range exists between the therapeutic dose and the toxic dose of lithium. Initially, blood levels may be drawn weekly or biweekly until therapeutic levels are reached (0.8 to 1.4 mEq/L). Actual maintenance blood levels should reach between 0.4 and 1.0 mEq/L. To avoid serious toxicity, lithium levels should not exceed 1.5 mEq/L (Lehne et al., 1994). See Table 8–2 for side effects and signs of lithium toxicity at various levels.

The client and family need to be instructed on the precautions when taking lithium. Use Box 8–3 as a guide for client and family teaching.

Before the administration of lithium, a medical evaluation is performed to assess the client's ability to tolerate the drug. Lithium should not be given to people who are pregnant, have brain damage, or have cardiovascular, renal, or thyroid disease. Lithium is often the drug of choice for bipolar clients; however, up to 40% of bipolar clients may not respond or may respond insufficiently to lithium (Post, 1992).

Other Antimanic Medications

Increasingly valproate (Depakote/Depakene) is becoming the drug of choice for bipolar clients, especially for clients who are newly diagnosed. Valproate seems to have a wider therapeutic range. Valproate is particularly useful in mixed-state and rapid-cycling bipolar clients (Schatzberg, De Battista, et al., 1997). Some clinicians find that valproate was better tolerated than lithium, and as effective in preventing subsequent bipolar episodes, over a 2-year period.

Table 8-2 ◆ Drug Information: Side Effects of Lithium and Signs of Toxicity

LEVEL	SIGN*	INTERVENTIONS
Expected Side Effects ≤0.4–1.0 mEq/L (therapeutic levels)	Fine hand tremors, polyuria, and mild thirst Mild nausea and general discomfort Weight gain	Symptoms may persist throughout therapy. Symptoms often subside during treatment. Weight gain may be helped with diet, exercise, and nutritional management.
Early Signs of Toxicity <1.5 mEq/L	Nausea, vomiting, diarrhea, thirst, polyuria, slurred speech, muscle weakness	Medication should be withheld, blood lithium levels drawn, and the dose reevaluated.
Advanced Signs of Toxicity 1.5–2.0 mEq/L	Coarse hand tremor, persistent gastrointestinal upset, mental confusion, muscle hyperirritability, electroencephalographic changes, incoordination	Use interventions outlined above or below, depending on severity of circumstances.
Severe Toxicity 2.0–2.5 mEq/L	Ataxia, serious electroencephalographic changes, blurred vision, clonic movements, large output of dilute urine, seizures, stupor, severe hypotension, coma. Death is usually secondary to pulmonary complications.	There is no known antidote for lithium poisoning. The drug is stopped and excretion is hastened. Gastric lavage and treatment with urea, mannitol, and aminophylline all hasten lithium excretion.
>2.5 mEq/L	Confusion, incontinence of urine or feces, coma, cardiac arrhythmia, peripheral circulatory collapse, abdominal pain, proteinuria, oliguria, and death.	Hemodialysis may also be used in severe cases.

*Careful monitoring is needed because the toxic levels of lithium are close to the therapeutic levels.
Data from Scherer, J.C. (1985). Nurses' Drug Manual. Philadelphia: JB Lippincott, pp. 631–632; Lehne et al. (1994), pp. 296–299.

❖

B O X   8 – 3

❖

Teaching Clients and Their Families About Lithium

The client and the client's family should be instructed about the following, encouraged to ask questions, and given the material in written form as well.

1. Lithium can treat your current emotional problem and will also help prevent relapse. So, it is important to continue with the drug after the current episode is resolved.

2. Because therapeutic and toxic dosage ranges are so close, your lithium blood levels must be monitored very closely, more frequently at first, then once every several months after that.

3. Lithium is not addictive.

4. Maintain a normal diet and normal salt and fluid intake (2500–3000 ml/day or six 12-ounce glasses). Lithium decreases sodium reabsorption by the renal tubules, which could cause sodium depletion. A low sodium intake causes a relative increase in lithium retention, which could lead to toxicity.

5. Withhold drug if excessive diarrhea, vomiting, or diaphoresis occurs. Dehydration can raise lithium levels in the blood to toxic levels. Inform your physician if you have any of these problems.

6. Diuretics (water pills) are contraindicated with lithium.

7. Lithium is irritating to the gastric mucosa. Therefore, take your lithium with meals.

8. Periodic monitoring of renal functioning and thyroid function is indicated with long-term use. Discuss your follow-up with your doctor.

9. Avoid taking any over-the-counter medications without checking first with your doctor.

10. If weight gain is significant, you may need to see a physician or nutritionist.

11. Many self-help groups have been developed to provide support for bipolar patients and their families. The local self-help group is (give name and phone number).

12. You can find out more information by calling (give name and phone number).

Data from Maxmen and Ward. (1995); Schatzberg, A.F., and Cole, J.O. (1991). Manual of Clinical Psychopharmacology. Washington, DC: American Psychiatric Press; Preston, J., and Johnson, J. (1995). Clinical Psychopharmacology Made Ridiculously Simple. Miami: MedMaster.

Table 8–3 ◆ Drug Information: Other Antimanic (Mood-Stabilizing) Medications

DRUG	DOSE	TYPE	MAJOR CONCERN/SIDE EFFECT
Carbamazepine (Tegretol)	200–1600 mg/day	Anticonvulsant	Agranulocytosis or aplastic anemia are most serious side effects. Blood levels should be monitored through first 8 weeks because drug induces liver enzymes that speed its own metabolism. Dose may need to be adjusted to maintain serum level of 6–8 mg/L. Sedation is most common problem; tolerance usually develops. Diplopia, incoordination, and sedation can signal excessive levels.
Valproate/valproic acid (Depakane, Depakote)	15–60 mg/kg/day	Anticonvulsant	**Baseline liver function tests should be done and monitored at regular intervals.** Hepatitis, although rare, has been reported with fatalities in children. Signs and symptoms to watch for: Fever, chills, right upper quadrant pain, dark-colored urine, malaise, and jaundice. Common side effects: Tremors, gastrointestinal upset, weight gain, and, rarely, alopecia.
Gabapentin Neurotin	900–2000 mg/day	Anticonvulsant	Tolerated well. Associated with somnolence, dizziness, gastrointestinal upset, headache, blurred or double vision, clumsiness and tremor.
Lamotrigine (Lamictal)	100–200 mg/day	Anticonvulsant	Tolerated well. Low-dose titration to reduce risk of rashes. **Rarely the rash can progress to a potentially life-threatening condition** (one person per 1000).
Clonazepam (Klonopin)	1–6 mg/day	Benzodiazepine	Used as an adjunct, can facilitate other antimanics. Same as those of all benzodiazepines (e.g., sedation, ataxia, and incoordination). Most expensive of all benzodiazepines.

Data from Schatzberg et al. (1997); Hodgson and Kizior (1999); Maxmen and Ward (1995).

Valproic acid blood levels can be monitored weekly until stable, until adequate levels are achieved. After stabilized, blood levels may be monitored monthly or less. The major worry with valproate is the risk of severe, even fatal, hepatotoxicity (see Table 8–3).

Other antimanic drugs include some anticonvulsant drugs, such as carbamazepine (Tegretol), and two newer drugs, lamotrigine (Lamictal) and gabapentin (Neurotin). *Lamotrigine* (Lamictal) seems effective in people with rapid-cycling bipolar disorder, hard-to-treat mixed states, and rapid cycling caused by antidepressants. *Gabapentin* (Neurotin) appears effective as an adjunct in the treatment of refractory bipolar clients.

Some benzodiazepines (e.g., clonazepam ([Klonopin]) and lorazepam ([Ativan]) have been found to be useful in treatment-resistant manic clients. See Table 8–3 for some of the major concerns and side effects of these medications.

◆ RESOURCES FOR NURSES, CLIENTS, AND FAMILIES—BIPOLAR DISORDER

Associations

National Alliance for the Mentally Ill (NAMI)
200 North Glebe Road, Suite 1015
Arlington, VA 22203-3754
1-703-524-7600; check 1-800-950-NAMI

Depressed Anonymous: Recovery from Depression
DSS, Inc.
P.O. Box 17471
Louisville, KY 40217
(502) 569-1989

National Foundation for Depressive Illness
P.O. Box 2257
New York, NY 10116
1-800-248-4344; 1-212-268-4260
http://www.depression.org

National Depressive & Manic-Depressive Association
730 N. Franklin #501
Chicago, IL 60610
1-800-82NDMDA
http://www.ndmda.org

Depression and Related Affective Disorders Association
Meyer #3-181
600 N. Wolfe St.
Baltimore, MD 21287-7381
1-410-955-4647
http://www.med.jhu.edu/drada/

Internet Sites

National Institute of Mental Health
List of publications on bipolar disorder
http://www.nimh.nih.gov/publicat/index.cfm

Bipolar Disorder Page
http://mentalhelp.net/disorders

Moodswing.org
Online resource for people with bipolar disorder
http://www.moodswing.org

Med Help International
Many good links
http://www.medhelp.org/

Bipolar Web Site
Good information and links
http://www.bipolar.com

Bipolar Disorder Guide at about.com
http://bipolar.about.com

CHAPTER 9

Schizophrenia and Other Psychotic Disorders

◆ SCHIZOPHRENIA

The schizophrenias are severe and persistent neurological diseases. These serious disorders affect a person's:

- Perceptions (hallucinations and delusions)
- Thinking (delusions, paranoia, disorganized thinking)
- Language (associative looseness, poverty of speech)
- Emotions (apathy, anhedonia, depression)
- Social behavior (aggressive, bizarre behaviors or extreme social withdrawal)

Schizophrenia affects about 1% of the population, and 95% of individuals who become schizophrenic have it throughout their lifetime. Schizophrenia is a relapsing psychotic disorder. A psychotic disorder is one in which people have difficulty with differentiating reality from fantasy (reality testing). Major symptoms seen in psychotic disorders are hallucinations, delusions, and disorganized thinking. Hallucinations and delusions can be very frightening, often terrifying for individuals. They can also be initially very disconcerting and even frightening to nurses and other health care individuals. These are the **positive symptoms** of schizophrenia. Nurses can greatly benefit from individual or peer supervision when dealing with these challenging phenomena. Communicating with clients who are delusional and hallucinatory and have disorganized thinking is a skill that is learned with guidance and practice. The **negative symptoms** of schizophrenia are more subtle and are the most damaging to the client's quality of life.

The symptoms of schizophrenia usually become apparent during adolescence or early adulthood (15 to 25 for men, 25 to 35 for women). Paranoid schizophrenia has a later onset. Schizophrenia is a severe biologically based mental illness. Current theories of schizophrenia involve neuroanatomical and neurochemical abnormalities, which may be induced either genetically or environmentally (virus, birth defects). Although schizophrenia is not caused by psychological events, stressful life events may trigger an exacerbation of the illness. Therefore, psychoeducational and family treatment modalities can be crucial in helping clients in a number of ways. Psychoeducational, family, group, and behavioral approaches, for example, can help clients increase their social skills, maximize their ability in self-care and independent living, maintain medical adherence, and, most important, increase the quality of their lives. Client and family education greatly improves the management of schizophrenia.

Schizophrenia is not a single disease, but rather a syndrome that involves cerebral blood flow, neuroelectrophysiology, neuroanatomy, and neurobiochemistry. The DSM-IV criteria for the diagnosis of schizophrenia are listed in Box 9–1.

Box 9–2 identifies five subtypes of schizophrenia.

◆ OTHER PSYCHOTIC DISORDERS

Schizophreniform Disorder

The essential features of this disorder are exactly those of schizophrenia except that:

- The total duration of the illness is at least 1 month but less than 6 months.
- Impaired social or occupational functioning during some part of the illness is not apparent (although it may appear).

This disorder may or may not have a good prognosis.

Brief Psychotic Disorder

This is a disorder in which there is a sudden onset of psychotic symptoms (delusions, hallucinations, disorganized speech) or grossly disorganized or catatonic behavior. The episode lasts at least 1 day but less than 1 month, and then the individual returns to his or her premorbid level of functioning. Brief psychotic disorders often follow extremely stressful life events.

Schizoaffective Disorder

This disorder is characterized by an uninterrupted period of illness during which time there is a major depressive, manic or mixed episode, concurrent with symptoms that meet the criteria for

---

❖   B O X   9 – 1   ❖
Diagnostic Criteria for Schizophrenia

---

1. *Characteristic symptoms:* Two (or more) of the following, each present for a significant portion of the time during a 1-month period (or less if successfully treated):
   - Delusions
   - Hallucinations
   - Disorganized speech (e.g., frequent derailment or incoherence)
   - Grossly disorganized or catatonic behavior
   - Negative symptoms, i.e., affective flattening, alogia, or avolition

   Note: Only one Criterion 1 symptom is required if delusions are bizarre or hallucinations consist of a voice keeping up a running commentary on the person's behavior or thoughts, or two or more voices conversing with each other.

2. *Social/occupational dysfunction:* For a significant portion of the time since the onset of the disturbance, one or more major areas of functioning such as work, interpersonal relations, or self-care are markedly below the level achieved prior to the onset (or when the onset is in childhood or adolescence, failure to achieve expected level of interpersonal, academic, or occupational achievement).

3. *Duration:* Continuous signs of the disturbance persist for at least 6 months. This 6-month period must include at least 1 month of symptoms (or less if successfully treated) that meet Criterion 1 (i.e., active-phase symptoms) and may include periods of prodromal or residual symptoms.

Adapted from American Psychiatric Association. (1994). Diagnostic and Statistical Manual of Mental Disorders, 4th ed. Washington, DC: American Psychiatric Press, p. 285; reprinted with permission. Copyright 1994 American Psychiatric Association.

---

schizophrenia. The symptoms must not be due to any substance use or abuse or general medical condition.

Delusional Disorder

This disorder involves nonbizarre delusions (situations that occur in real life, such as being followed, infected, loved at a distance, or deceived by a spouse, or having a disease) of at least 1 month's duration. The person's ability to function is not markedly impaired, nor is the person's behavior obviously odd or bizarre. Common

❖   B O X   9 – 2   ❖
                 Subtypes of Schizophrenia

Paranoid

Onset usually in the late 20s to 30s. People who develop this disorder usually function well before the onset of the disorder (good premorbid functioning). *Paranoia* (any intense and strongly defended irrational suspicion) is the main characteristic and the main defense is projection. *Hallucinations, delusions, and ideas of reference* are dominant.

Disorganized

The most *regressed and socially impaired* of all the schizophrenias. The person has highly disorganized speech and behavior and inappropriate affect. Bizarre mannerisms include grimacing along with other oddities of behavior.

Catatonia

The essential feature is abnormal motor behavior. Two extreme motor behaviors are seen in catatonia. One extreme is psychomotor agitation, which can lead to exhaustion. The other extreme is psychomotor retardation and *withdrawal* to the point of stupor. The onset is usually acute, and the prognosis is good with medications and swift interventions. Other behaviors may include autism, waxy flexibility, and negativism.

Undifferentiated (Mixed Type)

Clients experience active hallucinations and delusions, but no one clinical picture dominates (e.g., not paranoid, catatonic, or disorganized; rather the clinical picture is one of a *mixture* of symptoms).

Residual

A person who is referred to as having residual schizophrenia no longer has active symptoms of the disease, such as delusions, hallucinations, or disorganized speech and behaviors. However, there is a persistence of some symptoms—for example, marked social withdrawal; impairment in role function (wage earner, student, or homemaker); eccentric behavior or odd beliefs; poor personal hygiene; lack of interest, energy, initiative; and inappropriate affect.

types of delusions seen in this disorder are delusions of grandeur, persecution, or jealousy, or somatic or mixed delusions.

Shared Psychotic Disorder (*Folie à Deux*)

A shared psychotic disorder is an occurrence in which one individual, who is in a close relationship with another who has a psychotic disorder with a delusion, eventually comes to share the delusional beliefs either in total or in part. Apart from the shared delusion, the person who takes on the other's delusional behavior is not otherwise odd or unusual. Impairment of the person who shares the delusion is usually much less than the person who has the psychotic disorder with the delusion. The cult phenomenon is an example, as was demonstrated at Waco and Jonestown.

Induced or Secondary Psychosis

Psychosis may be induced by substances (drugs of abuse, alcohol, medications, or toxin exposure) or caused by the physiological consequences of a general medical condition (delirium, neurological conditions, metabolic conditions, hepatic or renal diseases, and many more). **Medical conditions and substances of abuse must always be ruled out before a primary diagnosis of a schizophrenia or other psychotic disorder can be made.**

◆ PHASES OF SCHIZOPHRENIA

Schizophrenia has been divided into three phases:

Phase I—Onset. This phase (acute phase) includes the prodromal symptoms (e.g., acute or chronic anxiety, phobias, obsessions, compulsions, dissociative features) as well as the acute psychotic symptoms of hallucinations, delusions, and/or disorganized thinking.

Phase II—Years following onset. Patterns that characterize this phase are the ebb and flow of the intensity and disruption caused by symptoms, which may, in some cases, be followed by complete or relatively complete recovery.

Phase III—Long-term course and outcome. This is the course that the severely and persistently mentally ill client follows when the disease becomes chronic. For some clients, the intensity of the psychosis may diminish with age; however, the long-term dysfunctional effects of the disorder are not so amenable to change.

Interventions During Phase I—Onset (Acute Phase)

- Intensive psychopharmacological treatment
- Supportive and directive communication
- Limit setting during times of escalating verbal or physical behavior
- Psychiatric, medical, and neurological evaluation

Interventions during the acute phase (Phase I) often require hospitalization, although currently more community-based settings and home care agencies are treating acute clients in the community because of shorter lengths of hospitalization than years ago.

Interventions During Phase II and Phase III

- Continued client and family teaching about the disease
- Medication teaching and side effect management
- Cognitive and social skills enhancement
- Identifying signs of relapse
- Attention to deficit in self-care, social, and work functioning

---

◆ ASSESSING PSYCHOTIC SYMPTOMS

History

1. Is there a history of schizophrenia or a family history of schizophrenia?
2. When did the symptoms begin: adolescence or early adulthood, or did they develop later?
3. Have other medical and mental disorders (e.g., bipolar disorder, delirium) been ruled out as a cause of the person's psychosis?
4. What medications or drugs/alcohol does the client currently take?
   a. How much?
   b. How often?
   c. For how long?

Assessment Tool

The Brief Psychotic Rating Scale (BPRS) (Table 9–1) is a useful tool for evaluating overall psychiatric functioning. It is particularly helpful in evaluating the degree to which psychotic symptoms affect a person's ability to function.

Table 9-1 ◆ Brief Psychiatric Rating Scale

DIRECTIONS: Place an X in the appropriate box to represent level of severity of each symptom

Patient Name _____ Physician _____

Patient SS# _____ UT# _____ HH# _____ Date _____

	Not Present	Very Mild	Mild	Moderate	Mod. Severe	Severe	Extremely Severe
SOMATIC CONCERN—preoccupation with physical health, fear of physical illness, hypochondriasis.	☐	☐	☐	☐	☐	☐	☐
ANXIETY—worry, fear, over-concern for present or future, uneasiness.	☐	☐	☐	☐	☐	☐	☐
EMOTIONAL WITHDRAWAL—lack of spontaneous interaction, isolation deficiency in relating to others.	☐	☐	☐	☐	☐	☐	☐
CONCEPTUAL DISORGANIZATION—thought processes confused, disconnected, disorganized, disrupted.	☐	☐	☐	☐	☐	☐	☐
GUILT FEELINGS—self-blame, shame, remorse for past behavior.	☐	☐	☐	☐	☐	☐	☐
TENSION—physical and motor manifestations of nervousness, over-activation.							
MANNERISMS AND POSTURING—peculiar, bizarre, unnatural motor behavior (not including tic).	☐	☐	☐	☐	☐	☐	☐
GRANDIOSITY—exaggerated self-opinion, arrogance, conviction of unusual power or abilities.	☐	☐	☐	☐	☐	☐	☐
DEPRESSIVE MOOD—sorrow, sadness, despondency, pessimism.	☐	☐	☐	☐	☐	☐	☐
HOSTILITY—animosity, contempt, belligerence, disdain for others.	☐	☐	☐	☐	☐	☐	☐
SUSPICIOUSNESS—mistrust, belief others harbor malicious or discriminatory intent.	☐	☐	☐	☐	☐	☐	☐
HALLUCINATORY BEHAVIOR—perceptions without normal stimulus correspondence.	☐	☐	☐	☐	☐	☐	☐
MOTOR RETARDATION—slowed weakened movements or speech, reduced body tone.	☐	☐	☐	☐	☐	☐	☐
UNCOOPERATIVENESS—resistance, guardedness, rejection of authority.	☐	☐	☐	☐	☐	☐	☐
UNUSUAL THOUGHT CONTENT—unusual, odd, strange, bizarre thought content.	☐	☐	☐	☐	☐	☐	☐
BLUNTED AFFECT—reduced emotional tone, reduction in formal intensity of feelings, flatness.	☐	☐	☐	☐	☐	☐	☐
EXCITEMENT—emotional tone, agitation, increased reactivity.	☐	☐	☐	☐	☐	☐	☐
DISORIENTATION—confusion or lack of proper association for person, place, or time.	☐	☐	☐	☐	☐	☐	☐

Global Assessment Scale (Range 0–100) _____

From Overall, J.R., and Gorham, D.R. (1962). The Brief Psychiatric Rating Scale. Psychological Reports 10:799–812; reprinted by permission. Copyright Southern Universities Press, 1962.

≡ | ASSESSMENT ALERTS

Assessing Positive Symptoms

1. Assess for command hallucinations (e.g., voices telling the person to harm self or another). **If yes:**
   • Do you plan to follow the command?
   • Do you believe the voices are real?
2. Assess if the client has fragmented, poorly organized, well-organized, systematized, or extensive system of beliefs that are not supported by reality (delusions). **If yes:**
   • Assess if delusions have to do with someone trying to harm the client, and if the client is planning to retaliate against a person or organization.
   • Assess if precautions need to be taken.
3. Assess for pervasive suspiciousness about everyone and their actions, for example:
   • Is on guard, hyperalert, vigilant
   • Blames others for consequences of own behavior
   • Is hostile, argumentative, often threatening verbalizations or behavior

Assessing Negative Symptoms

4. Assess for negative symptoms of schizophrenia (see Table 9–2 for definitions and suggested interventions).
5. Assess if client is on medications, what medications, and if treatment adherent with medications.
6. How does the family respond to increased symptoms? Overprotective? Hostile? Suspicious?
7. How do family members and client relate?
8. Assess support system. Is family well informed about the disease (e.g., schizophrenia)? Does family understand the need for medication adherence? Is family familiar with family support groups in the community, or where to go for respite and family support?

◆ **NURSING DIAGNOSES WITH INTERVENTIONS**

There are a number of complex phenomena the nurse encounters when dealing with psychotic clients. These phenomena are discussed in some detail in terms of assessment and interventions. Essentially, these phenomena are (1) hallucinations (**Sensory/Perceptual Alterations**), (2) delusions (**Altered Thought Processes**), and (3) paranoia (**Defensive Coping**). Other vital areas for assessment and intervention include working with the client to establish

Table 9–2 ◆ Negative (Deficit) Symptoms of Schizophrenia

SYMPTOMS	CLINICAL FINDINGS	TREATMENT
Apathy	Slow onset	The newer atypical antipsychotics may target some of the negative symptoms.
Poverty of speech or content of speech	Interferes with a person's life	The most used interventions include:
Poor social functioning	Positive premorbid history	1. Skill training interventions:
Anhedonia	Chronic deterioration	• Identify areas of skill deficit person is willing to work on.
Social withdrawal	Family history of schizophrenia	• Prioritize skills important to the person.
	Cerebellar atrophy and lateral and third ventricular enlargement on computed tomography scan	2. Working with person to identify stressors:
	Abnormalities on neuropsychological testing	• Identify which stressors contribute to maladaptive behaviors.
	Poor response to antipsychotics	3. Work with person on increasing appropriate coping skills.

a milieu that can maximize the client's level of functioning, medical adherence, and client and family teaching. People with schizophrenia and their significant others have exhaustive needs. Families and friends often have difficulty coping and maintaining close and nurturing relationships. Therefore, **Altered Family Processes** should always be assessed and referrals and teaching readily available.

The above are only some of the important areas needing interventions. Perhaps the most important area that involves the nurse in care planning is **Risk for Violence Directed at Self or Others** (refer to Chapters 13 and 14). Another important area is **Self-Care Deficit** related to disorganized thought processes (see Chapter 12, which covers most areas of self-care). One of the most challenging areas is clients' **Nonadherence** to medication or treatment (see Chapter 18). Refer to Table 9–3 for a list of potential nursing diagnoses.

Working with clients who are acutely psychotic is a challenge. Effective approaches for clients who are hallucinating, delusional, and defensive (paranoid) takes practice and skill. Therefore, interventions for these phenomena (hallucinations, delusions, and paranoia) are covered here.

Table 9–3 ♦ Potential Nursing Diagnoses: Schizophrenia

SYMPTOMS	NURSING DIAGNOSES
Positive Symptoms **Hallucinations:**	
• Hears voices (loud noises) that others do not hear.	**Sensory/Perceptual Alterations: Auditory/Visual**
• Hears voices telling them to hurt self or others (*command hallucinations*).	**Risk for Violence Directed at Self and Others**
Distorted thinking not based in reality, for example:	**Altered Thought Processes** **Defensive Coping**
• **Persecution:** thinking others are trying to harm them.	
• **Jealousy:** thinks spouse or lover is being unfaithful, or thinking others are jealous of them when not.	
• **Grandeur:** thinking they have powers they do not possess, or they are someone powerful or famous.	
• **Reference:** believing all events within the environment are directed at or hold special meaning for them.	

Table 9–3 ◆ Potential Nursing Diagnoses: Schizophrenia (*Continued*)

SYMPTOMS	NURSING DIAGNOSES
• Loose association of ideas (**looseness of association**).	**Impaired Verbal Communication**
• Uses words in a meaningless, disconnected manner (**word salad**).	**Alteration in Thought Processes**
• Uses words that rhyme in a nonsensical fashion (**clang association**).	
• Repeats words that are heard (*echolalia*).	
• Does not speak (**mutism**).	
• The person delays getting to the point of communication because of unnecessary and tedious details (**circumstantiality**).	
• **Concrete thinking:** The inability to abstract; uses literal translations concerning aspects of the environment.	

Negative Symptoms

Uncommunicative, withdrawn, no eye contact.	**Social Isolation**
Preoccupation with own thoughts.	**Impaired Social Interaction**
Expression of feelings of rejection or of aloneness (lies in bed all day . . . positions back to door.)	**Risk for Loneliness**
Talks about self as "bad" or "no good."	**Self-Esteem Disturbance**
Feels guilty because of "bad thoughts," extremely sensitive to real or perceived slights.	**Chronic Low Self-Esteem** **Risk for Violence: Self-Directed**
Lack of energy (**anergia**).	**Ineffective Individual Coping**
Lack of motivation (**avolition**); unable to initiate tasks (social contact, grooming, and other aspects of daily living).	**Self-Care Deficits (bathing, dressing, grooming and hygiene)**
	Constipation

Other

Families and significant others become confused, overwhelmed, lack knowledge of disease or treatment, feel powerless in coping with client at home.	**Ineffective Family Coping: Compromised or Disabling** **Altered Parenting** **Caregiver Role Strain** **Knowledge Deficit**
Nonadherence to medications and treatment: Client stops taking medication (often from side effects), stops going to therapy groups.	**Nonadherence**

◆ ASSESSING FOR HALLUCINATIONS

Hallucinations are false *sensory* experiences that have no basis in reality. The most common hallucinations in schizophrenia are **auditory** hallucinations. The client may hear voices that others do not hear. Often the voices are derogatory and demeaning to the client. **Command hallucinations** are when the voices tell the client to do something harmful or dangerous (jump from a window, hurt another person).

Presenting Symptoms

1. Clients state they hear voices.
2. Client denies hearing voices but observer notes client('s):
   a. Eyes following something in motion that observer cannot see
   b. Staring at one place in room
   c. Head turning to side as if listening
   d. Mumbling to self or conversing when no one else is present
   e. Inappropriate facial expressions, eyes blinking
3. If hallucinations are from other causes (e.g., drugs, alcohol, delirium), the underlying cause needs to be treated as soon as possible using accepted medical and nursing protocols.

ASSESSMENT ALERTS

1. Assess for command hallucinations (e.g., voices telling the person to harm self or another).
2. Assess when hallucinations seem to occur the most (e.g., times of stress, at night, etc.).

Sample Questions

The nurse uses a variety of therapeutic techniques to obtain the answers to the following questions. Use your discretion and decide which questions are appropriate to complete your assessment.

1. "When you are feeling very distressed, do your thoughts ever get so intense that they sound *almost like* a voice?"
   If yes, consider the following:
   a. "How would you describe the voices. Are the voices friendly, arguing, hateful, controlling, terrorizing, constant?"
   b. "What do the voices say? Do the voices tell you to harm yourself or others?"
      If yes:
      • "Have you ever done what they told?"
      • "Do you have plans to follow commands now?"

   c. "Describe the voices."
- "Was it your voice or someone else's?"
- "Whose voice? Men's or women's? How old were they?"
- "Was the voice speaking your own thoughts? Was there more than one voice?"
- "When does this happen? What brings the voices on?"
- "Are the voices loud or soft?"

   d. "What feelings do you have as you hear the voices?"

   e. "How do you usually cope with the voices?"

   If No, consider the following:

2. "Did you ever see or hear things others did not?"
3. "Have you ever heard noises in your head that disturb you?"

◆ NURSING DIAGNOSIS WITH INTERVENTIONS

Sensory/Perceptual Alterations: Auditory/Visual

A state in which the individual experiences a change in the amount or patterning of incoming stimuli (either internally or externally initiated) accompanied by a diminished, exaggerated, distorted, or impaired response to such stimuli

---

Related To (Etiology)

- ◆ Altered sensory reception: transmission or integration
- ◆ Biochemical imbalance
- ◆ Chemical alterations (e.g., drugs, electrolyte imbalances)
- ◆ Altered sensory perception
- ◆ Psychological stress
- ● Neurological/biochemical changes

As Evidenced By (Assessment Findings/Diagnostic Cues)

- ◆ Disorientation to time/place/person
- ◆ Auditory distortions
- ◆ Hallucinations
- ● Tilting the head as if listening to someone
- ● Frequent blinking of the eyes and grimacing
- ● Mumbling to self, talking or laughing to self
- ◆ Altered communication pattern

◆ NANDA accepted; ● In addition to NANDA.

◆ Change in problem-solving pattern
◆ Reported or measured change in sensory acuity
◆ Inappropriate responses

Outcome Criteria

Client will:

• State that the voices are no longer threatening, nor do they interfere with his or her life
• Demonstrate techniques that help distract him or her from the voices

Short/Intermediate Term Goals

Clients will:

• State, using a scale from 1 to 10, that "the voices" are less frequent and threatening when aided by medication and nursing intervention by (date)
• State three symptoms they recognize when their stress levels are high by (date)
• Identify two stressful events that trigger hallucinations by (date)
• Demonstrate one stress reduction technique by (date)
• Identify two personal interventions that decrease or lower the intensity or frequency of hallucinations (e.g., listening to music, wearing headphones, reading out loud, jogging, socializing) by (date)

Interventions and Rationales

Intervention	Rationale

1. If voices are telling the client to harm self or others, take necessary environmental precautions.
  a. Notify others and police, physician, and administration according to unit protocol.
  b. If in the hospital, use unit protocols for **suicidal** or **threats of violence** if client plans to act on commands.
	1. People often obey hallucinatory commands to kill self or others. Early assessment and intervention may save lives.

◆ NANDA accepted; ● In addition to NANDA.

c. If in the community, evaluate need for hospitalization.

Clearly document what client says and, if threat to another(s), who was contacted and notified (use agency protocol as a guide).

2. Decrease environmental stimuli when possible (low noise, minimal activity).

2. Decrease potential for anxiety that may trigger hallucinations. Helps calm client.

3. Accept the fact that the voices are real to the client, but you may explain that you do not hear the voices. Refer to the voices as "your voices" or "voices that you hear."

3. Validating that your reality does not include voices can help client cast "doubt" on the validity of his or her voices.

4. Stay with clients when they are starting to hallucinate, and direct them to tell the "voices they hear" to go away. Repeat often in a matter of fact manner.

4. Clients can sometimes learn to push voices aside when given repeated instruction, especially within the framework of a trusting relationship.

5. Keep to simple, basic, reality-based topics of conversation. Help client to focus on one idea at a time.

5. Client's thinking may be confused and disorganized, this helps client focus and comprehend reality-based issues.

6. Explore how the hallucinations are experienced by the client.

6. Exploring the hallucination and sharing the experience can help give the person a sense of power that he or she may be able to manage the hallucinatory voices.

7. Help the client to identify the needs that may underlie the hallucination. What other ways can these

7. Hallucinations may reflect needs for
   a. Power
   b. Self-esteem

Intervention	Rationale
needs be met?	c. Anger
	d. Sexuality
8. Help client to identify times that the hallucinations are most prevalent and frightening.	8. Helps both nurse and client identify situations and times that might be most anxiety producing and threatening to client.
9. Engage client in simple physical activities or tasks that channel energy (writing, drawing, crafts, noncompetitive sports, treadmill, walking on track, exercise bike).	9. Redirecting client's energies to acceptable activities can decrease the possibility of acting on hallucinations and help distract from voices.
10. Work with the client to find which activities help reduce anxiety and distract the client from hallucinatory material. **Practice new skills with client.**	10. If client's stress triggers hallucinatory activity, they may be more motivated to find ways to remove themselves from a stressful environment or try distraction techniques.
11. Be alert for signs of increasing fear, anxiety, or agitation.	11. May herald hallucinatory activity, which can be very frightening to client, and client may act upon command hallucinations (harm self or others).
12. Intervene with one-to-one, seclusion, or PRN medication (as ordered) when appropriate.	12. Intervene before anxiety begins to escalate. If client is already out of control, use chemical or physical restraints following unit protocols.

◆ ASSESSING FOR DELUSIONS

Delusions are *false fixed ideas* that have no basis in reality. In schizophrenia the most common types of delusions are those of **being controlled and persecutory and bizarre** delusions. Suspicious clients may believe that others intend to harm them (**paranoid delusions**). Or, they might believe that neutral things happening in the environment have special meaning for them (**ideas of reference**).

Presenting Symptoms

1. The client has fragmented, poorly organized, well-organized, systematized, or extensive system of beliefs that are not supported by reality.
2. The content of the delusions may be grandiose, persecutory, jealous, somatic, or based on guilt.

ASSESSMENT ALERTS
1. Assess if delusions have to do with someone trying to harm the client, or if the client is planning to retaliate against a person or organization. Assess threat to others, need to notify person and authorities. Confer with physician and administration if precautions need to be taken.
2. Assess when delusional thinking is the most prominent (e.g., when under stress, in presence of certain situations or people?).

Sample Questions

The nurse uses a variety of therapeutic techniques to obtain the answers to the following questions. Use your discretion and decide which questions are appropriate to complete your assessment.

1. "Do you think anyone has tried to control your mind?"
   If yes:
   a. "Did it seem as if someone tried to use unusual means to force thoughts into your mind?"
   b. "Tried to take some of your thoughts away?"
   c. "Tried to stop or block your thoughts?"
   d. "Tried to control your thoughts?"
2. "Are things on the TV/radio or in the papers, especially meaningful to you/contain special messages just for you?"
3. "Do you think that someone or something is out to get you? Is anyone plotting against you?"

◆ NURSING DIAGNOSIS WITH INTERVENTIONS

Altered Thought Processes

A state in which an individual experiences a disruption in cognitive operations and activities

Related To (Etiology)

- Biochemical/neurological imbalances
- Panic levels of anxiety
- Overwhelming stressful life event(s)
- Chemical alterations (e.g., drugs, electrolyte imbalances)

As Evidenced By (Assessment Findings/Diagnostic Cues)

- ◆ Inaccurate interpretation of environment
- ◆ Memory deficit/problems
- ◆ Egocentricity
- ◆ Inappropriate non–reality-based thinking
- Delusions

Outcome Criteria

- Client will refrain from acting on delusional thinking.
- Client will demonstrate satisfying relationships with real people.
- Client's delusions will no longer threaten or interfere with his or her ability to function in family, social, and work situations.

Short-Term Goals

Client will:

- State that the "thoughts" are less intense and less frequent with aid of medications and nursing interventions by (date)
- Talk about concrete happenings in the environment without talking about delusions by (date)
- Begin to recognize that his or her frightening (suspicious) "thinking" occurs most often at times of stress and when he or she is anxious

Interventions and Rationales

Intervention	Rationale
1. Utilize safety measures to protect clients or others, if clients believe they need to protect themselves against a specific person. Precautions are needed.	1. During acute phase, client's delusional thinking may dictate to them that they may have to hurt them or self in order to be safe. External controls may be needed.
2. Attempt to understand the significance of these beliefs	2. One may find important clues to underlying fears

---

◆ NANDA accepted; ● In addition to NANDA.

to the client at the time of their presentation.

3. Be aware that client's delusions represents the way that he or she experiences reality.

4. Identify feelings related to delusions. For example:
   a. If clients believe someone is going to harm them, client is experiencing fear.
   b. If clients believe someone or something is controlling their thoughts, client is experiencing helplessness.

5. Do not argue with the client's beliefs or try to correct false beliefs using facts.

6. Do not touch the client; use gestures carefully.

7. Interact with clients on the basis of things in the environment. Try to distract client from their delusions by engaging in reality-based activities (cards, simple board games, simple arts and crafts projects, cooking with another person, etc.).

and issues in the client's seemingly illogical fantasies.

3. Identifying the client's experience allows the nurse to understand the client's feelings.

4. When people believe that they are understood, anxiety may lessen.

5. Arguing will only increase clients defensive position, thereby reinforcing their false beliefs. This will result in the client feeling even more isolated and misunderstood.

6. A psychotic person may misinterpret touch as either aggressive or sexual in nature and may interpret gestures as aggressive moves. People who are psychotic need a lot of personal space.

7. When thinking is focused on reality-based activities, the client is free of delusional thinking during that time. Helps focus attention externally.

◆ ASSESSING FOR PARANOIA

Presenting Symptoms

1. Pervasive suspiciousness about one or more persons and their actions
2. On guard, hyperalert, vigilant
3. Blames others for consequences of own behavior
4. Hostile, argumentative, often threatening verbalizations or behavior
5. Poor interpersonal relationships
6. Delusions of influence, persecution, and grandiosity
7. Often refuses medications because "nothing is wrong with me"
8. May refuse food if believes it is poisoned

ASSESSMENT ALERTS
1. Assess for suicidal or homicidal behaviors.
2. Assess for potential for violence.
3. Assess need for hospitalization.

Sample Questions

The nurse uses a variety of therapeutic techniques to obtain the answers to the following questions. Use your discretion and decide which questions are appropriate to complete your assessment.

Ask clients if they ever believed:

1. "That there is anything about you that has made other people jealous of you or prejudiced against you?"
2. "That you have special powers or unusual strengths?"
3. "That you have ever received personal messages from God? Someone unusual?"
4. "That you are able to influence others/put thoughts in their mind?"
5. "That others are trying to hurt or kill you?"
6. "That drugs/poisons have been put in your food or drink?"

If clients answer **Yes** to any of these questions, ask them to tell you how such beliefs made them feel.

◆ NURSING DIAGNOSES WITH INTERVENTIONS

> ### Defensive Coping
>
> Repeated projection of falsely positive self-evaluation based on a self-protective pattern that defends against underlying perceived threats to positive self-regard

Related To (Etiology)

- Perceived threat to self
- Suspicions of the motives of others
- Perceived lack of self-efficacy/vulnerability

As Evidenced By (Assessment Findings/Diagnostic Cues)

- ◆ Projection of blame/responsibility
- ◆ Grandiosity
- ◆ Denial of obvious problems
- ◆ Rationalization of failures
- ◆ Superior attitude toward others
- ◆ Hostile laughter or ridicule of others
- ◆ Difficulty in reality testing of perceptions
- ◆ Difficulty establishing/maintaining relationships
- Hostility, aggression, or homicidal ideation
- Fearful
- False beliefs about the intentions of others

Outcome Criteria

Clients will:

- State they feel safe and more in control in their interactions with environment/with family/work/social gatherings
- Demonstrate decreased suspicious behaviors interacting with others

Short-Term Goals

Client will:

- Remain safe with the aid of medication and nursing interventions (either interpersonal, chemical, or seclusion), as will others in the client's environment

---

◆ NANDA accepted; ● In addition to NANDA.

- Focus on reality-based activity with the aid of medication /nursing intervention by (date)
- Demonstrate two newly learned constructive ways to deal with stress and feelings of powerlessness by (date)
- Demonstrate the ability to remove himself or herself from situations when anxiety begins to increase with the aid of medications and nursing interventions by (date)
- Identify one action that helps client feel more in control of his or her life

Nursing Intervention and Rationales

Intervention	Rationale
1. Use a nonjudgmental, respectful, and neutral approach with the client.	1. There is less chance for a suspicious client to misconstrue intent or meaning if content is neutral and approach is respectful and nonjudgmental.
2. Be honest and consistent with client regarding expectations and enforcing rules.	2. Suspicious people are quick to discern dishonesty. Honesty and consistency provide an atmosphere in which trust can grow.
3. Use clear and simple language when communicating with a suspicious client.	3. Minimize the opportunity for miscommunications and misconstruing the meaning of the message.
4. Explain to client what you are going to do before you do it.	4. Prepares the client beforehand and minimizes misinterpreting your intent as hostile or aggressive.
5. Be aware of client's tendency to have ideas of reference; do not do things in front of client that can be misinterpreted: a. Laughing b. Whispering c. Talking quietly when client can see but not hear what is being said	5. Suspicious clients will automatically think that they are the target of the interaction and interpret it in a negative manner (e.g., you are laughing at them, whispering about them, etc.).
6. Diffuse angry and hostile verbal attacks with a non-	6. When staff become defensive, anger of both client

defensive stand.

and staff escalates. A nondefensive and nonjudgmental attitude provides an atmosphere in which feelings can be explored more easily.

7. Assess and observe client regularly for signs of increasing anxiety and hostility.

7. Intervene before client loses control.

8. Provide verbal/physical limits when client's hostile behavior escalates: *We won't allow you to hurt anyone here. If you can't control yourself, we will help you.*

8. Often verbal limits are effective in helping a client gain self-control.

9. Maintain low level of stimuli and enhance a nonthreatening environment (avoid groups).

9. Noisy environments may be perceived as threatening.

10. Initially, provide solitary, noncompetitive activities that take some concentration. Later a game with one or more clients that takes concentration (e.g., chess, checkers, thoughtful card games such as bridge or rummy).

10. If a client is suspicious of others, solitary activities are the best. Concentrating on environmental stimuli minimizes paranoid rumination.

Altered Family Process

A change in family relationships and/or functioning

Related To (Etiology)

◆ Shift in health status of a family member
◆ Situational crisis or transition
◆ Family role shift

◆ NANDA accepted; ● In addition to NANDA.

◆ Developmental crisis or transition
● Mental or physical disorder of family member

As Evidenced By (Assessment Findings/Diagnostic Cues)

◆ Changes in participation in decision making
◆ Changes in mutual support
◆ Changes in stress reduction behavior
◆ Changes in communication patterns
◆ Changes in participation in problem solving
◆ Changes in expression of conflict in family
● Inability to meet needs of family and significant others (physical, emotional, spiritual)
● Knowledge deficit regarding the disease and what is happening with ill family member (may believe client is more capable than they are)
● Knowledge deficit regarding community and health care support

Outcome Criteria

Family members/significant others will:

• State they have received needed support from community and agency resources that offer support, education, coping skills training, and/or social network development (psychoeducational approach)
• Demonstrate problem-solving skills for handling tensions and misunderstanding within the family environment
• Recount in some detail the early signs and symptoms of relapse in their ill family member, and know whom to contact
• Know of at least two contact people when they suspect potential relapse
• Discuss the disease (schizophrenia) knowledgeably:
  • Understand the need for medical adherence
  • Support the ill family member in maintaining optimum health
  • Know about community resources (e.g., help with self-care activities, private respite)

Short-Term Goals

Family members/significant others will:

• Meet with nurse/physician/social worker the first day of hospitalization and begin to learn about this neurological/biochemical disease, treatment, and community resources

---

◆ NANDA accepted; ● In addition to NANDA.

- Attend at least one family support group (single family, multiple family) within 4 days from onset of acute episode
- Problem solve with nurse two concrete situations within the family all would like to change
- State what the medications can do for their ill member, the side effects and toxic effects of the drugs, and the need for adherence to medication at least 2 to 3 days before discharge
- Be included in the discharge planning along with client
- State and have written information identifying the signs of potential relapse and whom to contact before discharge
- Name and have complete list of community supports for ill family member and supports for all members of the family at least 2 days before discharge

Interventions and Rationales

Intervention	Rationale
1. Identify family's ability to cope (e.g., experience of loss, caregiver burden, needed supports).	1. Family's needs must be addressed to stabilize family unit.
2. Provide opportunity for family to discuss feelings related to ill family member and identify their immediate concerns.	2. Nurses and staff can best intervene when they understand the family's experience and needs.
3. Assess the family members' current level of knowledge about the disease and medications used to treat the disease.	3. Family may have misconceptions and misinformation about schizophrenia and treatment, or no knowledge at all. Teach at client's and family's level of understanding and readiness to learn.
4. Provide information on disease and treatment strategies at family's level of knowledge.	4. Meet family members' needs for information.
5. Inform the client and family in clear, simple terms about psychopharmacological therapy: dosage, the need to take medication as pre-	5. Understanding of the disease and the treatment of the disease encourages greater family support and client adherence.

Intervention	Rationale
scribed, side effects, and toxic effect. Written information should be given to client and family members as well. **See Table 9–4 as an example of a client and family teaching tool.**	
6. Provide information on family and client community resources for client and family for after discharge: support groups, organizations, day hospitals, psychoeducational programs, respite centers, etc. **See list of Associations and Internet Sites at end of chapter.**	6. Schizophrenia is an overwhelming disease for both the client and the family. Family groups, support groups, and psychoeducational centers can help: a. Develop family skills b. Access resources c. Access support d. Access caring e. Minimize isolation f. Improve quality of life for all family members
7. Teach family and client the warning symptoms of potential relapse.	7. Rapid recognition of early warning symptoms can help ward off potential relapse when immediate medical attention is sought.

◆ PSYCHOPHARMACOLOGY IN SCHIZOPHRENIA

Medications used to treat schizophrenia are called antipsychotic medications. Two groups of antipsychotic drugs exist: *standard* (traditional) and the newer *atypical* medications. The standard medications are covered here first; however, **many physicians urge the use of the *atypical* medications initially because of their better side effect profile and the fact that the atypical medications target the negative symptoms (apathy, lack of motivation) and anhedonia (lack of pleasure in life), thereby increasing the quality of life for clients.** Unfortunately, the atypical medications are more expensive than the standard medications and, in today's health care environment, this has become a consideration in planning care.

Atypical Medications

During the early 1990s new types of antipsychotics began appearing on the market, and they are presently used as first-line medications. (Clozapine [Clozaril] is the exception because of its tendency to cause agranulocytosis and its high incidence for seizures.) These drugs not only target the acute and disturbing symptoms seen in acute active episodes of schizophrenia (hallucinations, delusions, associative looseness, paranoia), called positive symptoms, but also target the negative symptoms, which allows for improvement in the quality of life for clients (increased motivation, improved judgment, increased energy, and ability to experience pleasure). These drugs also have a very low EPS profile and in general have a more favorable side effect profile. See Table 9–5 for a list of atypical antipsychotics, their dosages, and the side effects.

Standard Medications

The standard antipsychotic drugs target the more flagrant symptoms of schizophrenia (hallucinations, delusions, suspiciousness, associative looseness). These drugs can:

- Reduce disruptive and violent behavior
- Increase activity, speech, and sociability in withdrawn clients
- Improve self-care
- Improve sleep patterns
- Reduce the disturbing quality of hallucinations and delusions
- Improve thought processes
- Decrease resistance to supportive therapy
- Reduce rate of relapse
- Decrease intensity of paranoid reactions

Antipsychotic agents are usually effective 3 to 6 weeks after the regimen is started. Table 9–6 is a list of the standard antipsychotic medications, their usual doses, and some special considerations.

Side Effects

There are some troubling side effects of these drugs that can at times limit medical adherence. Some of these side effects respond to other medications. Table 9–7 identifies the extrapyramidal symptoms (EPS), cardiac side effects, and toxic effects of these drugs.

One of the most disturbing side effects to clients are the EPS. Common drugs used to treat the EPS caused by these standard antipsychotics are given in Table 9–8.

Text continued on page 254

Table 9–4 ◆ Client and Family Teaching Guide

CONTENT	RATIONALE
Medications*	Client compliance may be helped if:
What the medication can do to help client.	• Family is supportive and involved
Medication needs to be taken regularly. Schizophrenia is a relapsing disorder. It is extremely important to keep taking the drug even though things seem fine.	• Client knows what to expect • Client knows medication can be changed to decrease undesirable side effects
Side effects.	
• What to do to lessen severity if not harmful to client.	
Toxic effects. Medication should be discontinued. Client should call (give name) and take appropriate action until medical help is available.	
Stopping medications. Tolerance does not develop, but some clients report a rebound (e.g., nausea, vomiting, sleep disturbance) effect if drugs are stopped suddenly.	
Risk factors of tardive dyskinesia.	
Prolonged exposure to the sun should be avoided and client should wear sunscreen, sun glasses, long sleeves, and hats.	
These drugs (neuroleptics) are not addicting.	

Signs of Potential Relapse

Client and family need to be able to identify those symptoms that come before frank psychotic symptoms (unique to each client), for example:

- Feeling of tension
- Difficulty concentrating
- Trouble sleeping
- Increased withdrawal
- Increase in bizarre/magical thinking

Early warning signs recognized by both family and client may ward off psychotic relapse if immediate medical attention is sought.

Substances That Can Exacerbate a Psychotic Relapse

Marijuana

Alcohol

Psychomotor stimulants

- Amphetamine
- Crack cocaine
- Cocaine

Family support may influence client to minimize intake if client uses substances.

---

*Should be written down for client and family.

Table 9–5 ◆ Drug Information: Atypical Antipsychotic Medications

DRUG	ACUTE (mg/day)	MAINTENANCE (mg/day)	TOXIC/SIDE EFFECTS	SPECIAL CONSIDERATIONS
Clozapine (Clozaril)	300–900	200–400 (start with low doses)	Agranulocytosis (0.8–2% of patients) Seizures Hypersalivation Persistent tachycardia	Atypical antipsychotic, used when clients fail to respond to other neuroleptics. Can target the negative as well as the positive symptoms of schizophrenia. 1–2% incidence of agranulocytosis. Weekly white blood cell counts are required and sent to Clozaril National Registry. High incidence of dosage-related seizures. Can cause sedation, hypotension, tachycardia, and severe drooling.
Risperidone (Risperdal)		4–6	Insomnia (26%) Agitation (22%) EPS (17%) Headache (17%) Rhinitis (10%) Hypotension Anxiety (12%) Weight gain	Low EPS profile. Generally low side effects. Targets both positive and negative symptoms. Start at 5 mg/day and gradually increase dose to minimize orthostatic hypotension in the elderly. Effective first-line antipsychotic.
Olanzapine (Zyprexa)	10–20	7.5–12.5–20	Agitation Insomnia (10.4%) Headache Nervousness (5.6%) Drowsiness Dizziness	Low side effects profile, especially for cardiac and hematological problems. Targets both positive and negative symptoms. Effective first-line antipsychotic. Long half-life allows once-a-day dosage. Interactions with SSRIs and other antidepressants may occur.

| Quetiapine (Seroquel) | 300–400 (150 for some) | Akathisia (6.6%) Dry mouth (7.5%) Weight gain Agitation (20%) Headache (19%) Insomnia (19%) Somnolence (18%) Dizziness (10%) Dry mouth (8%) Orthostatic hypotension (5%) Syncope (1%) Weight gain Impaired motor skills | Caution in people with hepatic impairment. Caution in clients with history of cardiovascular disease. Start with 25 mg 2 times/day, then 25–50 mg 2–3 times on second day and third days, up to 300–400 mg the fourth day. |
| Sertindole (Serlect) | 12–20–24 | Rhinitis Decreased ejaculatory volume in men (17%) but not associated with erectile disturbance or decreased libido Orthostatic hypotension Tachycardia | Can cause a dose-related lengthening in the QT interval on ECG. ECG monitoring may be encouraged. Monitor for signs of dizziness or lightheadedness because of above ECG changes. Start with 4 mg/day and increase by 4 mg every 2–3 days to minimize orthostatic hypotension. |

Data From: Kaplan, H.I., and Sadock, B.J. (1995). Synopsis of Psychiatry, 6th ed. Baltimore: Williams & Wilkins; Kane, J.M. (1995). Clinical psychopharmacology of schizophrenia. In Goddard, G.O. (ed.), Treatment of Psychiatric Disorders, 2nd ed., Vol. 1. Washington, DC: American Psychiatric Press, pp. 970–986; Littrell, K. (1996). Olanzapine: An exciting new antipsychotic. Journal of American Psychiatric Nurse's Association, 8(4): 4; Marder, S.R., Wirshing, W.C., and Ames, D. (1997). New antipsychotic drugs. In Dunner, D.L. and Rosenbaum, J.F. (eds.), Psychiatric Clinic of North America Annual of Drug Therapy. Philadelphia: W.B. Saunders Company, pp. 195–207; American Psychiatric Association. (1997). Practice guidelines for the treatment of patients with schizophrenia. American Journal of Psychiatry (Suppl.) 154(4): 21–23; Hodgson and Kizior (1999).
Abbreviations: ECG, electrocardiogram; EPS, extrapyramidal side effects; SSRI, selective serotonin reuptake inhibitor.

Table 9–6 ◆ Standard Antipsychotics

DRUG	ROUTES	ACUTE (mg/day)*	MAINTENANCE (mg/day)*	SPECIAL CONSIDERATIONS
Phenothiazines				
Chlorpromazine (Thorazine)	PO, IM, R	200–1600	50–800	Increases sensitivity to sun (as with other phenothiazines). Highest sedation and hypotension effects; least potent.
Thioridazine (Mellaril)	PO	200–600	50–800	Known to cause retinitis pigmentosa in large doses; any diminished vision should be investigated. Low incidence of extrapyramidal side effects. High incidence of low blood pressure and cardiac effects. High incidence of decreased sexuality and retrograde ejaculation in men.
Trifluoperazine (Stelazine)	PO, IM	10–60	2–80	Low sedation—good for withdrawn or paranoid symptoms. High incidence of extrapyramidal side effects. Neuroleptic malignant syndrome may occur.
Perphenazine (Trilafon)	PO, IM, IV	12–32	8–64	Can help control severe vomiting and intractable hiccups.
Mesoridazine (Serentil)	PO, IM	75–300	25–400	Among the most sedative; severe nausea and vomiting may occur in adults.
Fluphenazine (Prolixin)	PO, IM, SC	2.5–20	2–40	Among the least sedative.

Drug	Route			Comments
Thioxanthenes				
Thiothixene (Navane)	PO, IM	10–120	6–30	High incidence of akathisia.
Chlorprothixene (Taractan)	PO, IM	50–600	50–400	Weight gain common.
Butyrophenones				
Haloperidol (Haldol)	PO, IM	5–50	1–15	Has low sedative properties; is used in large doses for assaultive patients, thus avoiding the severe side effect of hypotension. Appropriate for the elderly for the same reason as above; lessens the chance of falls from dizziness or hypotension
Dibenzoxazepines				High incidence of extrapyramidal side effects.
Loxapine (Loxitane)	PO, IM	60–100	20–250	Possibly associated with weight reduction.
Dihydroindolones				
Molindone (Moban)	PO	50–100	15–225	Possibly associated with weight reduction.
Decanoate: Long-acting				
Haloperidol decanoate (Haldol)	IM	50–100		Deep muscle Z-track IM; give every 4 weeks
Fluphenazine decanoate (Prolixin)	IM	25		Deep muscle Z-track IM; effective 1–2 weeks
Fluphenazine enanthate (Prolixin)	IM	25–75		Deep muscle Z-track IM; effective 3–4 weeks. Can cause acute dystonic reactions.

Data from Kaplan, H.I., and Sadock, B.J. (1995). Synopsis of psychiatry, 6th ed. Baltimore: Williams & Wilkins; Maxman and Ward (1995); Berkow, R., et al. (eds.). (1992). Merck Manual, 6th ed. Rahway, NJ: Merck Research Laboratories.

*Dosages vary with individual responses to antipsychotic agent employed.

Abbreviations: IM, intramuscular; IV, intravenous; PO, oral; R, rectal suppository; SC, subcutaneous.

Table 9–7 ◆ Drug Information: Nursing Measures for Side Effects of Antipsychotic Medications

SIDE EFFECTS	ONSET	NURSING MEASURES
Extrapyramidal Side Effects		
1. **Pseudoparkinsonism:** mask-like facies, stiff and stooped posture, shuffling gait, drooling, tremor, "pill-rolling" phenomenon.	5–30 days	1. Alert medical staff. Physician may lower dosage or switch to another phenothiazine. An anticholinergic agent (e.g., trihexyphenidyl [Artane] or benztropine [Cogentin]) may be used. Trihexyphenidyl and benztropine are used with caution because a "high" may result; benztropine has become a popular abused drug. Amantadine (Symetral) may also be prescribed.
2. **Acute dystonic reactions:** acute contractions of tongue, face, neck, and back (tongue and jaw first). • **Opisthotonos**—tetanic heightening of entire body, head back and belly up. • **Oculogyric crisis**—eye locked upward.	1–5 days	2. **First choice:** diphenhydramine hydrochloride (Benadryl) 25–50 mg IM/IV. Relief occurs in minutes. **Second choice:** benztropine (Cogentin) 1–2 mg IM/IV. **Prevent further dystonias** with any anticholinergic agent. Experience is very frightening. Take patient to quiet area, and stay with him or her until medicated.
3. **Akathisia:** motor inner-driven restlessness (e.g., tapping foot incessantly, rocking forward and backward in chair, shifting weight from side to side).	6–24 mos. or after several years	3. Physician may change antipsychotic or give antiparkinsonian agent. Tolerance does not develop to akathisia, but akathisia disappears when neuroleptic is discontinued. Propranolol (Inderal), lorazepam (Ativan), or diazepam (Valium) may be used.
4. **Tardive dyskinesia** • **Facial**—Protruding and rolling tongue, blowing, smacking, licking, spastic facial distortion, smacking movements. • **Limbs** **Choreic**—rapid, purposeless, and irregular movements.		4. **No known treatment.** Discontinuing the drug does not always relieve symptoms. Possibly 20% of patients taking the drug for >2 years may develop tardive dyskinesia. Nurses and doctors should encourage patients to be screened for tardive dyskinesia at least every 3 months.

Athetoid—slow, complex, and serpentine movement.
• **Trunk**—neck, shoulder, dramatic hip jerks and rocking, twisting pelvic thrusts.

Cardiovascular Effects

1. **Hypotension and postural hypotension**

1. Check blood pressure before giving; advise patient to dangle feet before getting out of bed to prevent dizziness and subsequent falls. A systolic pressure of 80 mm Hg when standing is indication to not give the current dose. This effect usually subsides when drug is stabilized in 1 to 2 weeks. Elastic bandages may prevent pooling. If condition serious, physician orders volume expanders or pressure agents.

2. Patients with existing cardiac problems should *always* be evaluated before the antipsychotic drugs are administered. Haloperidol is usually the preferred drug because of its low anticholinergic effects.

2. **Tachycardia**

Rare and Toxic Effects

1. **Agranulocytosis:** symptoms include sore throat, fever, malaise, and mouth sores. It is a rare occurrence, but one the nurse should be aware of; any flu-like symptoms should be carefully evaluated.

Usually occurs suddenly and becomes evident in the first 12 weeks

1. Notify medical staff STAT. Do not give medication. Physician may order blood work done to determine presence of leukopenia or agranulocytosis. If test results are positive, the drug is discontinued, and reverse isolation may be initiated. Mortality is high if drug is not ceased and treatment is not initiated.

2. **Cholestatic jaundice:** rare, reversible, and usually benign if caught in time; prodromal symptoms are fever, malaise, nausea, and abdominal pain; jaundice appears 1 week later.

2. Drug is discontinued; bed rest and high-protein, high-carbohydrate diet given. Liver function tests should be performed every 6 months.

(Table continued on following page)

Table 9–7 ◆ Drug Information: Nursing Measures for Side Effects of Antipsychotic Medications (*Continued*)

SIDE EFFECTS	ONSET	NURSING MEASURES
3. **Neuroleptic malignant syndrome (NMS):** somewhat rare, potentially fatal. • **Severe extrapyramidal symptoms:** such as severe muscle rigidity, oculogyric crisis, dysphasia, flexor-extensor posturing, cog wheeling. • **Hyperthermia:** elevated temperature (107°F) • **Autonomic Dysfunction:** hypertension, tachycardia, diaphoresis, incontinence.		3. • Stop neuroleptic. • Transfer STAT to medical unit. • Bromocriptine can relieve muscle rigidity and reduce fever. • Dantrolene may reduce muscle spasms. • Cool body to reduce fever. • Maintain hydration; oral/IV fluids. • Correct electrolyte imbalance. • Arrhythmias should be treated. • Small doses of heparin may decrease the possibility of pulmonary emboli. • Early detection increases patient's chance of survival.

Data from Schatzberg, A.F., and Cole, J.O. (1995). Manual of Clinical Psychopharmacology, 3rd ed. Washington, DC: American Psychiatric Press; Maxman and Ward (1995); Berkow, R., et al. (eds.). (1992). Merck Manual, 6th ed. Rahway, NJ: Merck Research Laboratories; Guze, B., Richeimer, S., and Szuba, M. (1995). The Psychiatric Drug Handbook. St. Louis: Mosby–Year Book.
Abbreviations: IM, intramuscular; IV, intravenous; STAT, immediately.

Table 9–8 ◆ Treatment of Neuroleptic-Induced Extrapyramidal Symptoms

DRUG	ORAL DOSE (mg)	INTRAMUSCULAR OR INTRAVENOUS DOSE (mg)	CHEMICAL GROUP
Amantadine hydrochloride (Symmetrel)	100 bid or tid	—	Dopaminergic agent
Benztropine mesylate* (Cogentin)	1–3 bid	1–2	ACA
Biperiden* (Akineton)	2 bid or qid	2	ACA
Trihexyphenidyl* (Artane)	2–5 tid	—	ACA
Diphenhydramine hydrochloride (Benadryl)	25–50 tid or qid	25–50	Antihistamine
Procyclidine hydrochloride (Kemadrin)	2.5–5 tid	—	ACA

*Antiparkinsonian drug.
Abbreviations: ACA, anticholinergic drugs (after 1 to 6 months of long-term maintenance antipsychotic therapy, most ACAs can be withdrawn); bid, twice a day; qid, four times a day; tid, three times a day.
From Maxman, J.S., and Ward, N.G. (1995). Psychotropic Drugs: Fast Facts, 2nd ed. New York: W.W. Norton, p. 69; reprinted with permission. Copyright © 1995 by Nicholas J. Ward and the Estate of Jerrold S. Maxem. Copyright © 1991 by Jerrold S. Maxem.

◆ CLIENT AND FAMILY RESOURCES— SCHIZOPHRENIA

Associations

National Alliance for the Mentally Ill (NAMI)
200 North Glebe Road, Suite 1015
Arlington, VA 22203-3754
1-800-950-NAMI (check this one out)
http://www.nami.org

Schizophrenia Anonymous
1209 California Road
Eastchester, NY 10709
1-914-337-2252; 1-810-557-6777 (check this one out!)

Recovery, Inc.
802 North Dearborn Street
Chicago, IL 60610
1-312-337-5661

Journey of Hope
(Free 12-week course for families sponsored by NIMH)
PO Box 2547
Baton Rouge, LA 70808
1-504-343-6928

Internet Sites (For Nurses and Families)

Doctors Guide to the Internet
Many articles; good site for schizophrenia information
http://www.pslgroup.com/SCHIZOPHR.HTM

Internet Mental Health
Vast amount of information/booklets/articles and general information
http://www.mentalhealth.com

National Alliance for Research on Schizophrenia and Depression
http://www.mhsource.com/narsad.html

Schizophrenia Home Page
http://www.schizophrenia.com/

C H A P T E R   1 0

Substance Abuse Disorders

When working with a substance-dependent client, the nurse keeps in mind that:

- Alcohol and drug dependence are among the most prevalent illnesses.
- Death from addictive disorders accounts for one fourth to one third of all deaths in the United States (Hurt et al., 1996).
- Addiction does not cure itself, and will worsen until it is treated.

Abuse of substances (alcohol/drugs) is divided into **substance abuse** and **substance dependence**. Box 10–1 presents the DSM-IV diagnostic criteria for substance abuse and substance dependence.

There are four important phenomena that need to be assessed in all clients with substance abuse problems. These are:

1. Tolerance and withdrawal
2. Polydrug use
3. Dual diagnoses
4. Medical comorbidity

Tolerance and Withdrawal

Tolerance and withdrawal are two characteristics of physiological addiction to a drug. When the body requires a larger and larger amount of the drug to achieve the same effect, the body builds up a **tolerance** to the drug. When the dose of the drug is reduced or the drug is no longer available, the lack of a certain level of the drug in the body produces **withdrawal symptoms**. Each drug has its own specific withdrawal syndrome.

Polydrug Abuse

Use of two or more substances of abuse (polydrug abuse) is not uncommon. Alcohol dependence in conjunction with other drug de-

---

❖   B O X   1 0 – 1   ❖
Diagnostic Criteria for Substance Abuse and Dependence

Substance Abuse

Maladaptive pattern of substance use leading to clinically significant impairment or distress, manifested by one or more of the following occurring within a 12-month period:

1. Inability to fulfill major role obligations at work, school, and home
2. Recurrent legal or interpersonal problems.
3. Continued use despite recurrent social or interpersonal problems.
4. Participation in physically hazardous situations while impaired (driving a car, operating a machine, exacerbation of symptoms, e.g., ulcers).

Substance Dependence

Maladaptive pattern of substance use leading to clinically significant impairment or distress, manifested by three or more of the following within a 12-month period:

1. Presence of tolerance to the drug
   or
2. Presence of withdrawal syndrome.
3. Substance is taken in larger amounts/for longer period than intended.
4. Reduction or absence of important social, occupational, or recreational activities.
5. Unsuccessful or persistent desire to cut down or control use.
6. Increased time spent in getting, taking, and recovering from the substance. May withdraw from family or friends.

Adapted from American Psychiatric Association. (1994). Diagnostic and Statistical Manual of Mental Disorders, 4th ed. Washington, DC: American Psychiatric Press, pp. 181–183; reprinted with permission. Copyright 1994 American Psychiatric Association.

---

pendence is very high, especially for people under 30 years of age. One study found that 80% of alcoholic individuals under 30 are dependent on another drug, most often marijuana, followed by cocaine, sedative-hypnotics, and opiates (Ries et al., 1997).

Dual Diagnosis

The co-occurrence of a substance use disorder with another psychiatric disorder is called dual diagnosis. The Epidemiologic Catchment

Area Study reported that more than 50% of substance-abusing individuals also were diagnosed with another psychiatric disorder (Beeder and Mellman, 1992). Common comorbid psychiatric disorders include personality disorders (borderline and antisocial), major depression, bipolar disorder, and schizophrenia. Dual diagnoses must always be identified and the comorbid disorder treated simultaneously if any change in drug-related behavior is to occur.

Medical Comorbidity

A number of serious and life-threatening medical problems are associated with the consequences of illicit injection drug use and its associated lifestyle. For example, systemic and organ-specific bacterial infections, viral hepatitis, tuberculosis, sexually transmitted disease, complications of pregnancy, pulmonary edema, and trauma are all found in injection drug users.

Another important consideration when working with substance-dependent individuals is that about 40% to 50% of clients with substance abuse problems have mild to moderate cognitive problems while actively using. These problems usually get better with long-term abstinence. However, it is best in the beginning to keep their treatment plan simple because these clients are not thinking or functioning at their optimum level (Zerbe, 1999).

Recovering is a lifetime process, and it comes about in steps. Because each client has different strengths, backgrounds, and supports, goals of treatment need to be tailored to the individual's immediate needs and abilities. Initially, however, a 12-step program based on Alcoholics Anonymous (**AA**) is the most effective treatment modality for all addictions. The 12 steps ("working the steps") are designed to help a person refrain from addictive behaviors as well as to foster individual change and growth.

Such support groups include **PA** (Pills Anonymous), **NA** (narcotics anonymous), **WFS** (Women for Sobriety), and **CA** (Cocaine Anonymous) to name a few. These groups help break down denial in an atmosphere of support, understanding, and acceptance. It is strongly advised that individuals find a reliable sponsor within the support group, especially for the early period of sobriety. A relationship has been established between a person's feelings of "belongingness" and treatment outcome. The more the client feels socially involved with peers, the greater the likelihood of successful treatment outcome, continuation of treatment, and lower relapse rates.

There are self-help groups for families and friends of an addicted person. They are also based on the 12 steps. These groups help clients, family, and friends work through accepting the disease model of addiction. This acceptance can remove the burdens of guilt, hostility, and shame from family members. They also offer pragmatic methods for identifying and avoiding enabling behaviors. Such support groups include **Al-Anon** (for friends and family members of an alcoholic), **Narc-Anon** (for friends and family members of a narcotic addict), and **ACOA** (for adult children of alcoholics).

NOTE: Be aware that several sessions over weeks or months may be necessary for the client to reach the point of accepting the reality of the problem and the need for treatment (Dunner, 1997).

◆ ASSESSMENT FOR DRUG/ALCOHOL ABUSE

Assessment for alcohol or drug intoxication, withdrawal, or overdose may be complex because many individuals use two or more substances simultaneously (**polydrug abuse**).

History

1. Does the client have a coexisting physical condition—for example, acquired immunodeficiency syndrome (AIDS) or central nervous system (CNS) disease (dementia, AIDS encephalopathy)?
2. Is there a history of psychiatric problems or comorbid psychiatric problems (**dual diagnosis**, e.g., depression, bipolar disorder, schizophrenia, borderline or antisocial personality disorder)?
3. Is there a history of physical abuse, sexual abuse, or family violence?
4. Is there a family history of alcohol or drug problems?
5. Is there a history of blackouts, delirium, or seizures?
6. Is there a history of withdrawal symptoms, overdoses, and complications from past alcohol or drug use?
7. Is there a police/criminal record or legal problems related to substance abuse problems (e.g., motor vehicle accidents, driving while intoxicated, physical violence)?
8. Does the client have a poor work record (e.g., absenteeism, poor performance) related to alcohol or substance use?
9. Does the client use coping styles that contribute to the maintenance of his or her drug/alcohol lifestyle? (See Table 10–1.)

When a person is unable to provide a drug history, the nurse attempts to get a history from accompanying family members or friends.

Table 10–1 ◆ Three Coping Styles That Contribute
to Substance Abuse Maintenance

Rationalization	Falsifying an experience by giving a contrived, socially acceptable, and logical explanation to justify an unpleasant experience or questionable behavior **Examples: "Sure I got a little angry with my boss. Everyone comes in late to work, so why does he have to pick on me all the time?"** **"My wife made such a big deal about me not showing up for our son's graduation. I had some business entertaining to do that night and we ran late. That happens to everyone."**
Projection	Attributing an unconscious impulse, attitude, or behavior to someone else (blaming or scapegoating) **Example: "Look, if it wasn't for the fact I can't find a job and my uncaring boyfriend, I wouldn't need coke to get through the day."**
Denial	Escaping unpleasant realities by ignoring their existence **Example: "I'm sick of everyone thinking I drink too much. I can control my drinking whenever I want . . . and stop whenever I want."**

Presenting Signs and Symptoms

1. Does the client have needle tracts in the antecubital fossa, wrist, or feet, or behind the knees?
2. Does the client have suicidal thoughts? If yes, assess for lethality of ideations. (**See Chapter 13 for discussion on assessment and interventions for suicidal individuals.**)
3. Does the client exhibit any of the signs and symptoms of **intoxication or withdrawal** for common substances of abuse?

Sample Questions

The nurse uses a variety of therapeutic techniques to obtain the answers to the following questions. Use your discretion and decide which questions are appropriate to complete your assessment.

If the client is impaired or unable to focus, friends and family members may be able to answer for the client.

1. "What drug(s) did you take before coming to the emergency room/hospital/clinic/session?"
2. "How did you take the drug(s) (e.g., intravenously, intramuscularly, orally, subcutaneously, smoking, intranasally)?"
3. "How much did you take (e.g., glasses of beer/wine/whisky)?"
4. "When was the last dose taken?"

❖   B O X   1 0 – 2   ❖
Michigan Alcohol Screening Test (MAST): Brief Version

Scoring Yes to 3 or more indicates alcoholism
1. Do you feel you are a normal drinker?
2. Do friends or relatives think you are a normal drinker?
3. Have you ever attended a meeting of Alcoholics Anonymous?
4. Have you ever gotten in trouble at work because of drinking?
5. Have you ever lost friends or girlfriends/boyfriends because of drinking?
6. Have you ever neglected your obligations, your family, or your work for 2 or more days in a row because of your drinking?
7. Have you ever had delirium tremens (DTs), severe shaking, or heard voices or seen things that were not there after heavy drinking?
8. Have you ever gone to anyone for help about your drinking?
9. Have you ever been in a hospital because of your drinking?
10. Have you ever been arrested for drunken drving or other drunken behavior?

From Pokorny, A.D., Miller, B.A., and Kaplan, H.B. (1972). The brief MAST: A shortened version of the Michigan Alcohol Screening Test. American Journal of Psychiatry 129:342–345; reprinted by permission. Copyright 1972 American Psychiatric Association.

5. "How long have you been using the substance? When did you start this last episode of use?"
6. "How often and how much do you usually use?"
7. "What kinds of problems has substance use caused for you? With your family/friends? Job? Health? Finances? The law?"

Sample Questions for Friends and Family Members

1. "Are you ever worried or embarrassed by this person's drinking/drug use?"
2. "Does he or she often promise to quit?"
3. "Do you lie to conceal the drinking/drug use?"
4. "Do you try to justify it?"
5. "Does he or she sometimes apologize after a drunken/drug-related episode?"

Assessment Guide

It is often less threatening to people when assessing their drug history to start with "safe" questions first, such as:

1. "What prescription drugs do you currently take?"
2. "What over-the-counter drugs do you currently take?"
3. "What social drugs do you currently take?"
   a. Start with nicotine and caffeine.
   b. Ask about alcohol.
   c. Ask about other social drugs (marijuana, cocaine, and heroin).

There are a number of helpful assessment tools that nurses can use to assess if the individual has an alcohol or drug problem. Two that may be very useful are:

1. **Alcohol problems**—The Brief Version of the Michigan Alcohol Screening Test (MAST) is a useful tool (see Box 10–2).
2. **For other drug-related problems**, the Drug Abuse Screening Test (DAST-10) (Box 10–3) can be a useful tool.

	ASSESSMENT ALERTS
	1. Is immediate medical attention warranted for a severe or major withdrawal syndrome? For example, alcohol and sedatives can be life-threatening during a major withdrawal.
	2. Is the client experiencing an overdose to a drug/alcohol that warrants immediate medical attention? For example, opioids or depressants can cause respiratory depression, coma, and death. Refer to Table 10–2 under Nursing Diagnoses for symptoms of drug overdose and treatments.
	3. Does client have any physical complications related to drug abuse (e.g., AIDS, abscess, tachycardia, hepatitis)?
	4. Does client have suicidal thoughts, or indicate through verbal or nonverbal cues a potential for self-destructive behaviors?
	5. Does the client seem interested in doing something about his or her drug/alcohol problem?
	6. Do the client and family have information about community resources for alcohol/drug withdrawal (detoxify safely) and treatment, for example: • Support groups • Treatment for psychiatric comorbidities • Family treatment to address enabling behaviors, support adaptive behaviors, and provide support for families and friends

❖   B O X   1 0 – 3   ❖
Drug Abuse Screening Test (DAST)

The following questions concern information about your involvement with drugs *not including alcoholic beverages* during the past 12 months.

In the statements, "drug abuse" refers (1) to the use of prescribed or OTC drugs in excess of the directions and (2) any nonmedical use of drugs. The various classes of drugs may include cannabis, solvents, antianxiety drugs, sedative-hypnotics, cocaine, stimulants, hallucinogens, and narcotics. Remember that the questions *do not include alcoholic beverages*.

These questions refer to the past 12 months.

Have you used drugs other than those required for medical purposes?	Yes ____ No ____
Do you abuse more than one drug at a time?	Yes ____ No ____
Are you always able to stop using drugs when you want to?	Yes ____ No ____
Have you had "blackouts" or "flashbacks" as a result of drug use?	Yes ____ No ____
Do you ever feel bad about your drug abuse?	Yes ____ No ____
Does your spouse (or parents) ever complain about your involvement with drugs?	Yes ____ No ____
Have you neglected your family because of your use of drugs?	Yes ____ No ____
Have you engaged in illegal activities in order to obtain drugs?	Yes ____ No ____
Have you ever experienced withdrawal symptoms (felt sick) when you stopped taking drugs?	Yes ____ No ____
Have you had medical problems as a result of your drug use (e.g., memory loss, hepatitis, convulsions, bleeding, etc.)?	Yes ____ No ____
Scoring: 1 positive response warrants further evaluation.	Yes ____ No ____

◆ NURSING DIAGNOSES WITH INTERVENTIONS

Nurses care for chemically impaired clients in a variety of settings and situations. Some interventions call for medical interventions and skilled nursing care, while others call for highly effective use of communication and counseling skills. The following sections offer the nurse guidelines for treatment.

Overdose

Drug overdoses can be medical emergencies needing timely medical interventions. Drug overdoses most often seen in hospital emergency rooms are CNS depressants (e.g., barbiturates, benzodiazepines, alcohol), stimulants (e.g., crack/cocaine), opiates (e.g., heroin), and to a lesser extent hallucinogens (e.g., phencyclidine [PCP]). Table 10–2 identifies the signs and symptoms of overdose for these drugs and identifies possible treatments.

Withdrawal

Withdrawal from alcohol and other CNS-depressant drugs is associated with severe morbidity and mortality, unlike withdrawal from other drugs. For example, a person experiencing severe alcohol withdrawal may have delirium tremens (DTs). Death from DTs may occur from volume depletion, electrolyte imbalance, cardiac arrhythmias, or suicide. Mortality rates range between 5% and 10% even with treatment (Dunner, 1997).

Therefore, individuals with severe alcohol withdrawal syndrome or withdrawal from a CNS depressant may need hospitalization and close medical attention. Other drug withdrawals may not hold the same dangers; however, the client may benefit from titrating the dose under medical supervision. The major nursing diagnosis that applies for an individual going through withdrawal of a substance of abuse is **Risk for Injury**.

Initial Drug Treatment and Active Treatment

People who are addicted to alcohol or drugs come from various environments, cultures, and sociological backgrounds. Therefore, people seeking treatment for drug addictions and related problems present with a variety of personal strengths and social backgrounds and have different economic supports. Many clients have legal problems, and certainly possible medical complications from the drug, as well as coexisting psychiatric problems. Therefore, one

Text continued on page 268

Table 10–2 ◆ Symptoms of Drug Overdoses and Possible Treatments

DRUG	OVERDOSE	POSSIBLE TREATMENTS
DEPRESSANTS		
Barbiturates (Amytal) Pentobarbital (Nembutal) Secobarbital (Seconal) **Benzodiazepines** Diazepam (Valium) Chlordiazepoxide (Librium) Lorazepam (Ativan) Oxazepam (Serax) Alprazolam (Xanax) **Chloral Hydrate** **Glutethimide** (Doriden) **Mephrobamate** (Equanil, Miltown) **Alcohol**	Cardiovascular or respiratory depression or arrest (mostly with barbiturates) Coma Shock Convulsions Death	**If Awake** Keep awake. Induce vomiting. Give activated charcoal to aid absorption of drug. Every 15 min, check vital signs (VS). **Coma** Clear airway—endotracheal tube. Intravenous (IV) fluids Gastric lavage with activated charcoal Frequent VS checks after client is stable for shock and cardiac arrest Seizure precautions Possible hemodialysis or peritoneal dialysis

STIMULANTS

Amphetamines (Long-Acting)	Respiratory distress	**Supportive Measures**
Dextroamphetamine (Dexedrine)	Ataxia	Acidify urine (ammonium chloride).
Methamphetamine (Methadrine)	Hyperpyrexia	Phenothiazines to treat psychotic reactions
Ice (synthesized for street use)	Convulsions	**Medical and Nursing Management for**
	Coma	Hyperpyrexia
	Death associated with hyperpyrexia,	Convulsions
	convulsions, cardiovascular shock	Respiratory distress
		Cardiovascular shock
Cocaine/Crack (Short-Acting)	Seizures	**Medical and Nursing Life-Saving Measure for**
Note:	Cardiac arrest	Convulsions (prescribe diazepam)
High obtained:	Respiratory depression/arrest	Hyperpyrexia (use hypothermia mattress)
Snorted, in 3 min	Convulsions	Respiratory depression/cardiac arrest
Injected, in 30 sec	Hyperpyrexia	
Smoked, in 4–6 sec (crack)	Death	
Average high lasts:		
For cocaine, 15–30 min		
For crack, 5–7 min		

(Table continued on following page)

Table 10–2 ◆ Symptoms of Drug Overdoses and Possible Treatments (*Continued*)

DRUG	OVERDOSE	POSSIBLE TREATMENTS
OPIATES		
Narcotics Opium (paragenic) Heroin Meperidine (Demerol) Morphine Codeine Methadone (Dolophine) Hydromorphone (Dilaudid) Fentanyl (Sublimaze) Fentanyl analogs	Pupils pinpoint *but* may be dilated as a result of anoxia Respiratory depression/arrest Coma Shock Convulsions Death	Narcotic antagonist (e.g., naloxone [Narcan]) quickly reverses central nervous system depression.
CANNABIS SATIVA (marijuana, hashish)	Fatigue Paranoia Psychois—rarely seen Anxiety/panic reactions	

HALLUCINOGENS

LSD (Lysergic Acid Diethylamide) **Mescaline (Peyote)** **Psilocybin**	Psychosis Brain damage Death	Keep client in room with low stimuli—minimal light, sound, activity. Have one person stay with client—reassure client, "talk down client." Speak slowly and clearly in low voice. Diazepam or chloral hydrate for extreme anxiety/tension. **NOTE: PCP and LSD-like drugs have different treatments.**
PCP (Phencyclidine Piperidine)	Psychosis Possible hypertensive crisis/cardio- vascular accident Respiratory arrest Hyperthermia Seizures	**If Alert** *Caution:* If gastric lavage is used, can lead to laryngeal spasms or aspiration. Acidify urine (cranberry juice, ascorbic acid); in acute stage, ammonium chloride—may continue for 10–14 days. Keep client in room with minimal stimuli. **Do not attempt to talk down!** Speak slowly, clearly, and in low voice. Diazepam may be used for agitation. Haloperidol may be used for severe behavioral disturbance. **Do not use a phenothiazine.** **Medical Intervention for** Hyperthermia High blood pressure Respiratory distress Hypertension

form of treatment for a specific substance will not be effective for everyone addicted to that specific substance. It is probably best to take a long-term view of addictions and remember that lapses or relapses are often part of the long-term course of recovering (Vaillart, 1988).

However, many nursing diagnoses may apply to the large majority of clients with substance abuse problems. For example, individuals who have been abusing drugs for a long period of time most likely have poor general health. These clients may have nutritional deficits, be susceptible to infections, or be at risk for AIDS and hepatitis. **Altered Health Maintenance** is often a nursing focus, and initially may be one of priority to clients when they present with life-threatening situations.

A common phenomenon shared among many addicted individuals is that people minimize their drug problems and have a tendency to deny having a "problem" (denial) or minimize the problem by blaming others (projection), rationalizing why they need the drug, or using other methods to deny responsibility for their drug-related behavior(s). Therefore, **Ineffective Denial** is present. Denial needs to be broken down in order for the client to begin to perceive how his or her life has changed in a negative way because of his or her drug use, and find motivation for change. Until individuals can admit that they have a problem, and are ready to start to take responsibility for their drug use, there is little incentive for change as long as they blame others for their problems and think their behavior is justified.

Relapse Prevention

Relapse prevention is part of most all treatment planning for medical as well as psychiatric mental health disorders. For people with addictions, the main thrust of relapse prevention is recognizing triggers for abuse and learning different ways to respond to these cues. Because new coping skills are needed, the nursing diagnosis **Ineffective Individual Coping** is used for relapse prevention.

There are many nursing diagnoses that may be a priority for your client(s). Certainly one area for assessment is **Violence Directed at Self or Others**. Assessment and intervention for **suicide is addressed in Chapter 13.** Suggestions for working with clients who are **angry and violent are found in Chapter 14.**

Addicted clients often have a lack of concern for the feelings of others and often act entitled or have a sense of grandiosity about them. Many clients who abuse substances learn to manipulate others (family, friends, and institutions) to get their needs met

Table 10–3 ◆ Potential Nursing Diagnoses: Substance Abuse

SIGNS AND SYMPTOMS	NURSING DIAGNOSES
Vomiting, diarrhea, poor nutritional and fluid intake	**Altered Nutrition** **Risk for Fluid Volume Deficit**
Audiovisual hallucinations, impaired judgment, memory deficits, cognitive impairments related to substance intoxication/withdrawal (problem solving, ability to attend to tasks, grasp ideas)	**Altered Thought Processes** **Sensory/Perceptual Alterations: Auditory-Visual**
Changes in sleep-wake cycle, interference with stage IV sleep, not sleeping or long periods of sleeping related to effects or withdrawal from substance	**Sleep Pattern Disturbance**
Lack of self-care (hygiene, grooming), not caring for basic health needs	**Altered Health Maintenance** **Self-Care Deficit** **Noncompliance (nonadherence to health care regimen)**
Feelings of hopelessness, inability to change, feelings or worthlessness, life has no meaning or future	**Hopelessness** **Helplessness** **Spiritual Distress** **Self-Esteem Disturbance** **Chronic Low Self-Esteem** **Increased Risk for Violence: Self-Directed**
Family crises and family pain, ineffective parenting, emotional neglect of others, increased incidence of physical and sexual abuse toward others, increased self-hate projected to others	**Altered Family Processes** **Altered Parenting** **Risk for Violence: Directed at Others**
Excessive substance abuse affects all areas of person's life: loses friends, poor job performance, illness rates increase, prone to accidents and overdoses	**Ineffective Individual Coping** **Impaired Verbal Communication** **Social Isolation** **Risk for Loneliness** **Anxiety** **Risk for Suicide**
Increased health problems related to substance used and route of use, as well as overdose	**Activity Intolerance** **Ineffective Airway Clearance** **Ineffective Breathing Pattern** **Altered Oral Mucous Membranes** **Risk for Infection** **Decreased Cardiac Output** **Sexual Dysfunction**
Total preoccupation and time consumed with taking and withdrawing from drug	**Altered Growth and Development** **Ineffective Individual Coping** **Impaired Social Interaction** **Ineffective Family Coping**

OVERALL GUIDELINES FOR NURSING INTERVENTION

1. Detoxify the client.
2. Assess for feelings of hopelessness, helplessness, and suicidal thinking.
3. Ascertain that the client is getting interventions for any comorbid medical and/or psychological condition (e.g., liver toxicity, infections, depression, anxiety attacks).
4. Intervene with the client's use of denial as well as rationalization, projection, and other defenses that stall motivation for change.
5. Enlist support of family members, confront any tendency on their part to minimize the problem or enable the client in maintaining his or her addiction.
6. Insist on abstinence.
7. Refer the client to self-help groups (AA, NA, CA, etc.) early on in treatment.
8. Teach client to avoid medications that promote dependence.
9. Encourage participation in psychotherapy (e.g., cognitive-behavioral strategies, motivational interviewing , solution-focused therapy).
10. Emphasize personal responsibility—placing control within the client's grasp removes the nurse from the all-knowing rescuer (Finfgeld, 1999).
11. Support residential treatment when appropriate, particularly for clients with multiple relapses.
12. Expect relapses.
13. Educate the client and the family on the medical and psychological consequences of taking the drug(s) of abuse.
14. Educate the client and family regarding pharmacotherapy for certain addictions (e.g., naltrexone or methadone to help prevent relapse in alcoholism and narcotic addiction).
15. Educate the client about the physical and developmental effects that taking the drug can have on future children (e.g., fetal alcohol syndrome, problems with school, social role performance).

Adapted from Zerbe, K.J. (1999). Women's Mental Health in Primary Care. Philadelphia: W.B. Saunders Company, p. 85; reprinted with permission.

(e.g., money for drugs, shift blame to others, make false promises). Setting limits is key to working with an addicted client or clients with dual diagnoses. Interventions for **manipulative behaviors are addressed in Chapter 17.**

People with a history of long-term substance abuse may have many other needs as well (e.g., medical, social, legal, job related, personal) warranting a variety of nursing diagnoses. See Table 10–3 for potential nursing diagnoses.

◆ WITHDRAWAL

Risk for Injury

A state in which the individual is at risk of injury as a result of internal or external environmental conditions interacting with the individual's adaptive and defensive resources

---

Related To (Etiology)

- ◆ Psychological (affective orientation)
- ◆ Sensory dysfunction
- ◆ Developmental age (psychological)
- ● Excess alcohol ingestion pattern
- ● Impaired judgment (disease, drugs, reality testing, risk-taking behaviors)
- ● Sensory-perceptual loss or disorientation
- ● Substance withdrawal
- ● Panic levels of anxiety and agitation
- ● Potential for electrolyte imbalance or seizures
- ● Unstable vital signs and temperature

As Evidenced By (Assessment Findings/Diagnostic Cues)

- ● Signs and symptoms of specific drug withdrawal
- ● Evidence of hallucinations (bugs, animals, snakes)
- ● Poor skin turgor
- ● Elevated temperature, pulse, respirations
- ● Agitation, trying to "get away" or climb out of bed
- ● Combative behaviors
- ● Misrepresentation of reality (illusions)

◆ NANDA accepted; ● In addition to NANDA.

Outcome Criteria

Client will:

- Remain free from injury while withdrawing from substance
- Be free of withdrawal symptoms within given time period for particular drug

Short-Term Goals

- Client's condition will stabilize within 72 hours.
- Client will be oriented during times of lucidity.
- Client will demonstrate decreased aggressive and threatening behavior within 24 hours using a scale of 1 to 5.

Interventions and Rationales

Interventions	Rationales
1. Vital signs need to be taken frequently, at least every 15 minutes until stable, then every hour for 4 to 8 hours according to hospital protocol or physician's order.	1. Pulse is the best indicator of impending DTs, signaling the need for more rigorous sedation.
2. Provide client with a quiet room free of environmental stimulation, a single room near the nurse's station if possible.	2. Lowers irritability and confusion.
3. Approach the client with a calm and reassuring manner.	3. Clients need to feel that others are in control and that they are safe.
4. Use simple, concrete language and directions.	4. Client is able to follow simple commands, and unable to process complex or abstract ideas.
5. Orient client to time/place and person during periods of confusion; inform client of his or her progress during periods of lucidity.	5. Fluctuating level of consciousness is the hallmark of delirium. Orientation can help reduce anxiety.
6. Institute seizure precautions according to hospital protocol.	6. Seizures may occur, and precautions for client safety are a priority.
7. Carefully monitor intake and output. Check for	7. Dehydration can aggravate electrolyte imbalance.

dehydration or over-hydration.

Overhydration can lead to congestive heart failure.

8. If the client is having **hallucinations**, reassure client that you do not see them, that you are there and you will see that he remains safe (e.g., "I don't see rats on the wall jumping on your bed. You sound frightened right now. I will stay with you for a few minutes.").

8. Don't argue with the hallucinations, but share your experience that you do not see anything frightening. Address the fear and let the client know that you and the staff are here to help him or her remain safe.

9. If client is experiencing **illusions**, correct the client's misrepresentation in a calm and matter-of-fact manner (e.g., "This is not a snake around my neck ready to strike you, it is my stethoscope . . . let me show you.").

9. Illusions can be explained to a client who is misinterpreting environmental cues. When client recognizes normal objects for what they are, anxiety is lessened.

10. Maintain safety precautions at all times; for example:
    a. Provide electric shaver.
    b. Take away all matches and cigarettes.
    c. Keep side-rails up at all times.
    d. Have client in private room where possible, near nurse's station.

10. During withdrawal, physical safety is the main priority.

11. Administer medications ordered for safe withdrawal.

11. Abrupt withdrawal from a CNS depressant can be fatal.

12. Use restraints with caution if client is combative and dangerous to others. Try to avoid mechanical restraints whenever possible. Always follow unit protocols.

12. In the past people have suffered myocardial infarctions, cardiac collapse, and death when fighting against the restraints during experiences of terror.

Interventions	**Rationales**
13. Keep frequent accurate records of client's vital signs, behaviors, medication, interventions and effects of interventions.	13. Monitor progress, identify what works best, identify potential complications.

◆ INITIAL AND ACTIVE DRUG TREATMENT

Altered Health Maintenance

Inability to identify, manage, and/or seek out help to maintain health

---

Related To (Etiology)

◆ Lack of ability to make deliberate and thoughtful judgments
◆ Ineffective individual coping
◆ Perceptual/cognitive impairment
● All activities of life focused on obtaining and taking drug
● Money spent on substance of abuse and none left for health care, nourishing food, or safe shelter
● Poor nutrition related to prolonged drug binges, taking drug instead of eating nourishing food, or diminished appetite related to choice of drug (e.g. cocaine)
● Inability to make or keep health care appointments (e.g., mammograms, dentist, yearly physicals) because of either being intoxicated, hung over, or withdrawing from an illicit substance
● Sleep deprivation related to decreased rapid eye movement (REM) sleep as a result of long-term stimulant, alcohol, or CNS depressant abuse
● Malabsorption of nutrients related to chronic alcohol abuse

As Evidenced By (Assessment Finding/Diagnostic Cues)

◆ History of lack of health-seeking behaviors
◆ Reported or observed inability to take responsibility for meeting basic health practices in any or all functional pattern areas
● Physical exhaustion
● Sleep disturbances

◆ NANDA accepted; ● In addition to NANDA.

- Unattended physical symptoms, for example:
  * Gastrointestinal problems
  * Extreme weight loss
  * Edema of extremities
  * Muscle weakness
  * Ascites
  * Abscesses on extremities
  * Bronchitis

Outcome Criteria

- Client will demonstrate responsibility in taking care of health care needs as evidenced by keeping appointments and adherence to medications and treatment.
- Client's medical tests will demonstrate a reduced incidence of medical complications related to substance abuse after 6 months.
- Client's weight is within normal range.
- Client's daily nutritional intake will include 5 servings from fruit and vegetables, 2 to 3 from dairy, 2 to 3 from meat/poultry/fish, and 6 from grains (pasta, bread, rice).
- Client will sleep at least 6 hours a night.
- Client keeps appointments for medical treatment and follow-up within 2 months of treatment.

Short-Term Goals

Client will:

- Go for medical checkup and treatment of any medical problems within 2 to 3 weeks of starting treatment
- Agree to go for nutritional counseling
- Identify three bodily effects of his or her substance abuse, and how these effects can affect self, loved ones, and unborn children within 1 to 2 weeks

Interventions and Rationales: If Hospitalized

Intervention	Rationale
1. Encourage small feedings if appropriate. Check nutritional status (e.g., conjunctiva, body weight, eating history).	1. If client is anorexic, small feedings will be better tolerated. Bland foods are often more appealing. Pale conjunctiva can signal an anemia.

◆ NANDA accepted; ● In addition to NANDA.

Intervention	**Rationale**
2. Monitor fluid intake and output. Check skin turgor. Check for ankle edema. Do urine specific gravity if skin turgor is poor.	2. Clients can have potentially serious electrolyte imbalances. Too little fluids may cause or signal renal problems. If client is retaining too much fluid there can be a danger of congestive heart failure.
3. When skin turgor is poor, offer fluids frequently containing protein and vitamins (e.g., milk, malts, juices).	3. Proteins and vitamins help build nutritional status.
4. Promote rest and sleep by placing client in a quiet environment.	4. Provide the client with long rest periods in between medical interventions.
5. Identify client's understanding of how the alcohol/drug(s) they are taking can cause possible future problems (e.g., fetal alcohol syndrome, hepatitis/AIDS, fertility issues).	5. Before teaching, nurse needs to identify what the client knows about the drugs, and evaluate his or her readiness to learn.
6. Review with clients their blood work and physical exam with physician's approval.	6. Lab results help the nurse identify possible causes of symptoms (e.g., infection) and initiate early counseling.
7. Set up an appointment for medical follow-up in the clinic or community.	7. Follow-up calls are important reminders.

Ineffective Denial

The state of conscious or unconscious attempt to disavow the knowledge or meaning of an event to reduce anxiety/fear to the detriment of health

Related To (Etiology)

- Physical and/or emotional dependence on substance(s) of abuse and need to maintain the status quo
- Fear of having to change and giving up substance(s) of dependence and taking responsibility for maladaptive past behaviors and chaotic life situations (legal, family, job problems)
- Underlying feelings of hopelessness and helplessness at having to cope with life without substance
- Long-term self-destructive patterns of behavior and lifestyle

As Evidenced By (Assessment Findings/Diagnostic Cues)

- ◆ Displays inappropriate affect.
- ◆ Minimizes symptoms and substance use.
- ◆ Does not perceive personal relevance of symptoms or danger.
  - * Continues to use substance/drug knowing it contributes to impaired functioning and exacerbation of physical symptoms.
  - * Uses substance/drug in potentially dangerous situations (e.g., driving while intoxicated).
- Uses rationalization and projection to explain irresponsible, aggressive, manipulative, and other maladaptive behaviors.
- Fails to accept responsibility for behaviors that result in disrupted family life, legal problems, serious problems at work/lack of work, disrupted relationships with others.
- Reluctant to discuss self or problems.

Outcome Criteria

Client will:

- Maintain abstinence from chemical substances
- Demonstrate acceptance or responsibility for own behavior at the end of 3 months
- Continue attendance for treatment and maintenance of sobriety (e.g., AA, CA, NA, or group therapy, cognitive-behavioral psychotherapy, or other)
- Demonstrate three alternative adaptive responses to stress in family, job, legal, and social situations
- Demonstrate three strategies to use in vulnerable situations
- Identify maladaptive behaviors used in the past and demonstrate three new adaptive behaviors used in the present
- Attend a relapse program during active course of treatment

◆ NANDA accepted; ● In addition to NANDA.

Short-Term Goals

Client will:

- Acknowledge that addiction does not cure itself; it will worsen until it is treated by third/fourth week of treatment
- Make a written contract to stay drug free one day at a time within the first week of treatment
- Participate in a support group at least three times a week by second week of treatment
- Agree to contact a support person when he or she feels the need to use substance by the end of the first session
- Identify and state when using denial, rationalization, and projection when speaking of drug use within the first month of treatment
- Identify at least three areas of his or her life that drugs have negatively affected within the first week
- Work with nurse, sponsor, chemical dependency counselor, therapist, or support group members on ways to change negative situations in his or her life
- Identify at least three positive role models, especially those that have overcome the same addiction themselves, within the first week
- Identify three vulnerable situations and give three strategies to employ
- Take advantage of cognitive-behavioral therapy to increase coping skills during active phase of treatment
- Work with nurse, therapist, chemical dependency counselor, sponsor (in support group) to develop a relapse program *or*
- Become a member of a relapse prevention group

Interventions and Rationales

INITIAL INTERVENTIONS

Intervention	**Rationale**
1. Initially, work with client on crisis situations and establishing a rapport with client.	1. People cannot work on issues when in crisis situations (e.g., practical living problems, family crisis).
2. Refer the client to appropriate social services, occupational rehabili-	2. Client may need help that the nurse cannot provide, but assistance that is

tation, or other resources as indicated.

3. Maintain an interested, nonjudgmental supportive approach.

4. Refrain from being pulled into power struggles, defending your position, preaching, or criticizing client's behaviors.

5. Continue to empathetically confront denial.

6. Forge an alliance with the client on some initial goals and what clients want to change in their lives.

7. Use of *miracle questions* can help identify what clients want to change (e.g., "What if your worst problem were miraculously solved overnight. What would be different about your life the next day?").

8. Help clients analyze specific pro's and con's of substance use/abuse.

9. Discourage the client's attempts to focus on only external problems (relationships, job related, and legal) without relating them to substance use/abuse.

needed if client is to focus on and make changes in drug-related problems and behaviors.

3. A nonjudgmental, supportive approach based on medical concern is most effective.

4. Will only make the client more defensive.

5. **Denial is the primary obstacle to receiving treatment.**

6. Initially, the client's goal may not be total abstinence. Identifying areas that the client wants to change gives both client and nurse a basis for working together.

7. Helps clients perceive their future without some of their problems. Gives direction to moving forward and identifying long- and short-term goals.

8. Helps clients look at what substances do and don't do for them in a clear light. Can help strengthen motives for change.

9. Helps clients see the relationship between their problems and their drug use. Helps break down denial.

Intervention	**Rationale**
10. Work with client to identify behaviors that have contributed to life problems (e.g., family problems, social difficulties, job-related problems, legal difficulties).	10. When clients take responsibility for maladaptive behaviors, they are more prepared to take responsibility for learning effective and satisfying behaviors.
11. Encourage client to stay in the "here and now" (e.g., *You can't change the fact that your mother put you down all your life. Let's focus on how you want to respond when you perceive that your boss puts you down.*).	11. Dwelling on past disappointments and hurt is not useful to working on new and more adaptive coping behaviors.
12. Refer and encourage client to attend a 12-step support group.	12. Research shows that such involvement is the most effective tool in countering addiction (Zerbe, 1999).
13. Encourage client to find a sponsor within the 12-step program, or other therapeutic mode.	13. Having a sponsor and being a sponsor according to some research, is important for success (Harvard Mental Health Letter, 1996).
14. Work with client to identify times they may be vulnerable to drinking/drugs and strategies to use at those times	14. Having thought out alternative strategies to drinking/drugs in vulnerable situations gives client ready choice.
15. Encourage family and friends to seek support, education, and ways to recognize and refrain from enabling client.	15. Enabling behavior supports the client's use of drugs by taking away incentive for change.
16. Educate family and client regarding the physical and psychological effects of the drug, the process of treatment, and aftercare.	16. An addicted family member greatly changes the dynamics and roles within families. Family and client need to make decisions based on facts.

17. Attend several open meetings in your local community.	17. Helps nurse understand how 12-step fellowship process works.
18. Realize that several sessions over weeks or months may pass before client accepts there is a problem and need for treatment.	18. When helpers push too hard and become impatient, the client may leave treatment before making a commitment.

ACTIVE TREATMENT

Intervention	**Rationale**
1. Expect sobriety. Work with clients to view their commitment to *one day at a time.* Thinking that he or she can NEVER take the drug again may seem like an overwhelming responsibility.	1. Client is not able to think rationally, make informed decisions, or learn while drug/alcohol impaired.
2. Give feedback constantly when client tries to rationalize, blame, or minimize effects of drug use.	2. As long as client believes that others are responsible or that his or her behavior is normal, or that there is really nothing wrong with his or her drug use, there will be no motivation for change.
3. Teach client alternative ways to deal with stress: a. Relaxation techniques b. Exercise c. Taking "time out" d. Getting proper rest and nutrition e. Strategies for vulnerable situations	3. Helps both client and nurse articulate what alternative skills can be identified, rehearsed, and practiced in social situations.
4. Have clients identify their stress level on a scale of 1 to 10. Then have them re-evaluate stress after using stress reduction technique(s), and discuss next session.	4. Helps client identify what works and what doesn't work. Nurse then works with client to try learning and trying alternative techniques.

Intervention	**Rationale**
5. Assess other coping skills that will help client maintain sobriety/abstinence; for example: a. Anger management b. Impulse control c. Maintaining relationships d. Problem-solving skills	5. Addicted client's usual method of getting all emotional needs met was through drugs. Problems with impulse control, anger, and problem solving are usually present. Relating to people in a drug-free environment can be very frightening.
6. Refer the client to social services, vocational rehabilitation, workshops, skills groups, or other resources when appropriate.	6. Client recovering from addictions may have a myriad of needs that must be addressed, which may be key for maintaining sobriety.
7. Continue to encourage group participation.	7. Group participation provides people with: a. Sense of belonging b. Source of friendships c. Reduction in feelings of isolation d. Reduction in feelings of despair and shame e. Alternatives to dealing with common situations and problems f. Increased motivation toward sobriety
8. Problem solve with client realistic future goals and identify life changes needed to meet these goals.	8. Drug-free activities and companions need to be established to take the place of usual drug-related activities and drug-abusing companions.
9. Discuss with client potential difficulty client may have relating to family and friends who continue to use substances of abuse.	9. Client needs to be prepared to communicate with impaired friends and family differently. Client also needs to identify ways to meet new friends to continue a drug-free lifestyle.

◆ RELAPSE PREVENTION

Ineffective Individual Coping

Inability to form a valid appraisal of the stressors, inadequate choices of practiced response, and /or inability to use available resources

Related To (Etiology)

◆ Inadequate opportunity to prepare for stressor
◆ Disturbance in pattern of appraisal of threat
◆ Disturbance in pattern of tension release
◆ Inadequate level of or perception of control
● Knowledge deficit
● Old coping styles no longer adaptive in present situations

As Evidenced By (Assessment Findings/Diagnostic Cues)

◆ Abuse of chemical agents
◆ Inadequate problem solving
◆ Destructive behavior toward self or others
◆ Inability to meet role expectations
◆ Risk taking
◆ Use of forms of coping that impede adaptive behavior
◆ Poor concentration

Outcome Criteria

Client will:

• Participate at least weekly in a relapse prevention program and/or 12-step program
• Continue counseling, cognitive-behavioral, interpersonal, or other therapy to deal with arising issues faced in sobriety
• Maintain total abstinence from all substances of abuse
• Verbalize cues or situations that pose increased risk of drug use
• Demonstrate strategies for avoiding and managing these cues
• State he or she has a stable group of drug-free friends and socialize with them at least three times a week

---

◆ NANDA accepted; ● In addition to NANDA.

- Participate in at least four drug-free activities on a routine basis that give satisfaction and pleasure
- State relationships among family members more enjoyable and stable; family members will agree

Short-Term Goals

- Client will identify at least three situations or events that serve as a source of vulnerability to relapse by (date).
- Client will demonstrate at least three cognitive-behavioral strategies to deal with sources of vulnerability to relapse by (date).
- Client will form relationships with at least four drug-free individuals that he or she enjoys spending time with in social activities by (date).
- Clients will increase their drug-free social circle by two new people by the end of each month within the first month of treatment.
- Clients will identify at least two drug-free activities that they enjoy that do not trigger drug cravings.
- Client will remain drug free each day at a time.
- Family members will state they feel supported in family counseling.

Interventions and Rationales

Intervention	Rationale
1. Work with client to keep treatment plan simple in the beginning.	1. About 40% to 50% of clients with substance abuse problems have mild to moderate cognitive problems while using substances.
2. Have clients write notes and self-memos in order to keep appointments and follow treatment plan.	2. Cognition usually gets better with long-term abstinence, but initially memory aids prove helpful.
3. Encourage client to join relapse prevention groups (**see Box 10–4, Relapse Prevention Strategies**).	3. Helps client anticipate and rehearse healthy responses to stressful situations.
4. Encourage client to find role models (counselors or other recovering people).	4. Role models serve as examples of how client can learn effective ways to make necessary life changes.

❖   B O X   1 0 – 4   ❖
Relapse Prevention Strategies

Basics
1. Keep the program simple at first; 40% to 50% of clients who abuse substances have mild to moderate cognitive problems while actively using.
2. Review instructions with health team members.
3. Use a notebook and write down important information and telephone numbers.

Skills
Take advantage of cognitive-behavioral therapy to increase your coping skills. Identify which important life skills are needed:
1. What situations do you have difficulty handling?
2. What situations are you managing more effectively?
3. What situations would you like to develop more skills to deal with more effectively?

Relapse Prevention Groups
Become a member of a relapse prevention group. These groups work on:
1. Rehearsing stressful situations using a variety of techniques
2. Finding ways to deal with current problems or ones that are likely to arise as you become drug free
3. Providing role models to help you make necessary life changes

Increase Personal Insight
Therapy—group therapy, individual, family therapy—can help you gain insight and control over a variety of psychological concerns, for example:
1. What drives your addictions?
2. What constitutes a healthy supportive relationship?
3. Increasing your sense of self and self-worth.
4. What does your addictive substance give you that you think you need and cannot find otherwise?

Adapted from Zerbe, K.J. (1999). Women's Mental Health in Primary Care. Philadelphia: W.B. Saunders Company, pp. 94–95; reprinted with permission.

Intervention	**Rationale**
5. Work with client on identifying triggers (people, feelings, situations) that help drive the client's addiction.	5. Mastering the issues that perpetuate substance use allows for effective change and targets areas for acquiring new skills.
6. Practice and role play with client alternative responses to triggers.	6. Increases client confidence of handling drug triggers effectively.
7. Give positive feedback when client applies new and effective responses to difficult "trigger" situations.	7. Validates client's positive steps toward growth and change.
8. Continue to empathetically confront denial throughout recovery.	8. Denial can surface throughout recovery, and can interfere with sobriety during all stages of recovery.
9. Continue work with client on the following three areas: a. **Personal issues** (relationship issue) b. **Social issues** (issues of family abuse) c. **Feelings of self-worth**	9. These areas of human life need to find healing in order for growth and change to take place.
10. Recommend family therapy.	10. Enhanced strategies for dealing with conflict in client's family are essential to recovery.
11. Stress substance abuse is a disease the entire family must conquer.	11. Family members also need encouragement to face their own struggles (Zerbe, 1999).
12. Expect slips to occur. Reaffirm that sobriety can be achieved as emotional pain becomes endurable.	12. Helps minimize shame and guilt, and rebuild self-esteem.

◆ CLIENT AND FAMILY TEACHING

Clients, families, and significant others all need support and information to guide them during early and middle phases of treatment. Box 10–5 offers the nurse some guidelines.

❖   B O X   1 0 – 5   ❖
Client and Family Education

- Teach clients and families that alcoholism and substance abuse are diseases, not moral weaknesses.
- Recognize that substance-related disorders affect all family members.
- Identify "enabling" behaviors, and teach families how to substitute healthier patterns.
- Tell families that they are not responsible for their member's substance abuse.
- Tell the client and family to report any worsening signs of depression or suicidal thoughts.
- Educate about the detrimental effects of alcohol and substance abuse, including depression and sleep disruption.
- Help the client and family identify community resources such as Adult Children of Alcoholics (ACOA), Al-Anon, and other self-help groups.
- Encourage clients to reveal their urges to use subtances before they can act on them.
- Educate clients about the risk of human immunodeficiency virus (HIV), hepatitis, and other diseases associated with substance abuse.

Adapted from Gorman, L.M., Sultan, D.F., and Raines, M.L. (1996). Davis's Manual of Psychosocial Nursing for General Patient Care. Philadelphia: F.A. Davis, pp. 283–289; reprinted with permission.

◆ NURSE, CLIENT, AND FAMILY RESOURCES— SUBSTANCE ABUSE DISORDERS

Associations

Alcoholics Anonymous World Services
475 Riverside
New York, NY 10115
1-212-870-3400

Narcotics Anonymous World Services Office
19737 Nordhoff Place
Chatsworth, CA
1-818-773-9999

Al-Anon Family Group Headquarters, Inc.
(for Al-Anon, Alateen, Alatots, ACOA)
P.O. Box 1822

Madison Square Station
New York, NY 10159
1-800-356-9996; Canada 1-613-722-1830

National Clearinghouse for Alcohol and Drug Information
P.O. Box 2345
Rockville, MD 20856
http://www.health.org

CSAT (Center for Substance Abuse Treatment)
National Drug Hotline (bilingual)
1-800-662-4357
http://www.samhsa.gov/csat/csat.htm

National Institute on Drug Abuse (NIDA)
American Self-Help Clearinghouse
1-201-625-7101
http://mentalhelp.net/selfhelp/

Internet Sites

National Addiction Technology Transfer Centers Home Page
http://www.nattc.org

Addiction Research Foundation/Centre for Addiction and Mental Health
http://www.arf.org

C H A P T E R   1 1

Eating Disorders

Anorexia nervosa and **bulimia nervosa** are both potentially fatal eating disorders. These disorders are severe and
disabling, and successful treatment entails long-term care
and follow-up. Unlike most psychiatric conditions, these disorders
can cause severe physiological damage (see Box 11–1 for some
medical complications of eating disorders). Because anorexia nervosa and bulimia nervosa are chronic complex disorders, nursing
interventions need to include actions to help minimize harm during
the acute phase and help prevent relapse. Predominately, these disorders affect adolescents, and cause great suffering and frustration
to the families, friends, and loved ones. Treating these disorders
can pose a formidable challenge to the health care system. The two
primary categories of eating disorders discussed in this section are
anorexia nervosa and bulimia nervosa. **Compulsive overeaters,** or
binge eaters, are a third category being considered for future edi-
tions of the DSM (Lyons, 1998). The suggested criteria for this
disorder address individuals who maintain patterns of overeating
resulting in obesity. **Eating disorders not otherwise specified**
(**NOS**) is the diagnosis often given when clients have signs and
symptoms of both categories.

◆ ANOREXIA NERVOSA

The diagnosis of anorexia nervosa is based upon psychological and
physical criteria. Psychological criteria include an intense fear of
gaining weight or becoming fat and a gross disturbance in body
image. Physiological requisites for the diagnosis of anorexia nervosa are maintenance of body weight less than 85% of that expected. Box 11–2 presents the DSM-IV diagnostic criteria for
anorexia nervosa.

The majority of cases of anorexia nervosa are seen in adolescent
women, with approximately 85% of cases developing between the

❖   B O X   1 1 – 1   ❖
Some Medical Complications of Eating Disorders

Complication	Laboratory Findings
Cardiovascular	Electrocardiographic abnormalities
Bradycardia	
Postural hypotension	
Dysrhythmias	
Metabolic	
Acidosis (laxatives)	$\downarrow K^+$
Alkalosis (vomiting)	$\uparrow$ Cholesterol
Hypokalemia	$\uparrow$ Liver function tests
Hypocalcemia	$\downarrow Mg^{2+}$
Hypomagnesemia	$\downarrow NA^+$
Osteoporosis	$\downarrow CA^{2+}$
Dehydration	$\downarrow$ Bone density
Renal	
Hematuria	$\uparrow$ Blood urea nitrogen
Proteinuria	
Gastrointestinal	
Hyperamylasemia	$\uparrow$ Serum amylase
Parotid swelling—hypertrophy	
Dental erosion (vomiting HCl)	
Esophagitis, esophogeal tears (vomiting)	
Pancreatitis	
Diarrhea (laxative abuse)	
Gastric dilation—bingeing	
Hematological	
Leukopenia	$\downarrow$ Erythrocyte sedimentation rate
Lymphocytosis	Abnormal complete blood count
Anemias (iron and vitamin B_{12} deficiency)	
Endocrine	
Amenorrhea	$\downarrow$ Follicle-stimulating hormone, luteinizing hormone, estradiol levels
$\downarrow$ Urinary and plasma gonadotropins	
Hypercortisolism	$\uparrow$ Corticotropin-releasing hormone
Abnormal thyroid function test	$\downarrow$ Tri-iodothyronine

---

❖   B O X   1 1 – 2   ❖
Diagnostic Criteria for Anorexia Nervosa

1. Refusal to maintain body weight over a minimum normal weight for age and height (e.g., weight loss leading to maintenance of body weight less than 85% of that expected, or failure to make expected weight gain during period of growth, leading to body weight less than 85% of that expected).
2. Intense fear of gaining weight or becoming fat, even though underweight.
3. Disturbance in the way in which one's body weight or shape is experienced, undue influence of body weight or shape on self-evaluation, or denial of the seriousness of the current low body weight.
4. In females, postmenarchal amenorrhea (i.e., the absence of at least three consecutive menstrual cycles). (A woman in considered to have amenorrhea if her periods occur only following hormone, e.g., estrogen, administration.)

Specify type:

Binge eating/purging type: During the episode of anorexia nervosa, the person engages in recurrent episodes of binge eating or purging behaviors.

Restricting type: During the episode of anorexia nervosa, the person does not engage in recurrent episodes of binge eating or purging behaviors.

Adapted from American Psychiatric Association. (1994). Diagnostic and Statistical Manual of Mental Disorders, 4th ed. Washington, DC: American Psychiatric Press, pp. 544–545; reprinted with permission. Copyright 1994 American Psychiatric Association.

---

ages of 13 and 20. Although the majority of anorectics are adolescents, anorexia is being diagnosed in preadolescents, in adults, and even in the elderly. Males account for about 5% of adolescents diagnosed with anorexia nervosa. The issues and the treatment modalities remain the same for both men and women.

There is evidence that the incidence of anorexia nervosa has been increasing in the past two decades in Western industrialized countries among young women between 15 and 24 years of age (Hoffman and Halmi, 1997). A large-scale English study revealed one severe case of anorexia nervosa per 200 girls ages 12 to 18 years old (Hoffman and Halmi, 1997).

Characteristically, anorectics are emaciated, but they still feel "fat" and want to hide their "ugly, fat body." Anorectics may have ritualistic eating patterns and compulsive behaviors; often feel hopeless, helpless, and depressed; and may feel the only control they can exert in their life is through what food they will eat. Suicide is a real concern.

People with this disorder use two methods to control weight:

1. **Bulimic** approach alternates bingeing and starvation (including purging and laxative and/or diuretic abuse). Purging may occur in up to 70% of young clients (binge eating/purging type).
2. **Restrictive** approach uses low calorie intake and exercise (restricting type).

The course of anorexia varies from (Hoffman and Halmi, 1997):

- a single episode with weight and psychological recovery, to
- nutritional rehabilitation with relapses, to
- an unremitting course resulting in death.

The disease has a mortality rate of 5% (most studies) to 20% (long-term studies looking at ultimate mortality rate over 20 years or longer) (Hoffman and Halmi, 1997). Death occurs from starvation, fluid and electrolyte imbalance, or suicide in chronically ill clients. Goldberg (1995) has identified favorable and negative prognostic indicators for anorexia nervosa:

1. **Favorable prognostic indicators:**
    a. Earlier age at onset
    b. Return of menses
    c. Good premorbid school/work history
2. **Negative prognostic indicators:**
    a. Recurrent illness
    b. Multiple hospitalizations
    c. Male
    d. Family pathology
    e. Premorbid personality difficulties and poor social adjustment in childhood

Box 11–3 identifies the most effective therapeutic modalities for anorectic clients.

◆ ASSESSING FOR ANOREXIA NERVOSA

History

1. Does client have a history of being overweight at 11 or 12 years of age? If yes, was there a pattern of restricting calories with subsequent spiraling weight loss?
2. Does client report prior hospitalizations?

Effective Therapeutic Modalities
for Anorectics

Behavioral Therapy

Behavioral therapy is effective in inducing short-term weight gain in anorectic clients, and this approach is incorporated into most structured treatment programs for anorexia using an operant conditioning paradigm.

Cognitive Therapy

Cognitive therapy helps clients challenge the validity of distorted beliefs and perceptions that are perpetuating their illness. The modification of cognitive techniques for the treatment of anorexia nervosa includes examining underlying assumptions, modifying basic assumptions, reinterpreting body image misperceptions, and using the "what if" technique (Dunner, 1997).

Family Therapy

Family therapy is advocated not as a single mode of treatment, but as an adjunct therapy, especially for anorectic clients with an early age of onset (younger than 18 years). The most commonly found dysfunctional difficulties are enmeshment, rigidity, and failure to resolve conflict. These issues are usually compounded by the pathological family dynamics that usually develop around the eating problems.

Individual Psychotherapy

Although most therapists who work with anorectic clients advocate some form of individual psychotherapy, the traditional psychoanalytic approach is thought to be *ineffective* with these clients. Successful psychotherapy needs to be highly interactive, explore relevant issues, educate, negotiate, challenge assumptions underlying anorectic behavioral, and encourage the client directly and openly (Dunner, 1997). Themes that are common when treating anorectic clients are:

- Low self-esteem
- Self-hatred
- Perfectionist strivings
- Inner emptiness
- Profound sense of ineffectiveness

3. Is there a history or evidence of physical and/or sexual abuse?
4. Are the boundaries in these families loose and unclear? Are the relationships within the family chaotic or unstable?
5. Do any first-degree relatives have a history of depression or substance abuse?
6. Have other *medical disorders* been ruled out? (**hypothalamic disease, diabetes mellitus, Addison's disease, gastrointestinal [GI] disorders, genetic disorders**)
7. Have other *psychiatric disorders* been ruled out? (**major depression, obsessive-compulsive disorders, psychotic disorder** where food is feared as part of a delusion, **phobic disorder** where food is avoided, **somatization disorder**, **substance abuse, or personality disorders [antisocial, borderline]**)

Presenting Symptoms

Psychosocial

1. Extreme fear of gaining weight
2. Poor social adjustment with some areas of high functioning (e.g., intellectual)
3. Odd food habits (hoarding, hiding food, e.g., in pockets or under plate)
4. Hyperactivity (compulsive and obsessive exercise and/or secretive physical activity in order to burn calories)
5. Mood and/or sleep disturbances
6. Obsessive-compulsive behaviors (e.g., eating only one pea at a time, arranging and rearranging food on plate before each bite, cutting food into tiny pieces and chewing each piece excessively)
7. Perfectionist
8. Introverted; avoids intimacy and sexual activity
9. Denies feelings of sadness or anger and will often appear pleasant and compliant
10. Although cachectic, clients see themselves as fat, underlying an unrealistic body image
11. Families often have rigid rules and have high expectations for their members

Physiological and Endocrine Symptoms

1. Emaciated physical appearance
2. Changes in cardiac status (e.g., bradycardia, hypotension, arrhythmia)

3. Dry, yellowish skin
4. Amenorrhea, infertility
5. Hair loss, possible presence of lanugo (fine body hair covering)
6. Decreased metabolic rate
7. Chronic constipation
8. Fatigue and lack of energy
9. Insomnia
10. Loss of bone mass, osteoporosis
11. In clients who vomit or use laxatives to purge, may see loss of tooth enamel and scarring of the back of the hand from inducing vomiting, and enlarged salivary glands. Serum amylase level is often elevated.
12. Dehydration, edema
13. Laboratory abnormalities and medical complications (refer to Box 11–1)

Sample Questions

The nurse uses a variety of therapeutic techniques to obtain the answers to the following questions. Use your discretion and decide which questions are appropriate to complete your assessment.

1. "On a scale of 1 to 10 (1 the least and 10 the most), how would you rate the seriousness of your low body weight?"
2. "How would you describe your appearance?"
3. "Do you think of yourself as having a great deal of control over your life?" (explain)
4. "Is it easy or difficult for you to make decisions?" (give an example)
5. "Describe how you feel about situations where people can see your body." (communal changing rooms, swimming baths, and intimate situations)

◆ ASSESSMENT GUIDE

The nurse needs to be able to make a comprehensive nursing assessment as well as be able to assess when a medical or psychological emergency warrants hospitalization and alert the medical staff. Box 11–4 helps the nurse assess if the client with an eating disorder warrants hospitalization.

ASSESSMENT ALERTS—ANOREXIA NERVOSA

Determine if:

1. The client has a medical or psychiatric situation that warrants hospitalization (see Box 11–4).
2. The family has information about the disease and knows where to get support.
3. The client is amenable to attending, or compliant with appropriate therapeutic modalities.
4. Family counseling has been offered to the family or individual family members for support, or to target a family or individual family member's problem.
5. A thorough physical exam with appropriate blood work has been done.
6. Other medical conditions have been ruled out.
7. The family and client need further teaching or information regarding client's treatment plan (e.g., psychopharmacological interventions, behavioral therapy, cognitive therapy, family therapy, individual psychotherapy). If the client is a candidate for partial hospitalization, can the family/client discuss their function?
8. The client and family desire a support group; if yes, provide referrals.

◆ NURSING DIAGNOSES WITH INTERVENTIONS

Eating disorders have both physiological and psychological components. The aims of treatment are survival based (Hill, 1998):

- Regain a healthy weight.
- Restore healthy eating habits.
- Treat physical complications.
- Address dysfunctional beliefs.
- Intervene in those dysfunctional thoughts, feelings, and beliefs.
- Deal with affective and behavioral issues.
- Include family therapy when appropriate and possible.
- Teach relapse prevention.

The first steps in treating the anorexic client include nutritional rehabilitation and weight restoration. Psychotherapy is not appropriate at this phase because there are profound psychological effects on mood and behavior from self-starvation. Hospitalization is warranted when emaciation is severe, vomiting is present, outpatient treatment has failed, or there is severe depression or suicidal feelings or physical complications (see Box 11–4).

❖   B O X   1 1 – 4   ❖
Criteria for Hospital Admission for Clients with an Eating Disorder

---

Physical Criteria

1. Weight loss over 30% over 6 months
2. Rapid decline in weight
3. Severe hypothermia as a result of loss of subcutaneous tissue, or dehydration (T <36°C or 96.8°F)
4. Inability to gain weight repeatedly with outpatient treatment
5. Heart rate less than 40 beats/min
6. Systolic blood pressure less than 70 mm Hg
7. Hypokalemia (K^+ under 3 mEq/L) or other electrolyte disturbances not corrected by oral supplementation
8. ECG changes (especially arrhythmias)
9. Inability to gain weight repeatedly with outpatient treatment

Psychiatric Criteria

1. Suicidal or severely out-of-control self-mutilating behaviors
2. Out-of-control use of laxatives, emetics, diuretics, or street drugs
3. Failure to comply with treatment contract
4. Severe depression
5. Psychosis
6. Family crisis/dysfunction

During hospitalization, treatment goals include the following:

- Weight restoration
- Normalizing eating behavior
- Change in the pursuit of thinness
- Prevention of relapse

Therefore, **Altered Nutrition: Less Than Body Requirements** is a primary nursing diagnosis.

Because clients with anorexia have extreme distortions of their body (seeing themselves as fat when emaciated) and an intense fear of being fat, **Body Image Disturbance** is an important nursing diagnosis; a realistic perception of body size is important to help the client refrain from compulsive need to lose weight. There is real threat for self-harm, therefore, **Risk for Self-Harm** may be appropriate for some young clients. **Refer to Chapter 13 for guidelines to assessment and care.** Clients with anorexia are terrified about gaining weight and will do anything to prevent gaining weight. Therefore, they frequently try to manipulate staff. Although briefly addressed here, **refer to Chapter 17 for dealing with manipulative behaviors**, because anorectic clients are desperate in their quest to avoid gaining weight.

Understand that anorectics are notoriously disinterested in treatment. Gaining trust and cooperation can be difficult. Table 11–1 offers potential nursing diagnoses for people with eating disorders.

Table 11–1 ◆ Potential Nursing Diagnoses—Eating Disorders

SYMPTOMS	NURSING DIAGNOSES
Emaciated, dehydrated, fatigue and lack of energy, edema	**Altered Nutrition: Less Than Body Requirements** **Risk for Fluid Volume Deficit** **Risk for Impaired Skin Integrity** **Risk for Altered Body Temperature** **Activity Intolerance** **Fatigue** **Risk for Infection** **Decreased Cardiac Output**
Chronic constipation or diarrhea, use of laxatives	**Constipation** **Diarrhea**
Sees self as fat (even when emaciated), extreme fear of gaining weight, denies feelings of sadness or anger, obsessive thoughts around food	**Altered Thought Processes** **Ineffective Denial** **Body Image Disturbance**
Poor social adjustment, introverted, compulsive behaviors (sexual acting out, shoplifting, bingeing, substance use), perfectionistic, manipulates to avoid calorie intake	**Ineffective Individual Coping** **Social Isolation** **Impaired Social Interaction**
Feelings of helplessness, worthlessness, feelings of being out of control, mood and sleep disturbances	**Hopelessness** **Powerlessness** **Chronic Low Self-Esteem** **Risk for Violence: Self-Directed** **Risk for Self-Mutilation** **Spiritual Distress** **Risk for Loneliness** **Anxiety**
Disrupted family, family in crisis, family confusion	**Ineffective Family Coping** **Compromised Family Coping** **Disabling Family Coping** **Knowledge Deficit**
Resistance to treatment, denial of problems, shame over bingeing, extreme fear of gaining weight, nonadherence to medications or treatment	**Noncompliance** **Anxiety**

OVERALL GUIDELINES FOR NURSING INTERVENTION

1. Gaining an anorectic's cooperation is best accomplished by acknowledging his or her desire for thinness and control and stimulating motivation for change.

2. Do a self-assessment and be aware of your own reactions that may hinder your ability to help the client. Some nurses may (Gorman et al., 1996):
   - Feel shocked or disgusted by the client's behavior or appearance.
   - Resent the client, believing that the disorder is self-inflicted.
   - Feel helpless to change the client's behavior, leading to anger, frustration, and criticism.
   - Become overwhelmed by the client's problems, leading to feelings of hopelessness or setting rigid limits to feel more in control of the client's behavior.
   - Be swept up into power struggles with the client, resulting in angry feelings in the nurse toward the client.

   When any of these or other negative feelings toward the client arise, supervision and/or peer review is needed to help shape the nurses perspective, and lessen feelings of helplessness, guilt, need for control, frustration, or hopelessness.

3. When problems in the family contribute to the feeling of loss of control, family therapy has provided a significant improvement rate.

4. Individual and group therapy are essential in treating client with eating disorders. Treatment for anorectic clients often includes a behavior modification program, especially initially. Family therapy and family education are often key to a client's success.

5. Behavior therapy is often used to change the eating patterns of an anorexic who is seriously close to death. This is usually implemented after the anorexic has been tube-fed to prevent death.

6. Refrain from focusing on the anorectic's need to eat; recognize that other, nonfood factors are the heart of the problem.

7. Monitor lab values and report abnormal values to primary clinician.

Altered Nutrition: Less Than Body Requirements

The state in which an individual experiences an intake of nutrients insufficient to meet metabolic needs

Related To (Etiology)

◆ Inability to ingest or digest food or to absorb nutrients because of biological, psychological, or economic factors
● Excessive fear of weight gain
● Restricting caloric intake or refusing to eat
● Excessive physical exertion resulting in caloric loss in excess of caloric intake
● Self-induced vomiting related to self-starvation

As Evidenced By (Assessment Findings/Diagnostic Cues)

◆ Weight loss (with or without adequate intake):15% or more under ideal body weight
◆ Reported or observed food intake less than recommended minimum daily requirements
◆ Excessive hair loss or increased growth of hair on body (lanugo)
◆ Poor muscle tone
◆ Fatigue
◆ Diarrhea and/or steatorrhea, abdominal cramping, pain
● Emaciated appearance
● Serious medical complications resulting from starvation (e.g., electrolyte imbalances, hypothermia, bradycardia, hypotension, cardiac arrythmias, edema)

Outcome Criteria

• Client's electrolytes will be within normal limits.
• Client's cardiac status will be within normal limits.
• Client will achieve 85% to 90% of ideal body weight.
• Client will commit to long-term treatment to prevent relapse.
• Client will demonstrate regular, independent, nutritional eating habits.

◆ NANDA accepted; ● In addition to NANDA.

Short-Term Goals

Client will:

- Increase caloric and nutritional intake, showing gradual increases on a weekly basis
- Gain no more than 1 to 2 pounds in the first week of refeeding, and no more than 3 to 5 pounds per week afterward
- Exercise in limited amounts only when assessed to be both nutritionally and medically stable
- Formulate with the nurse a *nurse-client contract* facilitating a therapeutic alliance and a commitment on the part of the client to treatment

Interventions and Rationales

THE SEVERELY MALNOURISHED
CLIENT—**NUTRITIONAL REHABILITATION**

Intervention	**Rationale**
1. When severely malnourished and refusing nourishment, client may require tube feedings, either alone or in conjunction with oral or parenteral nutrition.	1. Tube feedings may be the only means available to maintain client's life. Client may be unable to tolerate solid foods at first. The use of nasogastric tube feedings decreases the change of vomiting.
2. Tube feedings or parenteral nutrition is often given at night.	2. Using nighttime administration may diminish drawing attention or sympathy from other clients, and allows the client to participate more fully in daytime activities.
3. After completion of tube feeding, it is best to supervise client for 90 minutes initially, then gradually reduce to 30 minutes, after administration of nasogastric tube feeding.	3. Helps to minimize the client's chance of vomiting or siphoning off feedings.
4. Vital signs at least tid until stable, then daily. Repeat electrocardiogram (ECG) and laboratory tests (electro-	4. As client begins to increase in weight, cardiovascular status improves to within normal range, and moni-

Intervention	**Rationale**
lytes, acid-base balance, liver enzymes, albumin, and others) until stable.	toring is needed less frequently.
5. Administer tube feedings in a matter-of-fact, non-punitive manner. Tube feedings are not to be used as threats, nor are they something to be bargained about.	5. Tube feedings are medical treatments, not a punishment or a bargaining chip. Being consistent and enforcing limits lowers the chance of manipulation and the use of power struggles.
6. Give the client the chance to take foods or liquid supplements orally, and supplement insufficient intake through tube feedings.	6. Allows the client some control over whether he or she needs tube feedings or not. The client's life is the priority, however.
7. Weigh the client weekly or biweekly at the same time of day each week. Use the following guidelines: • Before the morning meal • After the client has voided • Weigh client in hospital gown or bra and pants only.	7. Clients are terrified about gaining weight. Staff need to guard against clients trying to manipulate their weight by drinking lots of water before being weighed, having a full bladder, putting heavy objects in their pockets or on their person.
8. Use a matter-of-fact manner, neither approving nor disapproving.	8. Keep issues of approval and disapproval separate from issues of health. Weight gain/loss is a health matter, not an area that has to do with the staff's pleasure or disapproval.

THE LESS SEVERELY MALNOURISHED CLIENT—**NUTRITIONAL MAINTENANCE**

Intervention	**Rationale**
1. When possible, set up a contract with the client regarding treatment goals and outcome criteria.	1. When clients do agree to take part in establishing goals, clients are in a position to have some control over their care.

2. Provide a pleasant, calm atmosphere at mealtime. Mealtime should be structured. Clients need to be told the specific times and duration of a meal (e.g., 30 minutes).

2. Mealtimes become episodes of high anxiety, and knowledge of regulations decreases tension in the milieu, particularly when the client has given up so much control by entering treatment.

3. Observe client *during* meals to prevent hiding or throwing away food. Accompany to the bathroom if purging is suspected. Observe client for at least 1 hour *after* meals/snacks to prevent purging.

3. These behaviors are difficult for the client to stop. A power struggle may emerge around issues of control.

4. Observe client closely for using physical activity to control weight.

4. Clients are often discouraged from engaging in planned exercise programs until their weight reaches 85% of ideal body weight.

5. Closely monitor and record:
   • Fluid and food intake
   • Vital signs
   • Elimination pattern: discourage the use of laxatives, enemas, or suppositories.

5. Fluid and electrolyte balance is crucial to client's well-being and safety. Abnormal data may alert staff to potential physical crises.

6. Continue to weigh client as above.

6. Monitor progress.

7. As clients approach their target weight, gradually encourage client to make own choices for menu selection.

7. Fosters a sense of control and independence.

8. Privileges are based on weight gain (or loss) when setting limits. When weight *loss* occurs, decrease privileges. Use this time to focus on circumstances surrounding the weight loss and feelings of the client.

8. By not focusing on eating, physical activity calorie counts, and the like, there is more emphasis on the client's feelings and perceptions.

Intervention

9. When weight gain occurs, increase privileges.

Rationale

9. Client receives positive reinforcements for healthy outcomes and behaviors.

MAINTENANCE

Intervention

1. Continue to provide a supportive and empathetic approach as client continues to meet target weight.

2. The weight maintenance phase of treatment challenges the client. This is the ideal time to address more of the issues underlying the client's attitude toward weight and shape.

3. Use a cognitive-behavioral approach to client's expressed fears regarding weight gain. Identify dysfunctional thoughts.

4. Emphasize social nature of eating. Encourage conversation that does not have the theme of food during mealtimes.

5. Focus on the client's strengths, including his or her good work in normalizing weight and eating habits.

6. Encourage client to apply all the knowledge, skills, and gains made from the various individual, family, and group therapy sessions.

Rationale

1. Eating regularly for the anorectic client, even within the framework of restoring health, is extremely difficult.

2. At a healthier weight, the client is cognitively better prepared to examine emotional conflicts and themes.

3. Confronting dysfunctional thoughts and beliefs is crucial to changing eating behaviors.

4. Eating is a social activity, shared with others, and participating in conversation serves both as a distraction from obsessional preoccupation and as a pleasurable event.

5. The client has achieved a major accomplishment and should be proud. Explore noneating activities as a source of gratification.

6. The client should have been receiving intensive therapy (cognitive-behavioral) and education, which have provided tools and techniques

7. Teach and role model assertiveness.

useful in maintaining healthy eating and living behaviors.

7. Client learns to get his or her needs met appropriately. Helps lower anxiety and acting-out behaviors.

FOLLOW-UP CARE

Intervention

1. Involve the client's family and significant others with teaching, treatment, and discharge and follow-up plans. Teaching includes nutrition, medication if any, and the dynamics of the illness (Schultz and Videbeck, 1998).
2. Make arrangements for follow-up therapy for both the client and the family.
3. Offer referrals to the client and family to local support groups or national groups. (See list at end of chapter for suggestions.)

Rationale

1. Family involvement is a key factor to client success. Family dynamics are usually a significant factor in the client's illness and distress.

2. Follow-up therapy for both family and client is key to prevention of relapse.
3. Support groups offer emotional guidance and support, resources, and important information, and help minimize feelings of isolation, and encourage healthier coping strategies.

Body Image Disturbance

Disruption in the way one perceives one's body image; negative self-evaluation and feelings about self-capabilities, which may be directly or indirectly expressed

---

Related To (Etiology)

◆ Cognitive/perceptual factors
◆ Psychosocial factors

◆ NANDA accepted; ● In addition to NANDA.

- Morbid fear of obesity
- Low self-esteem
- Feelings of helplessness
- Chemical/biological imbalances

As Evidenced By (Assessment Findings/Diagnostic Cues)

◆ Verbalized negative feelings about body (e.g., dirty, big, unsightly)
◆ Verbalized feelings of helplessness, hopelessness, and /or powerlessness in relation to body and fear of rejection/reaction of others
◆ Self-destructive behavior (purging, refusal to eat, abuse of laxatives)
● Sees self as fat even though body weight is normal, or client severely emaciated
● High to panic levels of anxiety over potential for slight weight gain, even though grossly underweight to the point of starvation

Outcome Criteria

Client will:

- Describe a more realistic perception of body size and shape in line with height and body type
- Refer to body in a more positive way
- Improve grooming, dress, and posture and present self in more socially acceptable and appropriate manner

Short-Term Goals

Client will:

- Challenge dysfunctional thoughts and beliefs about weight with help of nurse after acute phase of treatment has passed
- State three positive aspects about self

Interventions and Rationales

Intervention	Rationale
1. Establish a therapeutic alliance with client.	1. Anorexic clients are highly resistant to giving up their distorted eating behaviors.

◆ NANDA accepted; ● In addition to NANDA.

2. Give the client factual feedback about the client's low weight and resultant impaired health. However, do not argue or challenge the client's distorted perceptions (Ibrahim, 1998).

2. Focuses on health and benefits of increased energy. Arguments or power struggles will only increase the client's need to control.

3. Recognize that the client's distorted image is real to the client. Avoid minimizing client's perceptions (e.g., "I understand you see yourself as fat. I do not see you that way.")

3. Acknowledges client's perceptions, and helps the client feel understood even if your perception is different. This kind of feedback is easier to hear than a negation of client's beliefs.

4. Encourage expression of feelings regarding how the client thinks and feels about self and body.

4. Promotes a clear understanding of client's perceptions and lays the groundwork for working with client.

5. Assist the client to distinguish between thoughts and feelings. Statements such as "I feel fat" should be challenged and reframed (Ibrahim, 1998).

5. It is important for the client to distinguish between feelings and facts. The client often speaks of feelings as if they are reality.

6. Nurses who have training in cognitive-behavioral therapeutic interventions can encourage client to keep a journal of thoughts and feelings and teach client how to identify and challenge irrational beliefs.

6. Cognitive and behavioral approaches can be very effective in helping client challenge irrational beliefs about self and body image.

7. Encourage client to identify positive personal traits. Have client identify positive aspects of personal appearance.

7. Helps client refocus on strengths and actual physical and other attributes. Encourages breaking negative rumination.

8. Educate family regarding the client's illness and encourage attendance at

8. Reactions of others often become triggers for dysphoric reactions and

Intervention	**Rationale**
family and group therapy sessions.	distorted perceptions. Relationships with others, while not casual, are the context in which the eating disorder exists and thrives.
9. Encourage family therapy for family members and significant others.	9. Families and significant others need assistance in how to communicate and share a relationship with the anorexic client (Ibrahim, 1998).

◆ PSYCHOPHARMACOLOGY

Although there have been many drugs used to treat anorexia nervosa, no medication has been shown to be effective in maintaining weight gain, change anorectic attitudes, or preventing relapse either by itself or as an adjunct for treating anorexia nervosa (Maxmen and Ward, 1995).

Neuroleptics have been used in the past with anorectic clients; however, double-blind studies fail to show significant drug effect on weight gain, weight habits, or body distortion. *Lithium carbonate*, in the only single-blind trial, was also found to have minimal effect on facilitating weight gain. The marginal results versus the toxicity of this drug do not seem to justify the use of lithium for these clients (Dunner, 1997).

Antidepressants have had some success with anorectic clients. Although amitriptyline has had marginal success, it is associated with significant side effects. Clomipramine (Anafranil), however, seems to have had more success. Fluoxetine (Prozac) has also been used with some success, resulting in diminishing depression, encouraging weight gain, and a diminution in preoccupation with food and weight. What is needed is a controlled double-blind study on the efficacy of fluoxetine in the treatment of anorexia nervosa to establish optimal dosage and duration of treatment.

Cyproheptadine hydrochloride (Periactin), an *antihistamine*, has also been found to be effective in emaciated anorectic clients in decreasing depression and in inducing weight gain among the anorexic restrictors (but not the bulimic subgroups).

One challenge is that often teenagers are nonadherent with medication and treatment. This knowledge is best factored into the nurse's approach to the anorectic.

♦ BULIMIA NERVOSA

Bulimics might be slightly overweight, normal weight, or slightly below. The hallmark feature of bulimia nervosa is an excessive intake of food (binge eating) with purging behaviors to maintain body weight. Purging behaviors may include self-induced vomiting or the excessive use of laxatives, diuretics, or enemas. Other behaviors directed at maintaining body weight might include prolonged fasting, excessive exercise, or misuse of diet pills. Purging is used by 80% to 90% of individuals who present for treatment at eating disorder clinics (APA, 1994).

Bulimics who use purging behaviors are referred to as having **bulimia nervosa–purging type**. Similarly, **bulimia nervosa–nonpurging type** represents people who use inappropriate compensatory behaviors (fasting, excessive exercise, misuse of diet pills), but do not engage in the above-mentioned purging behaviors. (See the DSM-IV diagnostic criteria in Box 11–5.)

Women considered most at risk for bulimia in the United States are Caucasian females between the ages of 14 and 40 years old, although the majority are in late adolescence or their early 20s. Bulimia occurs rarely in men, about 0.1% to 0.5% (Pages, 1997). Some bulimic features are present in 5% to 25% of the young adult population (Goldberg, 1995).

Depressive symptoms may often complicate the picture. Associated with depression may be suicidal behaviors or self-mutilation behaviors. Depression usually follows the development of bulimia nervosa (up to 70% of the time). However, in some cases depression precedes bulimia. Substance abuse (particularly alcohol and stimulants such as cocaine) are often present. Between one third and one half of bulimic clients may have personality features of one or more personality disorders, frequently borderline personality disorder (APA, 1994). This may account for the prevalence of bulimic individuals who present with dysfunctional personal relationships.

Individuals with bulimia are often more socially skilled and may be sexually active as compared to clients with anorexia nervosa. The bulimic's bingeing is usually done alone and in secret. In one episode of bingeing, a bulimic can consume over 5000 calories. Excessive vomiting may lead to severe dehydration and electrolyte imbalance, particularly hypokalemia. Teeth may appear discolored or rotten as a result of erosion by gastric acid related to excessive vomiting. Calluses on fingers result from inducing vomiting.

A sense of being out of control accompanies the excessive and/or compulsive consumption of large amounts of food. Binges

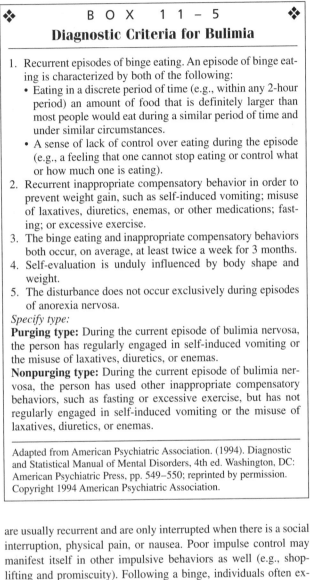

❖   B O X   1 1 – 5   ❖
Diagnostic Criteria for Bulimia

1. Recurrent episodes of binge eating. An episode of binge eat-
    ing is characterized by both of the following:
    - Eating in a discrete period of time (e.g., within any 2-hour
      period) an amount of food that is definitely larger than
      most people would eat during a similar period of time and
      under similar circumstances.
    - A sense of lack of control over eating during the episode
      (e.g., a feeling that one cannot stop eating or control what
      or how much one is eating).
2. Recurrent inappropriate compensatory behavior in order to
    prevent weight gain, such as self-induced vomiting; misuse
    of laxatives, diuretics, enemas, or other medications; fast-
    ing; or excessive exercise.
3. The binge eating and inappropriate compensatory behaviors
    both occur, on average, at least twice a week for 3 months.
4. Self-evaluation is unduly influenced by body shape and
    weight.
5. The disturbance does not occur exclusively during episodes
    of anorexia nervosa.

Specify type:
Purging type: During the current episode of bulimia nervosa,
the person has regularly engaged in self-induced vomiting or
the misuse of laxatives, diuretics, or enemas.

Nonpurging type: During the current episode of bulimia nervosa, the person has used other inappropriate compensatory
behaviors, such as fasting or excessive exercise, but has not
regularly engaged in self-induced vomiting or the misuse of
laxatives, diuretics, or enemas.

Adapted from American Psychiatric Association. (1994). Diagnostic
and Statistical Manual of Mental Disorders, 4th ed. Washington, DC:
American Psychiatric Press, pp. 549–550; reprinted by permission.
Copyright 1994 American Psychiatric Association.

are usually recurrent and are only interrupted when there is a social
interruption, physical pain, or nausea. Poor impulse control may
manifest itself in other impulsive behaviors as well (e.g., shoplifting and promiscuity). Following a binge, individuals often experience tremendous guilt, depression, or disgust with themselves.
Young women with bulimia nervosa have an obsessive and persistent overconcern with body shape and weight and experience
a distortion of body image. That is, they see themselves as too

fat or large even when they may be near or below normal body weight.

Treatment is provided in an outpatient setting unless there is a physical or psychological emergency. (Refer to Box 11–4 to identify criteria for hospital admittance.)

The clinical course of bulimia nervosa may be either chronic or intermittent, with waxing and waning of symptoms. Many individuals may also experience the development of other psychiatric or medical problems. Up to 50% of bulimics recover; about 25% remain unimproved in follow-up. Mortality may be 5% to 15% (Goldberg, 1995).

◆ ASSESSING FOR BULIMIA NERVOSA

History

1. Assess if the client has a history of a mood disorder, suicidal behavior, or self-mutilating behavior.
2. Identify if the client has a substance abuse problem. Is there a family history of substance abuse?
3. Assess if client has been diagnosed with a personality disorder (borderline/obsessive-compulsive/panic disorder).
4. What are the client's previous eating behaviors? Is there a history of dieting behavior?
5. Identify other medical complications related to bulimia nervosa (refer to Box 11–1).
6. Have other diagnoses been ruled out? (anorexia nervosa, major depression, bipolar disorder, adjustment disorder, Klein-Levin syndrome [hypersomnia and hyperphagia])

Presenting Signs and Symptoms

1. Enlarged parotid glands
2. Dental erosion, caries
3. Calluses on dorsum of hands (from manually stimulating vomiting) and/or finger calluses
4. Electrolyte imbalance, especially hypokalemia
5. Irregular menses
6. Fluid retention and/or dehydration
7. Hypotension
8. Ulcerations around mouth and cheeks (from emesis splashback)
9. Chronic hoarseness, chronic sore throat
10. Possible cardiac arrhythmias secondary to electrolyte imbalance
11. Fatigue and lack of energy

12. GI problems (e.g., constipation, diarrhea, reflux, and esopha-
    gitis)
13. Alkalosis

Sample Questions

*The nurse uses a variety of therapeutic techniques to obtain the an-
swers to the following questions. Use your discretion and decide
which questions are appropriate to complete your assessment.*

1. Does the client acknowledge:
   a. Eating normal amounts in public, but bingeing in private
   b. Using purging behaviors after binges (e.g., self-induced
      vomiting; overusing laxatives, diet pills, or diuretics; fasting
      or excessive exercise)
   c. Maintain secrecy regarding eating habits or amounts eaten
   d. Suicidal thoughts
2. Do clients admit to:
   a. Feeling powerless over binge-purge cycle
   b. Believing they are unable to change
   c. Being preoccupied with appearance, weight
   d. Drug or alcohol abuse, especially cocaine as a means of
      keeping weight down

◆ ASSESSMENT GUIDE

Refer to Table 11–2 for a comparison of assessment features between anorexia and bulimia.

ASSESSMENT ALERTS—BULIMIA NERVOSA
1. Medical stabilization is the first priority. Problems re-sulting from purging are disruptions in electrolyte and fluid balance and cardiac function. Therefore, a thorough medical exam is vital.   2. Medical evaluation usually includes a thorough phys-ical, as well as pertinent lab values: • Electrolytes   • Glucose   • Thyroid function tests   • Neuroimaging of pituitary   • Complete blood count   • ECG   3. Psychiatric evaluation is advised because treatment of psychiatric comorbidity is important to outcome.

Table 11–2 ◆ Comparison of Characteristics of Anorexia and Bulimia

CHARACTERISTIC	ANOREXIA—RESTRICTING TYPE	BULIMIA
Prevalence	About 0.5%–1.0% for presentations that meet full criteria. Those who are subthreshold for the disorder (Eating Disorder NOS) are more common.	About 1%–3% among adolescent and young adult females. The disorder in males is about one tenth that in females.
Appearance	Below 85% of ideal body weight	Normal weight range, may be slightly above or below
Onset of Illness	Early adolescence with peaks at 14 and 17 years of age	Late adolescence, early adult
Physical Signs	Thin, emaciated	Altered thyroid and cortisol function
	Amenorrhea	Enlarged parotid glands
	Slight yellowing of skin	Dental erosion, caries
	Bradycardia	Calluses on dorsum of hands from inducing vomiting
	Hypotension, hypothermia	Electrolyte imbalance, especially hypokalemia
	Peripheral edema	Fluid retention
	Bradycardia, ECG abnormalities	Cardiac problems (heart failure, ECG change, cardiomyopathy)
		↑ Blood urea nitrogen
Familial Patterns	Increased incidence of mood disorders in first-degree relatives	Increased incidence of mood disorders, substance abuse, dependence in first-degree relatives
Personality Traits	Perfectionism	Poor impulse control
	Social isolation	Low self-esteem
Insight Into Illness	Denies seriousness of illness; eating disordered behaviors are egosyntonic	Aware of illness; disturbed behaviors are egodystonic

Data from APA (1994).

◆ NURSING DIAGNOSES AND INTERVENTIONS

Individuals with uncomplicated bulimia nervosa are usually treated as outpatients in a clinic setting, a partial hospitalization program, or in private practice. However, hospitalization may be necessary when purging is so severe that it is out of the client's control, or it is causing severe electrolyte and metabolic disturbances. Psychiatric emergencies such as suicidal ideation or uncontrolled substance abuse may also indicate a need for hospitalization.

Because electrolyte and fluid balance and cardiac function can all be affected, there is a serious potential for **Risk for Injury**. Because bingeing and purging are often felt to be out of the individual's ability to control, **Powerlessness** is an area that needs to be targeted. **Comorbidity with personality disorders** may play a part in treatment, and the reader is encouraged to refer to Chapter 5. If there are issues of **substance abuse**, Chapter 10 may offer some guidelines for care. Because depression is usually present, there is always the concern with the **potential for suicide**. Please refer to Chapter 13 for intervention strategies. Refer to Table 11–1 for potential nursing diagnoses for people with bulimia nervosa.

OVERALL GUIDELINES FOR NURSING INTERVENTION

1. Cognitive-behavioral psychotherapy has been shown to be useful.
2. Often coexisting disorders complicate the clinical picture (depression, substance use, personality disorders), and these may warrant additional psychotherapy (psychodynamic, interpersonal, family therapy).
3. Group therapy with other individuals suffering from bulimia is often part of successful therapy.
4. Because anxiety and feelings of stress often precede bingeing, alternative ways of dealing with anxiety and alternative coping strategies to lessen anxiety are useful tools.
5. Family therapy is helpful and encouraged.

Risk for Injury

A state in which the individual is at risk of injury as a result of environmental conditions interacting with the individual's adaptive and defensive resources

Related To (Etiology)

- Uncontrollable binge-purge cycles
- Inadequate coping mechanisms to deal with anxiety and stress
- Coexisting conditions, when not addressed, could cause injury or self-injury (suicidal thoughts, self-mutilation, substance abuse)
- Poor impulse control

As Evidenced By (Assessment Findings/Diagnostic Cues)

- Medical Complications
  * Electrolyte imbalances (hypokalemia, hypomagnesemia, hyponatremia, hypocalcemia)
  * Esophageal tears
  * Cardiac problems
  * Altered thyroid and cortisol function
- Overuse of laxatives, diet pills, or diuretics
- Self-destructive behaviors
- Denial of feelings, illness, or problems

Outcome Criteria

Client will:

- Demonstrate at least four newly learned skills for managing stress and anxiety, shame and guilt, and other triggers that induce compulsive eating
- Abstain from binge-purge behaviors
- Obtain and maintain normal electrolyte balance
- Be free of self-directed harm
- Demonstrate ability to recognize and refute dysfunctional thoughts and record in journal
- Obtain and maintain normal electrocardiogram readings
- Verbalize a desire to participate in an ongoing treatment program (support groups or therapy as indicated)
- Express feelings in non–food-related ways

Short-Term Goals

Client will:

- Remain free of self-directed harm
- Identify and role play with nurse three alternative ways to deal with anxiety and stress by (date)

◆ NANDA accepted; ● In addition to NANDA.

- Identify dysfunctional thoughts that may precede a binge-purge episode, and learn to challenge and refute these thoughts with aid of nurse within 2 weeks
- Identify signs and symptoms of low potassium level and other medical complication that would warrant immediate medical attention within 2 days

Interventions and Rationales

Intervention	Rationale
1. Assess for suicidal thoughts and other self-destructive thoughts and behaviors.	1. Always be on guard for psychiatric and medical emergencies, which take precedence over other forms of treatment.
2. Educate the client regarding the ill effects of self-induced vomiting (low potassium level, dental erosion, cardiac problems)	2. Health teaching is crucial to treatment. The client needs to be reminded of the benefits of normal eating behavior.
3. Educate the client about the binge-purge cycle and its self-perpetuating nature.	3. The compulsive nature of the binge-purge cycle is maintained by the cycle of restricting, hunger, bingeing, then purging accompanied by feelings of guilt. Then the cycle begins again.
4. Identify client triggers that induce compulsive eating and purging behaviors.	4. Work with client to find alternative ways to think and behave when triggers are present.
5. Explore with the client dysfunctional thoughts that precede the binge-purge cycle. Teach clients to refute these thoughts and to reframe them in healthier ways.	5. Strong rebuttals and non-judgmental reframing can balance and combat distorted thinking. More rational thinking can lead to healthier behaviors to combat issues of self-esteem, body image, self-worth, and feelings of alienation.
6. Have client record thoughts and refutes in journal and share with nurse.	6. Recognizing and reviewing with nurse helps reinforce learning.

7. Work with the client to identify problems and mutually establish short- and long-term goals.

7. Clients need to develop tools for dealing with personal problems, rather than turning to automatic binge-purge behaviors.

8. Assess and teach problem-solving skills when dealing with client's problem.

8. Gives the client alternative means of dealing with problems other than binge-purge behaviors.

9. Arrange for the client to learn ways to increase interpersonal communication, socialization, and assertiveness skills.

9. Client is often isolated from close relationships, and lack appropriate skills for getting their needs met.

10. Encourage attendance at support group or therapy groups with other bulimic individuals. Provide information for family members as well.

10. The eating disorders are chronic diseases, and long-term follow-up therapy is critical for success.

Powerlessness

Perception that one's own actions will not significantly affect an outcome; a perceived lack of control over a current situation or immediate happening

---

Related To (Etiology)

◆ Lifestyle of helplessness
◆ Interpersonal interaction
● Inability to control binge-eating and purging behavior
● Severe distortion of body image that perpetuates dysfunctional behavior
● Feelings of low self-worth
● Insufficient coping skills in dealing with stress and anxiety

As Evidenced By (Assessment Findings/Diagnostic Cues)

◆ Verbal expressions of having no control or influence over situations

---

◆ NANDA accepted; ● In addition to NANDA.

◆ Nonparticipation in care or decision making when opportunities are provided
◆ Expression of doubt regarding role performance
◆ Reluctance to express true feelings
● Guilt over uncontrollable behavior
● Distorted perceptions and beliefs regarding eating and self-image (e.g., "If I gain an ounce, I'll feel fat. Being thin is crucial to my success.")

Outcome Criteria

Clients will:

• Verbalize increased feelings of security and autonomy over their life
• Identify people and resources in the community for support and follow-up
• State that they feel better able to cope with stress and anxiety
• Demonstrate ability to refrain from binge-purge behaviors

Short-Term Goals

Client will:

• Keep a journal of thoughts and feelings and learn to identify automatic thoughts and beliefs that trigger binge-purge behaviors by (date)
• Review journal with nurse/counselor on a weekly basis (clinic)
• Demonstrate the ability to dispute dysfunctional negative thoughts about self and abilities by (date)
• Demonstrate ability to do a realistic self-appraisal of strengths by (date)

Interventions and Rationales

Intervention	Rationale
1. Explore the client's experience of out-of-control eating behavior.	1. Listening in an empathetic, nonjudgmental manner helps clients feel understood and that someone understands their experience.
2. Encourage the client to keep a journal of thoughts and feelings surrounding	2. Automatic thoughts and beliefs maintain the binge-purge cycle. A journal is an

◆ NANDA accepted; ● In addition to NANDA.

binge-purge behaviors.

3. Teach or refer to a counselor who can teach client how to challenge dysfunctional thoughts and beliefs in a systematic manner.

4. Review with the client the kinds of cognitive distortions that affect feelings, beliefs, and behavior.

5. Encourage client's participation in decisions and client's responsibility in his or her care and future.

6. Teach client alternative stress reduction techniques and visualization skills to improve self-confidence and feelings of self-worth.

7. Role play new skills. Encourage client to apply new skills in individual and group therapy in communications with others, particularly family.

8. Teach the client that a lapse is not a relapse. One slip of control does not eliminate all positive accomplishments.

excellent way to identify these dysfunctional thoughts and underlying assumptions.

3. These automatic dysfunctional thoughts must be examined and challenged if change in client thinking and behavior is to occur.

4. Cognitive distortions reinforce unrealistic views of self in terms of strengths and future potential. Realistic self-views are necessary for change to occur.

5. Helps clients gain a sense of control over their lives, and that there are options they can take to make important changes in their lives.

6. Visualizing a positive self-image and positive outcomes for life goals stimulates problem solving toward desired goals.

7. Role-play allows the opportunity for client to become comfortable with new and different ways of relating and responding to others in a safe environment.

8. At time of lapse, it is helpful to examine what led to the lapse, knowing that one lapse does not eliminate all positive accomplishments.

◆ PSYCHOPHARMACOLOGY

No single drug has been proven effective by itself or as an adjunct for treating bulimia nervosa. *Antidepressants* have been used with bulimia nervosa. In particular, the SSRIs have been well studied.

Fluoxetine has been shown to affect positively the binge-purge cycle in some bulimic clients. In particular, the SSRIs can be effective with highly obsessional clients as well as clients who are depressed. The SSRIs may also help carbohydrate craving and mood disturbance that are associated with bulimia nervosa and obesity (Schatzberg et al., 1997).

◆ NURSE, CLIENT, AND FAMILY TEACHING FOR EATING DISORDERS

The National Association of Anorexia Nervosa and Associated Disorders (ANAD) has put out information that families and friends might find helpful in their dealings with a person with an eating disorder (Box 11–6).

◆ CLIENT AND FAMILY RESOURCES—EATING DISORDERS

Self-Help Groups

American Anorexia/Bulimia Association
293 Central Park West, #R
New York, NY 10024
1-212-891-8686
(for people with eating disorders)

National Association of Anorexia Nervosa and Associated Disorders (ANAD)
P.O. Box 7
Highland Park, IL 60035
1-847-831-3438
(for people with eating disorders)

National Eating Disorders Organization
6655 South Yale Avenue
Tulsa, OK 74136
1-918-481-4044
(for people with eating disorders, their families, and friends)

Eating Disorders Awareness and Prevention
603 Stewart Street, Suite 803
Seattle, WA 98101
1-206-382-3587

Internet Sites

Mirror Mirror Eating Disorders Home Page
http://www.mirror-mirror.org/eatdis.htm

❖   B O X   1 1 – 6   ❖
Do's and Don'ts in Helping Someone Recover from an Eating Disorder

This information is provided by the National Association of Anorexia Nervosa and Associated Disorders (ANAD).

Do:
- Gently encourage her to eat properly.
- Express your love and support.
- Try to understand, even though this seems impossible.
- Take time to listen, even though the talk may seem trivial or insignificant to you.
- Try to see how she (and each family member) perceive the situation.
- Realize that she is terrified of gaining weight and being fat even though she may actually be underweight. These irrational fears are real to her.
- Emphasize the positive and all her good characteristics, and compliment her on all the things she does right.
- Encourage her to accept support and honestly express her feelings.
- Talk honestly and sincerely with love and understanding.
- Recognize that other, non-food factors are at the heart of the problem.
- Help her find someone to support her, who knows what she is going through.
- Realize that, while she must have help from others, she must want to get better and she needs to love herself.

Don't:
- Try to force her to eat or stop exercising.
- Get angry or punish her.
- Be impatient (this is really tough) and don't lecture.
- Be too busy, even if you have to give up "important" things.
- Jump to conclusions or see things only through your eyes and mind.
- Make her feel bad or guilty for having an eating disorder and don't spy on her.
- Place the blame on anyone.
- Be afraid to talk about problems.
- Pretend it will all just go away.
- Expect an instant recovery.
- Let her feel she is the only one with this problem.

Do all that you can to help her realize what a beautiful person she really is.

MSI-ANAD014
©1994–1998 National Association of Anorexia Nervosa and Associated Disorders, licensed to Medical Strategies, Inc. (MSI); ANAD, Box 7, Highland Park, IL 60035, 1-847-831-3438; reprinted by permission.

The Center for Eating Disorders
http://www.eatingdisorder.org

Anorexia Nervosa and Related Eating Disorders, Inc.
http://www.anred.com

Academy for Eating Disorders
http://www.acadeatdis.org

Health*touch* Online
http://www.healthtouch.com

CHAPTER 12

Cognitive Disorders

DELIRIUM AND DEMENTIA

Delirium is usually characterized by a sudden disturbance of consciousness and a change in cognition, such as impaired attention span and disturbances of consciousness (APA, 1994). Delirium is always secondary to another condition such as a general medical condition (i.e., infections, diabetes), or is substance induced (drugs, medications, or toxins); delirium may also have multiple causes. Delirium is usually a transitory condition and reversed when interventions are timely. Prolonged delirium can lead to dementia.

Dementia develops more slowly and is characterized by multiple cognitive deficits that include impairment in short-term and long-term memory. Dementia is usually irreversible. Dementia can be primary, or secondary to another condition. Refer to Table 12–3 in the second half of the Chapter for a side by side comparison of the characteristics of delirium and dementia.

◆ DELIRIUM

Box 12–1 presents the DSM-IV diagnostic criteria for delirium.

Because delirium is always secondary to medical disorder or toxicity, delirium is often seen on medical and surgical units. Delirium is often experienced by elderly clients, children with high fevers, postoperative clients, and clients with cerebrovascular disease and congestive heart failure. Delirium may occur in people with infections, metabolic disorders, drug intoxications and withdrawals, medication toxicity, neurological diseases, tumors, and certain psychosocial stressors. Delirium is important to recognize because, if it continues without intervention, irreversible brain damage may occur.

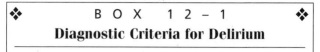

❖   B O X   1 2 – 1   ❖
Diagnostic Criteria for Delirium

1. Disturbance of consciousness (i.e., reduced clarity of awareness of the environment with reduced ability to focus, sustain, or shift attention).
2. A change in cognition (memory deficit, disorientation, language disturbance) or the development of a perceptual disturbance that is not better accounted for by a preexisting, established, or evolving dementia.
3. The disturbance develops over a short period of time (usually hours to days) and tends to fluctuate during the course of the day.
4. The disturbance is due to:
   • A general medical condition, *or*
   • Substance-induced (intoxication or withdrawal), *or*
   • Multiple etiologies (both of the above causes), *or*
   • Not known (not otherwise specified).

Adapted from American Psychiatric Association. (1994). Diagnostic and Statistical Manual of Mental Disorders, 4th ed. Washington, DC: American Psychiatric Press, pp. 129, 131–133; reprinted with permission. Copyright 1994 American Psychiatric Association.

◆ ASSESSING FOR DELIRIUM

History

A positive history includes:

1. A history of episodes of delirium
2. A thorough medical evaluation revealing abnormal lab results
3. An electroencephalogram (EEG)–confirmed cerebral dysfunction
4. The underlying cause of the delirium has been identified.
5. The client has been examined more than once at different times of day to detect fluctuations in levels of consciousness that characterize the syndrome
6. Delirium is often misdiagnosed as depression, anxiety, dementia, or personality disorder. These have been ruled out.

Presenting Signs and Symptoms

1. Fluctuating levels of consciousness. The individual may be disoriented and severely confused at night and during early morning hours (**sundowning**), and remain lucid during the day.
2. Impaired ability to reason and carry out goal-directed behavior

3. Alternating patterns of *hyperactivity* to *hypoactivity* (slow down activity to stupor or coma)
4. Behaviors seen when **hyperactive** include:
    a. Hypervigilance
    b. Restlessness
    c. Incoherent, loud, or rapid speech
    d. Irritability
    e. Anger and/or combativeness
    f. Profanity
    g. Euphoria
    h. Distractibility
    i. Tangentiality
    j. Nightmares
    k. Persistent abnormal thoughts (delusions)
5. Behaviors seen when **hypoactive** include:
    a. Lethargy
    b. Speaks and moves little or slowly
    c. Has spells of staring
    d. Reduced alertness
    e. Generalized loss of awareness of the environment
6. Impaired attention span
7. Cognitive changes not accounted for by dementia:
    a. Memory impairment
    b. Disorientation to time and place
    c. Language disturbance, may be incoherent
    d. Perceptual disturbance (hallucinations and illusions)
8. Alterations in sleep-wake patterns
9. Fear and high levels of anxiety

Sample Questions to Ask

The nurse uses a variety of therapeutic techniques to obtain the answers to the following questions from either the client when lucid, or client's family and friends. Use your discretion and decide which questions are appropriate to complete your assessment.

1. Describe the onset of confusion and disorientation: Sudden? Gradual over a long period of time?
2. Does the individual's confusion and disorientation of time change during the day or night? What time of day or night is it the worst?
3. What medications or recreational drugs does the client take? How much did he or she last take and how much of each drug or medication was taken?

4. Describe previous episodes that were similar to this one. What were you told that caused this reaction?
5. What does the client (if lucid at that time) or family/friends think might be responsible from their knowledge of client's recent history?
6. What does the client (if lucid at that time) or family/friends believe will help or hinder the problem?

Assessment Guide

When assessing individuals with confusional states, it is helpful to use structured cognitive screening tests. A useful tool is the Folstein Mini Mental State examination (Box 12–2).

—	ASSESSMENT ALERTS

1. Assess for fluctuating levels of consciousness, which is **key** in delirium.
2. Interview family or other caregivers.
3. Assess for past confusional states (e.g., prior dementia diagnosis).
4. Identify other disturbances in medical status (e.g., dyspnea, edema, presence of jaundice).
5. Identify any EEG, neuroimaging, or lab abnormalities in client's record.
6. Assess potential for injury (is the client safe from falls, wandering).
7. Assess need for comfort measures (pain, cold, positioning).
8. Are immediate medical interventions available to help prevent irreversible brain damage?

◆ NURSING DIAGNOSIS AND INTERVENTIONS

Individuals experiencing delirium often misinterpret environmental cues (**illusions**) or imagine they see things (**hallucinations**) that they most likely believe are threatening or harmful. When clients act on these interpretations of their environment, they are likely to demonstrate a **Risk for Injury**. The symptoms of confusion usually fluctuate, and nighttime is the most severe (this is often called sundowning). Therefore, these clients often have **Sleep Pattern Disturbances**. During times of severe confusion, individuals are usually terrified, and are not able to care for their needs or interact appropriately with others, so **Fear, Self-Care Deficit**, and **Im-**

❖　　　　B O X　　1 2 – 2　　　　❖

Folstein's Mini Mental State Examination

Patient's Name: _____
Social Sec. #: _____
Examiner's Name: _____
Date Administered: _____

Assess the patient's level of consciousness along this continuum

Alert	Drowsy	Stupor	Coma

Maximum Score	Patient Score	
		Orientation
5	_____	What is the (year) (season) (date) (day) (month)?
5	_____	Where are we (state) (county) (town) (hospital) (floor)?
		Registration
3	_____	Remember these three words: cup pencil airplane Asked the patient to say all three. If patient fails to say one or more of the words, repeat all three again up to a maximum of 6 repetitions. Number of repetitions _____
		Attention and Calculation
5	_____	I want you to count backwards from 100 by sevens. Stop after 5 subtractions (93, 86, 79, 72, 65). Score one point for each correctly placed number.
		If patient refuses or will not attempt serial sevens, ask the patient to spell the word 'WORLD' backwards (D-L-R-O-W).
		Recall
3	_____	Please tell me the three words I gave you earlier.
		Language *Naming*
2	_____	Point to a pencil and a watch. Have the patient name them as you point.

Continued

1	_____	*Repetition* Ask the patient to repeat the following: "No ifs ands or buts"
3	_____	*Three Stage Command* Place a piece of paper in front of the patient and say: "Take the paper in your right hand, fold it in half and put it on the floor."
1	_____	*Reading* Ask the patient to read and obey the sentence on the bottom of the page.

"CLOSE YOUR EYES"

| 1 | _____ | *Writing*
On the following page ask the patient
to write a sentence. |
| 1 | _____ | *Copying*
Ask the patient to copy
the intersecting 5-angle
designs and give one
point if all sides and
angles are preserved
and if the intersecting
sides form a quadrangle. |

30	_____	**Total Score**
Maximum	**Patient**	
Score	**Score**	

Scoring: 0–12 (severe), 12–22 (moderate), 23–24 (mild),
25–30 (none). These ranges vary.

From Folstein, M., Folstein, S., and McHugh, P. (1975). Mini-Mental State: A practical method of grading the cognitive state of patients for the clinician. Journal of Psychiatric Research 12:189; reprinted with permission. © 1975, 1998 MiniMental LLC.

paired Social Interactions are also potential diagnoses. This section on delirium will deal with **Acute Confusion**, which covers many of the above problems.

Please note that many of the interventions, especially those for communication with the client with dementia, are also applicable to the delirious client when confused. These are discussed in the second half of the chapter. Table 12–1 identifies potential nursing diagnoses useful for all confused clients (delirium or dementia).

OVERALL GUIDELINES FOR NURSING INTERVENTIONS

1. Delirium, unlike dementia, is transitory when interventions are instituted and if delirium does not last a prolonged period of time. Therefore, **immediate intervention** for the underlying cause of the delirium is needed to prevent irreversible damage to the brain. Medical interventions are the first priority.
2. When clients are confused and frightened and are having a difficult time interpreting reality, they may be prone to accidents. Therefore, **SAFETY** is a high priority.
3. Delirium is a terrifying experience for many clients. When some individuals recover to their premorbid cognitive function, they are left with frightening memories and images. Some clinicians advocate preventive counseling and education after recovery from acute brain failure (Borson, 1997).
4. Refrain from using restraints. Encourage one or two significant others to stay with client to provide orientation and comfort by their presence.

Acute Confusion

The abrupt onset of a cluster of global, transient changes and disturbances in attention, cognition, psychomotor activity, level of consciousness, and/or sleep-wake cycle

Related To (Etiology)

- ◆ Over 60 years of age
- ◆ Dementia
- ◆ Alcohol abuse
- ◆ Drug abuse
- ◆ Delirium
- ● Metabolic disorder, neurological disorder, chemicals, medications, infections, fluid and electrolyte imbalances

As Evidenced By (Assessment Findings/Diagnostic Cues)

- ◆ Fluctuation in cognition
- ◆ Fluctuation in sleep-wake cycle
- ◆ Fluctuation in level of consciousness

◆ NANDA accepted; ● In addition to NANDA.

**Table 12–1 ◆ Potential Nursing Diagnoses—
Confused Client**

SYMPTOMS	NURSING DIAGNOSES
Wandering, unsteady gait, acts out fear from hallucinations or illusions, forgetting things (leaves stove on, doors open)	**Risk for Injury**
Awake disoriented during the night (**sundowning**), frightened at night	**Sleep Pattern Disturbance** **Fear** **Acute Confusion**
Too confused to take care of basic needs:	**Self-Care Deficit** **Ineffective Individual Coping** **Functional Incontinence** **Altered Nutrition** **Fluid Volume Deficit**
Sees frightening things that are not there (**hallucinations**), mistakes everyday objects for something sinister and frightening (**illusions**), may become paranoid thinking that others are doing things to confuse them (**delusions**)	**Sensory/Perceptual Alterations** **Impaired Environmental Interpretation Syndrome** **Altered Thought Processes**
Does not recognize familiar people or places, has difficulty with short- and/or long-term memory, forgetful and confused	**Impaired Memory** **Impaired Environmental Interpretation Syndrome** **Acute/Chronic Confusion**
Difficulty with communication, can't find words, difficulty in recognizing objects and/or people, incoherence	**Impaired Verbal Communication**
Devastated over losing their place in life as they know it (during lucid moments), fearful and overwhelmed by what is happening to them.	**Spiritual Distress** **Helplessness/Hopelessness** **Self-Esteem Disturbance** **Grieving**
Family and loved ones overburdened and overwhelmed, inability to care for client's needs.	**Ineffective Family Coping** **Altered Family Processes** **Impaired Home Maintenance** **Caregiver Role Strain**

◆ Agitation or restlessness
◆ Misperceptions of the environment (e.g., illusions, hallucinations)
◆ Lack of motivation to initiate and/or follow through with goal-directed or purposeful behavior

◆ NANDA accepted; ● In addition to NANDA.

Outcome Criteria

- Client will correctly state time/place and person within a few days.
- Client and others will remain free of harm throughout client's periods of confusion.

Short-Term Goals

- Client and others will remain safe during client's periods of agitation or aggressive behaviors.
- Clients will respond positively to staff efforts to orient them to time/place and person throughout periods of confusion.
- Clients will take medication as offered to help alleviate their condition.

Interventions and Rationales

Interventions	Rationale
1. Introduce self and call client by name at the beginning of each contact.	1. With short-term memory impairment, person is often confused and needs frequent orienting to time, place, and person.
2. Maintain face-to-face contact.	2. If client is easily distracted, he or she needs help to focus on one stimulus at a time.
3. Use short, simple, concrete phrases.	3. Client may not be able to process complex information.
4. Briefly explain everything you are going to do before doing it.	4. Explanation prevents misinterpretation of action.
5. Encourage the family and friends (one at a time) to take a quiet, supportive role.	5. Familiar presence lowers anxiety and increases orientation.
6. Keep room well lit.	6. Lighting provides accurate environmental stimuli to maintain and increase orientation.
7. Keep head of bed elevated.	7. Helps provide important environmental cues.
8. Provide clocks and calendars.	8. These cues help orient client to time.

Interventions	**Rationale**
9. Encourage client to wear prescribed eyeglasses or hearing aid.	9. Helps increase accurate perceptions of visual, auditory stimuli.
10. Make an effort to assign the same personnel on each shift to care for client.	10. Familiar faces minimize confusion and enhance nurse-client relationships.
11. When *hallucinations* are present, assure clients they are safe (e.g., "I know you are frightened. I'll sit with you a while and make sure you are safe.").	11. Client feels reassured that he or she is safe, and fear and anxiety often decrease.
12. When *illusions* are present, clarify reality (e.g., "This is a coat rack, not a man with a knife . . . see? You seem frightened. I'll stay with you for a while.").	12. With illusion, misinterpreted objects or sounds can be clarified, once pointed out.
13. Inform client of progress during lucid intervals.	13. Consciousness fluctuates: client feels less anxious knowing where he or she is and who you are during lucid periods.
14. Ignore insults and name calling, and acknowledge how upset the person may be feeling. For example: *Client*: You incompetent jerk, get me a real nurse, some one who knows what they are doing. *Nurse*: What you are going through is very difficult. I'll stay with you.	14. Terror and fear are often projected onto the environment. Arguing or becoming defensive only increases client's aggressive behaviors and defenses.
15. If client behavior becomes physically abusive: a. *First*, set limits on behavior (e.g., "Mr. Jones, you are not to hit me or anyone else. Tell me how you feel." *or*	15. Clear limits need to be set to protect client, staff, and others. Often client can respond to verbal commands. Chemical and physical restraints are used as a last resort, if at all.

"Mr. Jones, if you have difficulty controlling your actions, we will help you gain control.").

b. *Second*, check orders for use of chemical restraint.

16. After client returns to pre-morbid cognitive state, educate client and offer counseling for client's recollection of terrifying, frightening memories and images.	16. Client can believe his or her illusions or hallucinations were real, and it may take time for client to come to terms with the experience.

◆ DEMENTIA

Dementia is marked by progressive deterioration in intellectual function, memory, and ability to solve problems and learn new skills. Judgment and moral and ethical behaviors decline as personality is altered. Box 12–3 presents the DSM-IV diagnostic criteria for Dementia.

Unlike delirium, dementia may be of a primary nature and is usually NOT reversible. Dementia is usually a slow and insidious process progressing over months or years. Dementia affects memory and ability to learn new information, or to recall previously learned information. Dementia also compromises intellectual functioning and the ability to solve problems.

The most prevalent primary dementia is **dementia of the Alzheimer's type (DAT).** The second most common form of dementia is vascular dementia, which is caused by multiple strokes. Substances can also cause dementia (alcohol, inhalants, phencyclidine, piperidine), as can other medical conditions.

◆ ASSESSING FOR DEMENTIA

History

1. Assess for a history of depression. Depression can masquerade as dementia.
2. Does client have a medical condition that, if treated, could reverse some of the symptoms of dementia? (For example: Korsakoff's syndrome—treat with thiamine (B_1); pernicious anemia—treat with vitamin B_{12}; folic acid deficiency—supplement with folic acid.)

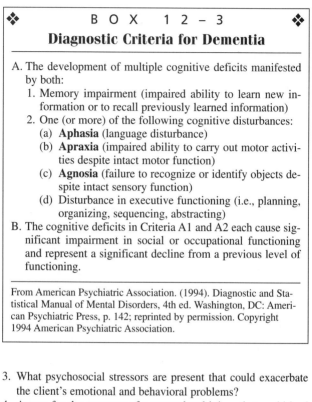

❖   B O X   1 2 – 3   ❖
Diagnostic Criteria for Dementia

A. The development of multiple cognitive deficits manifested by both:
  1. Memory impairment (impaired ability to learn new information or to recall previously learned information)
  2. One (or more) of the following cognitive disturbances:
    (a) **Aphasia** (language disturbance)
    (b) **Apraxia** (impaired ability to carry out motor activities despite intact motor function)
    (c) **Agnosia** (failure to recognize or identify objects despite intact sensory function)
    (d) Disturbance in executive functioning (i.e., planning, organizing, sequencing, abstracting)
B. The cognitive deficits in Criteria A1 and A2 each cause significant impairment in social or occupational functioning and represent a significant decline from a previous level of functioning.

From American Psychiatric Association. (1994). Diagnostic and Statistical Manual of Mental Disorders, 4th ed. Washington, DC: American Psychiatric Press, p. 142; reprinted by permission. Copyright 1994 American Psychiatric Association.

3. What psychosocial stressors are present that could exacerbate the client's emotional and behavioral problems?
4. Assess for the presence of a recent head injury that could lead to a subdural hematoma.
5. What does the neuropsychiatric examination show? Is there evidence of memory and concentration deficits?
6. Is delirium superimposed on a dementia, since they often coexist?
7. Because other medical conditions can often masquerade as dementia, a thorough examination is needed. Box 12–4 lists lab tests that can be used to help rule out all other pathophysiological conditions.

Presenting Signs and Symptoms

1. Memory impairment, usually short term first
2. Cognitive impairment (Goldberg, 1995):
  a. **Aphasia:** language disturbance, difficulty finding words, using words incorrectly

---

❖   B O X   1 2 – 4   ❖
Basic Work-up for Dementia

- Chest and skull x-ray studies
- Electroencephalography
- Electrocardiography
- Urinalysis
- Sequential multiple analyzer: 12-test serum profile
- Thyroid function tests
- Folate levels
- Venereal Disease Research Laboratories (VDRL), HIV tests
- Serum creatine assay
- Electrolyte assessment
- Vitamin B_{12} levels
- Vision and hearing evaluation
- Neuroimaging (when diagnostic issues are not clear)

---

   b. **Apraxia:** inability to carry out motor activities despite motor functions being intact (e.g., putting on ones pants, blouse, etc.)

   c. **Agnosia:** loss of sensory ability; inability to recognize or identify familiar objects, such as a toothbrush, or sounds, such as the ringing of the phone; loses ability to problem solve, plan, organize, or abstract

3. A significant decline in previous level of functioning; poor judgment

4. Mood disturbances, anxiety, hallucinations, delusions and impaired sleep often accompany dementia

Sample Questions

The nurse uses a variety of therapeutic techniques to obtain the answers to the following questions from the client, family members, and friends. Use your discretion and decide which questions are appropriate to complete your assessment.

1. Can the client manage complex tasks (e.g., balancing a checkbook)?

2. Does the client remember telephone numbers, names of family and friends, dates of important events?

3. Does the client complain of forgetting the location of familiar objects or forgetting information the client just heard?

4. Does the client try to hide the signs of impaired memory loss by using confabulation or anger or by rambling off of the topic?

5. Does the client exhibit mood swings, agitation, anger, anxiety, or other symptoms that are outside the client's usual personality profile?
6. Does the client experience **catastrophic reactions** (extreme over-reaction in clients with dementia to a seemingly neutral situation)?
7. Does the client wander or have an intense need to keep walking?
8. Does the client have difficulty finding and using the bathroom?

Assessment Guides

A variety of other medical problems may masquerade as dementia. For example, depression in the elderly is often misdiagnosed as dementia. Table 12–2 highlights the difference between dementia and depression and can be a useful guide for assessment.

At times it is important to distinguish dementia from delirium. Table 12–3 helps the nurse identify differences in the symptoms between one and the other. One always has to keep in mind that delirium may coexist with dementia, and that often clouds the picture.

	ASSESSMENT ALERTS
	1. Identify the underlying cause.
	2. How well is the family prepared and informed about the progress of the client's dementia (e.g., the phases and course of Alzheimer's disease, vascular dementia, AIDS-related dementia, multiple sclerosis, lupus, brain injury)?
	3. How is the family coping with the client? What are the main issues at this time?
	4. What resources are available to the family? Does the family get help from other family members, friends, and community resources? Is(are) the caregiver(s) aware of community support groups and resources?
	5. Obtain the data necessary to provide appropriate safety measures for the client.
	6. How safe is the client's home environment (e.g., wandering, eating inedible objects, falls, provocative behaviors toward others)?
	7. For what client behaviors could the family use teaching and guidance (e.g., catastrophic reaction, lability of mood, aggressive behaviors, nocturnal delirium [increased confusion and agitation at night; sundowning])?

Table 12–2 ◆ Dementia Versus Depression

DEMENTIA	DEPRESSION
1. Recent memory is impaired. In early stages, patient attempts to hide cognitive losses; is skillful at covering up.	1. Patient readily admits to memory loss; other cognitive disturbances may or may not be present.
2. Symptoms progress slowly and insidiously; difficult to pinpoint onset.	2. Symptoms are of relatively rapid onset.
3. Approximate or "near-miss" answers are typical; tries to answer.	3. "Don't know" answers are common; client does not try to recall or answer.
4. Client struggles to perform well but is frustrated.	4. Little effort to perform; is apathetic; seems helpless and pessimistic.
5. Affect is shallow or labile.	5. Depressive mood is pervasive.
6. Attention and concentration may be impaired.	6. Attention and concentration are usually intact.
7. Changes in personality (e.g., from cheerful and easygoing to angry and suspicious).	7. Personality remains stable.

From Varcarolis, E. (1998). Foundations of Psychiatric Mental Health Nursing, 3rd ed. Philadelphia: W.B. Saunders Company, p. 694; reprinted with permission.

◆ NURSING DIAGNOSES WITH INTERVENTIONS

The care of a client with dementia requires a great deal of patience and creativity. These clients have enormous needs, and put enormous demands on staff caring for demented clients, and on families who carry the burden at home. As some of these diseases progress, most notably Alzheimer's disease, so do the demands on the staff, caregivers, and family. Safety is always a major concern. **Risk for Injury** may be related to impaired mobility, sensory deficits, history of accidents, or lack of knowledge of safety precautions.

As time goes on, the person loses the ability to perform tasks that were once familiar and routine. The inability of the person to care for basic needs covers all areas (e.g., bathing, hygiene, grooming, feeding, and toileting). Therefore, **Self-Care Deficit** usually involves many functions. The goals are set up so that individuals can do as much for themselves as possible during each phase of the dementia.

Impaired Verbal Communication is often related to diminished comprehension, difficulty recognizing objects, aphasia, cerebral impairment, and severe memory impairment. Therefore, family and health care workers need to know ways to interact with a person with this nursing diagnosis.

Table 12–3 ◆ Nursing Assessment: Delirium Versus Dementia

	DELIRIUM	DEMENTIA
Onset	Acute impairment of orientation, memory, intellectual function, judgment, and affect.	Slow insidious deterioration in cognitive functioning.
Essential Feature	Disturbance in consciousness, fluctuating levels of consciousness, and cognitive impairment.	Progressive deterioration in memory, orientation, calculation, and judgment; symptoms do not fluctuate.
Cause	The syndrome is secondary to many underlying disorders that cause temporary, diffuse disturbances of brain function.	The syndrome is either *primary* in etiology or *secondary* to other disease states or conditions.
Course	The clinical course is usually brief (hour to days); prolonged delirium may lead to dementia.	Progresses over months or years; often irreversible.
Speech	May be slurred; reflects disorganized thinking.	Generally normal in early stages; progressive aphasia; confabulation.
Memory	Short-term memory impaired.	Short-term, then long-term, memory destroyed.
Perception	Visual or tactile hallucinations; illusions.	Hallucinations not prominent.
Mood	Fear, anxiety, and irritability most prominent.	Mood labile; previous personality traits become accentuated (e.g., paranoid, depressed, withdrawn, and obsessive-compulsive).
EEG	Pronounced diffuse slowing or fast cycles.	Normal or mildly slow.

From Varcarolis, E. (1998). Foundations of Psychiatric Mental Health Nursing, 3rd ed. Philadelphia: W.B. Saunders Company, p. 694; reprinted with permission.

The burden of caring for a family member with dementia can be enormous, especially over prolonged periods of time. Family members need a great deal of support, education, and guidance from community agencies and well-informed health care workers if they are to survive as a family. Families may experience **Compromised** or even **Disabling Ineffective Family Coping**, and this should always be addressed when it is recognized. Therefore, **Risk for** and/or **Caregiver Role Strain** needs to be part of the initial assessment, and must be continuously assessed as the dementia progresses. Most all families will need information, support, and periods of respite.

There are numerous nursing diagnoses that may be appropriate. Refer to Table 12–1 for nursing diagnoses for confused clients.

Risk for Injury

A state in which the individual is at risk of injury as a result of environmental conditions interacting with the individual's adaptive and defensive resources

---

Related To (Etiology)

- ◆ Sensory dysfunction
- ◆ Cognitive or emotional difficulties
- ◆ Chemical (drugs, alcohol)
- ◆ Biochemical
- ● Confusion, disorientation
- ● Faulty judgment
- ● Loss of short-term memory
- ● Lack of knowledge of safety precautions
- ● Previous falls
- ● Unsteady gait
- ● Wandering
- ● Provocative behavior

As Evidenced By (Assessment Findings/Diagnostic Cues)

- ● Getting into fights with others
- ● Choking on inedible object
- ● Wandering
- ● Burns
- ● Falls

◆ NANDA accepted; ● In addition to NANDA.

- Getting lost
- Poisoning—wrong medication, wrong dose

Outcome Criteria

- Client will remain free of fractures, bruises, contusions, and burns.
- With guidance and environmental manipulation, clients will not hurt themselves if a fall occurs.
- With the aid of identification bracelet and neighborhood or hospital alert and enrollment in Safe Return Program, client will be returned within 3 hours of wandering.
- Client will ingest only correct doses of prescribed medication and appropriate food and fluids.

Short-Term Goal

- Client will remain injury free whether at home or in the hospital with the aid of environmental manipulation and family or nursing staff precautions and interventions.

Interventions and Rationales

SAFE ENVIRONMENT

Intervention	**Rationale**
1. Restrict the use of car.	1. Impaired judgment can lead to accidents.
2. Remove throw rugs and other objects.	2. Minimizes tripping and falling.
3. Minimize sensory stimulation.	3. Decreases sensory overload, which can increase anxiety and confusion.
4. If clients become verbally upset, listen briefly, give support, then change the topic.	4. When attention span is short, clients can be distracted to more productive topics and activities.
5. Label all rooms and drawers with pictures. Label often-used objects (e.g., hairbrushes and toothbrushes).	5. May keep client from wandering into other client's rooms. Increases environmental clues to familiar objects.
6. Install safety bars in bathroom.	6. Prevents falls.

◆ NANDA accepted; ● In addition to NANDA.

7. Supervise clients when they smoke.	7. Danger of burns is always present.
8. If client wanders during the night, put mattress on the floor.	8. Prevents falls when client is confused.
9. Have client wear Medic Alert bracelet that cannot be removed (with name, address, and telephone number). Provide police department with recent pictures.	9. Client can easily be identified by police, neighbors, or hospital personnel.
10. Alert local police and neighbors about wanderer.	10. May reduce time necessary to return client to home or hospital.
11. Put complex locks on door.	11. Reduces opportunity to wander.
12. Place locks at top of door.	12. In moderate and late DAT, ability to look up and reach upward is lost.
13. Encourage physical activity during the day.	13. Physical activity may decrease wandering at night.
14. Explore the feasibility of installing sensor devices.	14. Provides warning if client wanders.
15. Enroll the client in the Alzheimer's Association's *Safe Return program (www.alz.org).*	15. Helps track individuals with dementia who wander and are at risk of getting lost or injured.

Self-Care Deficit

Inability to complete feeding, bathing, toileting, dressing, and grooming of self

---

Related To (Etiology)

◆ Perceptual or cognitive impairment
◆ Neuromuscular impairment
◆ Decreased strength and endurance
◆ Confusion

◆ NANDA accepted; ● In addition to NANDA.

- Apraxia (inability to perform once routine tasks)
- Severe memory impairment

As Evidenced By (Assessment Findings/Diagnostic Cues)

- ◆ Inability to wash body or body parts
- ◆ Impaired ability to put on or take off necessary items of clothing
- ◆ Inability to maintain appearance at a satisfactory level
- ◆ Inability to get to toilet or commode
- ◆ Inability to carry out proper toilet hygiene

Outcome Criteria

- Client's self-care needs will be met with optimal participation by client.
- Client will participate in self-care at optimal level with supervision and guidance.
- Client's skin will remain intact despite incontinence or prolonged pressure.
- Client will maintain nutrition, hygiene, dress, and toileting activities with appropriate support from others (caregivers, family, staff).

Short-Term Goals

Client will:

- Be able to follow step-by-step instructions for dressing, bathing, and grooming
- Put on own clothes appropriately with aid of fastening tape (Velcro) and supervision
- Participate in toilet training procedures
- Ingest adequate calories (1500 to 2200 calories/day)
- Maintain an adequate fluid intake (2400 to 3200 ml /day)

Interventions and Rationales

DRESSING AND BATHING

Intervention	**Rationale**
1. Always have clients perform all tasks that they are capable of.	1. Maintains self-esteem, uses muscle groups, and minimizes further regression.
2. Always have client wear own clothes, even if in the hospital.	2. Helps maintain client's identity and dignity.

◆ NANDA accepted; ● In addition to NANDA.

3. Use clothing with elastic, and substitute fastening tape (Velcro) for buttons and zippers.

3. Minimizes client's confusion and increases independence of functioning.

4. Label clothing items with client's name and name of item.

4. Helps identify client if they wander and gives clients additional clues when aphasia or agnosia occurs.

5. Give step-by-step instructions whenever necessary (e.g., "Take this blouse . . . put in one arm . . . now the next arm . . . pull it together in the front . . now . . .").

5. Client can focus on small pieces of information more easily; allows client to perform at optimum level.

NUTRITION

Intervention

Rationale

1. Monitor food and fluid intake.

1. Client may have anorexia or be too confused to eat.

2. Offer finger food that client can walk around with.

2. Increases input throughout the day; client may eat only small amounts at meals.

3. During period of hyperorality, watch that client does not eat nonfood items (e.g., ceramic fruit or food-shaped soaps).

3. Client puts everything into mouth; may be unable to differentiate inedible objects.

BOWEL AND BLADDER FUNCTION

Intervention

Rationale

1. Begin bowel and bladder program early; start with bladder control.

1. Same time of day for bowel movements and toileting—in early morning, after meals and snacks, and before bedtime—can help prevent incontinence.

2. Evaluate use of adult disposable undergarments.

2. Prevents embarrassment if incontinent.

3. Label bathroom door, as well as doors to other rooms, with a picture.

3. Additional environmental clues can maximize independent toileting. Pictures are more readily interpreted.

SLEEP

Intervention	**Rationale**
1. Because client may awaken frightened, and/or cry out at night, keep area well lit.	1. Reinforces orientation, minimizes possible illusions.
2. Nonbarbiturates may be ordered (e.g., chloral hydrate).	2. Barbiturates can have a paradoxical reaction, causing agitation.
3. Avoid the use of restraints.	3. Can cause client to become more terrified and fight against restraints until exhausted to a dangerous degree.

Impaired Verbal Communication

The state in which an individual experiences a decreased or absent ability to use or understand language in human interaction

---

Related To (Etiology)

◆ Decrease in circulation to the brain
◆ Physical barrier (e.g., brain tumor, subdural hematoma)
◆ Deterioration or damage to the neurological centers in the brain that regulate speech and language
◆ Biochemical changes in the brain/physiological conditions
● Severe memory impairment
● Escalating anxiety
● Delusions or illusions

As Evidenced By (Assessment Findings/Diagnostic Cues)

◆ Difficulty forming words or sentences
◆ Difficulty expressing thoughts verbally
◆ Speaks or verbalizes with difficulty
◆ Does not or cannot speak
◆ Has difficulty finding the right word for objects (aphasia)
● Has difficulty identifying objects (agnosia)
● Inability to focus or concentrate on a train of thought
● Impaired comprehension
● Refers back to first language

◆ NANDA accepted; ● In addition to NANDA.

Outcome Criteria

- Client will communicate basic needs with the use of visual and verbal clues when needed.
- Client will communicate important thoughts with the use of visual and verbal clues when needed.
- Client's family and caregivers demonstrate ability to minimize client's agitation and fear when client is delusional or having illusions.

Short-Term Goals

- Client's basic needs will be met when in the hospital (hydration and nutrition, hygiene, dress, bowel and bladder function).
- Client will learn to adopt alternative modes of communication with the use of nonverbal techniques (e.g., writing, pointing, demonstrating an action [pantomime]).
- Client's anxiety and fear will be decreased when delusions or illusions occur through the use of appropriate nursing techniques.

Interventions and Rationales

Follow the guidelines for intervention with a confused client in the first half of this chapter. Communication techniques **specific for dementia** follow.

Intervention	Rationale
1. Use a variety of nonverbal techniques to enhance communication: a. Point, touch, or demonstrate an action while talking about it. b. Ask clients to point to parts of their body or things that they want to communicate about. c. When client is searching for a particular word, guess at what is being said and ask if you are correct (e.g., "You are pointing to your mouth saying pain. Is it your dentures? No. Is your	1. Both delirium and dementia can pose huge communication problems, and often alternative nonverbal or verbal methods have to be used.

Intervention	Rationale
mouth sore? Yes. OK, let me take a look to see if I can tell what is hurting you."). Always ask client to confirm whether your guess is correct.	
d. Use of cue cards, flash cards, alphabet letters, signs, and pictures on doors to various rooms is often helpful for many clients and their families (e.g., bathroom, "Charles' bedroom"). Use of pictures is helpful when ability to read decreases.	
2. Encourage reminiscing about happy times in life.	2. Remembering accomplishments and shared joys helps distract client from deficit and gives meaning to existence.
3. If a client gets into an argument with another client, stop the argument and get them out of each other's way. After a short while (5 minutes), explain to each client matter-of-factly why you had to intervene.	3. Prevents escalation to physical acting out. Shows respect for client's right to know. Explaining in an adult manner helps maintain self-esteem.
4. Reinforce client's speech through pictures, nonverbal gestures, X's on calendars, and other methods used to anchor client in reality.	4. When aphasia starts to hinder communication, alternate methods of communication need to be instituted.

Burnside (1988) suggests useful guidelines for implementing nursing interventions or teaching a severely cognitively impaired person (see Box 12–5).

Caregiver Role Strain

A caregiver's felt or exhibited difficulty in performing the family caregiver role

❖   B O X   1 2 – 5   ❖
Guidelines for Caring for the Cognitively Impaired

1. Provide only one visual clue (object) at a time.
2. Know that the client may lack understanding of the task assigned.
3. Remember that relevant information is remembered longer than irrelevant information.
4. Break tasks into very small steps.
5. Give only one instruction at a time.
6. Report, record, and document all data.

Related To (Etiology)

◆ Severity of the care receiver's illness
◆ 24-hour care responsibility
◆ Duration of caregiving
◆ Lack of support from significant others
◆ Lack of respite and recreation for the caregiver
◆ Inadequate physical environment for providing care
◆ Family's and/or caregiver's isolation

As Evidenced By (Assessment Findings/Diagnostic Cues)

◆ Difficulty in performing required activities
◆ Altered caregiver health status (hypertension, cardiovascular disease, etc.)
◆ Inability to complete caregiving tasks
● Expressions by caregiver(s) of:
  • Feelings of stress in relationship with client
  • Feelings of anger and/or depression
  • Family conflict regarding issues of providing care
  • Feelings that caregiving interferes with other important roles in their lives

Outcome Criteria

Caregivers will:

• State that they have help from family and/or friends, and /or the community that has helped stabilize their situation
• Demonstrate adaptive coping strategies for dealing with the stress of the caregiver role

---

◆ NANDA accepted; ● In addition to NANDA.

- Demonstrate effective problem-solving techniques they use to deal with issues of caring for their family member
- Identify resources they can use when new situations arise that appear to need new coping strategies
- State that they now maintain social relationships with other individuals and families as evidenced by involvement in community groups, with extended family members, and with friends

Short-Term Goals

Caregivers will:

- State they understand and have written information on their family member's/friend's type of dementia (e.g., Alzheimer's disease, multi-infarct dementia) and appropriate caregiving techniques by (date)
- Know and discuss the available resources in their community, national resources, and sites on the Internet that will provide information, support, and how to arrange respite by (date)
- Identify at least three steps they can take to relieve some of the family stress and enhance well-being to all members of the family unit by (date)
- Learn at least three new coping strategies and coping mechanisms to diffuse the tension and strain on caregiver and family by (date)
- Care for their own needs through diet, exercise and plenty of rest and give five examples of healthy changes by (date)
- Be aware of where to go to get legal and financial planning advice early in the disease process by (date)
- Acknowledge realistic goals of treatment for their family member by (date)

Interventions and Rationales

Intervention	Rationale
1. Assess what caregivers and family know about client's dementia, and educate regarding the client's specific illness.	1. Point out areas that will benefit from planning and preparation (e.g., legal issues, financial issues, additional caregiving techniques, and knowing what they can and what they cannot change or accomplish).
2. Provide a list of community agencies and support groups where family and primary	2. Help diminish a sense of hopelessness and increase a sense of empowerment.

caregiver can receive support, further education, and information regarding how to arrange respite.

3. Help the caregiver and family to identify areas that need intervention, and those areas that are presently stable.

3. Identify specific areas needing assistance, and those that will need assistance in the future.

4. Teach the caregiver and family specific interventions to use in response to behavioral or social problems brought on by the dementia.

4. Caregivers need to learn many new ways to intervene in situations that are common with demented clients (agitation, catastrophic reactions, sleep-wake disturbances, wandering).

5. Safety is a major concern. Box 12–6 identifies some steps that caregiver(s) and family can take to make the home a safer place.

5. These steps prepared by the Alzheimer's Association can help make the home safe for the person with dementia.

6. Encourage spending non-stressful time with the client at client's present level of functioning (e.g., watching a favorite movie together, reading with client a simple book with pictures, performing simple tasks like setting the table, washing dishes, washing the car).

6. Encourages the client to participate as much as possible in family life. Helps diminish feelings of isolation and alienation temporarily.

7. Encourage caregiver/family members to follow family traditions (church activities, holidays, and vacations).

7. Helps family maintain their family rituals and helps client's sense of belonging.

8. Encourage caregiver(s)/family members to use respite care during regular intervals (e.g., vacations).

8. Regular periods of respite can help caregivers/family prevent burnout, allow caregivers to continue participating in their life

❖   B O X   1 2 – 6   ❖
Home Safety

Make Potentially Dangerous Places Less Accessible
- Install door locks out of sight
- Use special safety devices, such as child-proof locks and door knobs, to limit access to places where knives, appliances, equipment and cleaning fluids are stored

Accommodate Visual Changes
- Add extra lighting in entries, outside landings, areas between rooms, stairways and bathrooms because changes in level of light can be disorienting
- Place contrasting colored rugs in front of doors or steps to help the individual anticipate staircases and room entrances

Avoid Injury During Daily Activities
- Monitor the temperature of water faucets and food because the person may have a decreased sensitivity to temperature
- Install walk-in showers, grab bars, and decals to slippery surfaces in the bathroom to prevent falls
- Supervise the person in taking prescription and over-the-counter medications

Beware of Hazardous Objects and Substances
- Limit the use of certain appliances and equipment such as mixers, grills, knives and lawnmowers
- Supervise smoking and alcohol consumption
- Remove objects, such as coffee tables, floor lamps, to create safe wandering areas and to reduce the possibility of injury

Be Prepared for Emergencies
- Keep a list of emergency phone numbers and addresses for the local police departments, hospitals and poison control help lines
- Check fire extinguishers and smoke alarms, and conduct fire drills regularly
- If the person with Alzheimer's tends to wander, enroll him or her in the **Safe Return program**.

Intervention	Rationale
	and can help minimize feelings of resentment.
9. Identify financial burdens placed on caregiver/family. Refer to community, national associations, or other resources that may help.	9. Any kind of long-term illness within a family can place devastating financial burdens on all members.

◆ PSYCHOPHARMACOLOGY FOR DEMENTIA

Alzheimer's disease is the most common dementia accounting for 70% of all dementias (Goldberg, 1995), and is the fourth most prevalent cause of death in the adult population. Cholinesterase inhibitors can help in Alzheimer's dementia. One example is tacrine (Cognex), which can modestly help mild to moderate dementia by reversing 6 months of dementia's progression. Significant effects can be seen in 6 weeks. The most serious side effect and the main reason for discontinuation of the drug is elevation of liver chemistries (aspartate transaminase, alanine transaminase). The drug may also alter hematocrit, hemoglobin, and electrolytes.

Donepezil (Aricept), another cholinesterase inhibitor, also appears to cut down deterioration in cognitive functions in individuals with mild to moderate dementia, but without the serious liver toxicity attributed to tacrine.

Other Agents Used for Targeting Specific Symptoms in Dementia

Agitation and Aggression (Maxmen and Ward, 1995)

- **Hypoanxiolytics (lorazepam 0.5 mg PO)** have less drug accumulation and induce less confusion than do longer-acting anxiolytics. Watch for sedation/falls.
- **Trazodone (Desyrel; doses between 25 and 500 mg/day)**, and **buspirone (Buspar; doses between 10 and 60 mg/day)** can decrease agitation and aggression without decreasing cognitive performance.

Anxiety

Buspirone (Buspar) is not a sedative and does not produce many unwanted side effects, such as psychomotor impairment, drowsiness, or cognitive impairment. For this reason many prefer this drug to the benzodiazepines.

Depression

The **SSRIs** are effective and are tolerated better than drugs with high anticholinergic side effects, such as the TCAs. Tricyclics also produce orthostasis (leading to falls or fractures) and cardiac conduction delays (Goldberg, 1995). Useful medications included in this group are fluoxetine (Prozac), paroxetine (Paxil), sertraline (Zoloft), and nefazodone (Serzone)

Psychotic Features (Hallucinations and Delusions)

The newer atypical antipsychotics have been found to help clear client's thinking but do not have the more troubling and potentially serious side effect profile of the standard (phenothiazine-like). Appropriate atypical drugs include: olanzapine (Zyprexa), quetiapine (Seroquel), and risperidone (Risperdal)

♦ NURSE, CLIENT, AND FAMILY RESOURCES — COGNITIVE DISORDERS

Associations

Alzheimer's Disease and Related Disorders Association
919 North Michigan Avenue, Suite 1000
Chicago, IL 60611-1676
1-312-335-8700; 1-800-272-3900
(For caregivers of Alzheimer's clients)

Alzheimer's Disease Education and Referral Center
Hotline: 1-800-438-4380
(Information, referrals, publications regarding clinical trials)

Internet Sites

Alzheimer's Association
http://www.alz.org

Alzheimer Society of Canada
http://www.alzheimer.ca

Yahoo's Alzheimer's Disease Links
http://www.yahoo.com

Infoseek's Alzheimer's Disease Links
http://www.infoseek.com

PART III

PHENOMENA THAT MAY REQUIRE CLINICAL INTERVENTION

# CHAPTER 13

Suicide Behaviors

lthough suicide is a behavior that needs careful assessment in depression, alcoholism/substance abuse, schizophrenia, and personality disorders (borderline, paranoid, and anti-social), suicide is not necessarily synonymous with mental disorders. Up to 50% of all suicidal individuals seen in therapy do not qualify for a DSM-IV disorder (Axis I or II disorder) (Chiles and Strosahl, 1997).

Physical illness may play a role in suicide behavior (pain, recent surgery, chronic physical illness). Suicide seems to be most prevalent among clients with diseases that result in suffering and dependency, such as AIDS and cancer. Therefore, we as nurses may encounter suicidal individuals in outpatient settings, intensive care units, nursing homes, or medical/surgical units; during home visits; or even among one's own circle of family and friends. People who are taking medications that contribute to depression and psychotic symptoms could also be at risk.

Suicide does seem to cluster in some families; therefore, family history is pertinent. This could be the result of inherited markers for depression, learned problem-solving behavior within the family, inherited low cerebrospinal fluid levels of 5-hydroxyindole-acetic acid (low levels of which are associated with higher risk of attempted suicide), or some other genetic factor associated with suicide.

Suicidal people may share other commonalities. They are often poor problem solvers, have troubled emotional lives (depression, anger, anxiety, guilt, and/or boredom), have a low threshold for emotional pain, are often impulsive, and may engage in extreme solutions sooner than non–suicide-prone individuals (Chiles and Strosahl, 1997). People who are isolated (have poor social supports) and people who are experiencing severe life stress at any age may also be at risk. Risk factors for age were compiled by the National Institute of Mental Health (1995) as follows:

355

- The strongest risk factors for *youth* are alcohol or other drug use disorders and aggressive or disruptive behaviors. Depression and social isolation are also risk factors. Suicide in youths is the second leading cause of death following accidents.
- The strongest risk factors for *adults* are depression, alcohol abuse, cocaine use, and separation or divorce.
- Most *elderly* suicides have visited their primary care physician in the month before suicide. Recognition and treatment of depression in the medical setting is a promising way to prevent suicide in the elderly. Other risk factors include social isolation, solitary living arrangements, widowhood, lack of financial resources, and poor health. The elderly commit suicide more than any other group in the United States.

◆ ASSESSING POTENTIAL FOR SUICIDE

History

1. Past history of suicidal attempts or self-mutilation
2. Family history of suicide attempts or completion
3. History of a mood disorder, drug or alcohol abuse, or schizophrenia
4. History of chronic pain, recent surgery, or chronic physical illness
5. Client has a history of personality disorder (borderline, paranoid, antisocial)
6. Client is experiencing a bereavement or other significant loss (divorce, job, home)

Presenting Symptoms

1. Presents with:
   a. Suicidal ideation—thoughts of harming self
   b. Suicidal threat—communicates desire to harm/kill self
   c. Suicide attempt, failed—attempted to kill self
   d. Deliberate self-harm syndrome—clients who mutilate their bodies
2. A high degree of hopelessness, helplessness, and anhedonia, which are crucial factors in suicide

Assessing Risk Factors for Suicide

There are a number of tools one can use to assess for risk factors when assessing for potential suicidal behaviors. An acronym can facilitate the health care worker's recall when in the midst of crisis situations. One such acronym, the SAD PERSONS Scale (Patterson et al., 1983), is presented in Table 13–1.

Table 13–1 ◆ Nursing Assessment: SAD PERSONS Scale

S	Sex	Men kill themselves three times more than women, although women make attempts three times more often than men.
A	Age	High-risk groups: 19 years or younger; 45 years or older, especially the elderly 65 years or over.
D	Depression	Studies report that 35–79% of those who attempt suicide manifested a depressive syndrome.
P	Previous attempts	Of those who commit suicide, 65–70% have made previous attempts.
E	ETOH	ETOH (alcohol) is associated with up to 65% of successful suicides. Estimates are that 15% of alcoholics commit suicide. Heavy drug use is considered to be in this group and is given the same weight as alcohol.
R	Rational thinking loss	People with functional or organic psychoses (schizophrenia, dementia) are more apt to commit suicide than those in the general population.
S	Social supports lacking	A suicidal person often lacks significant others (friends, relatives), meaningful employment, and religious or spiritual supports. All three of these areas need to be assessed.
O	Organized plan	The presence of a specific plan for suicide (date, place, means) signifies a person at high risk.
N	No spouse	Repeated studies indicate that people who are widowed, separated, divorced, or single are at greater risk than those who are married.
S	Sickness	Chronic, debilitating, and severe illness is a risk factor. Suicide risk is two times higher among people with cancer and is high among AIDS clients; clients on hemodialysis or with DTs and respiratory diseases are all at high risk.

POINTS	GUIDELINES FOR INTERVENTION
0–2	Treat at home with follow-up care.
3–4	Closely follow up and consider possible hospitalization.
5–6	Strongly consider hospitalization.
7–10	Hospitalize.

Adapted from Patterson, W., et al. (1983). Evaluation of suicidal patients. The SAD PERSONS Scale. Psychosomatics, 24(4):343; reprinted with permission.

If individuals state they do have a *plan* of how to kill themselves, it is important to ascertain concrete behavioral information in order to assess the measure of lethality. Shea (1998) suggests the following steps:

1. Find out what plans have been contemplated.
2. Determine how far the person took actions or plans to take action on these plans.
3. Determine how much of the person's time is spent on these plans and accompanying ruminations about suicide.
4. Determine how accessible and lethal the mode of action is.

Sample Questions

The nurse uses a variety of therapeutic techniques to obtain the answers to the following questions. Use your discretion and decide which questions are appropriate to complete your assessment.

1. "When was the first time you thought about hurting/killing yourself?"
2. "Do you believe now that you want to die?"
3. "Have you recently/in the last month made any plans to hurt/kill yourself?" If yes, "Tell me about this."
4. "When you have suicidal thoughts, how long do they last?"
5. "How much control do you have over these thoughts?"
6. "Has something specifically happened that brings (brought) on these thoughts?" (e.g., a loss [separation, divorce, death, job], move, drugs, physical abuse, financial disaster)
7. "Have you planned how you might hurt yourself?"
8. "Do you have the means to carry out your plan?"
9. "What would keep you from taking your life at this point?"
   a. Lack of a reason to live or lack of any future planning implies higher risk.
   b. Reasons to live (children, religion, future plans) mitigates the risk.

	ASSESSMENT ALERTS
	1. Assess risk factors, including history of suicide (family, client, friends), degree of hopelessness, helplessness, and anhedonia; and lethality of plan.
	2. Determine the appropriate level of suicide precautions for the client (physician or nurse clinician), even in the emergency room. If client is at a high risk, hospitalization may be necessary.

Continued

3. A red flag goes up if the client suddenly goes from sad/depressed to happy and seemingly peaceful. Often a decision to suicide "gives a way out of severe emotional pain."
4. If the client is to be managed on an outpatient basis, then:
   • Assess social supports.
   • Assess friends' and family's knowledge of signs and symptoms of potential suicidal behavior (e.g., increasing withdrawal, preoccupation, silence, and remorse).
   • Identify community supports and groups the client and family could use for support.

◆ NURSING DIAGNOSES WITH INTERVENTIONS

A sound assessment provides the framework for determining the level of protection the client warrants at that time. Therefore, **Risk for Violence: Self-Directed** is the first area of concern.

Believing that one's situation or problem is intolerable, inescapable, and interminable leads to feelings of hopelessness. Therefore, **Hopelessness** is most often a crucial phenomenon requiring intervention.

A third area of intervention is to tackle the phenomenon of "tunnel vision" that suicidal clients have during times of acute stress and pain. That is, problem-solving skills are poor, and suicidal people have difficulty in performing flexible cognitive operations. Therefore, teaching the client, or reinforcing the client's own, effective problem-solving skills and helping him or her reframe life difficulties as events over which control can be exercised is a strategic part of the counseling process with suicidal clients. Thus, **Ineffective Individual Coping** can be viewed as the third leg of intervention. Other potential nursing diagnoses include **Helplessness, Loneliness, Low/Chronic Low Self-Esteem, Knowledge Deficit, Social Isolation, and Ineffective Family Coping**.

OVERALL GUIDELINES FOR NURSING INTERVENTIONS

Hospitalized: Put on Suicide Precautions

• Suicide precautions range from arms'-length constraint (one-to-one with staff member at arms length at all times), to one-to-one contact with staff at all

Continued

times but may attend activities off the unit maintaining one-to-one contact, to knowing the client's whereabouts at all times on the unit and accompanied by staff while off the unit.

- If there is fear of imminent harm, restraints may be required.
- ***Follow unit protocols and keep detailed records in client chart.***

Outside the Hospital

- If a client is to be managed outside the hospital, the family, significant other, or friends should be alerted to the risk and treatment plan and informed of signs of deepening depression, such as a return or worsening of hopelessness.
- When the client is to be managed on an outpatient basis (Slaby, 1994), then:
  - * Social support should be rallied.
  - * Appropriate psychopharmacotherapy, psychotherapy, or sociotherapy should be initiated.
  - * Clients and their family and friends should be given the psychiatric clinician's telephone number as well as that of a backup clinician or emergency room where they can go if the clinician is unavailable.
  - * A return visit (even the next day if it is felt the decision to not hospitalize may need to be reconsidered) should be scheduled.
  - * Friends and family should be alerted to signs such as increasing withdrawal, preoccupation, silence, remorse, and sudden change from sad to happy and "worry-free."
  - * Careful records should be kept in all instances documenting specific reasons why a client was or was not hospitalized.
- If the client is to be managed on an outpatient basis, then medication should be given in limited amount (e.g., 5-day supply with no refill).

If an Accepted Procedure at Your Facility/Clinic:

- Form a written no-suicide contract with the client, such as "I will not kill myself for any reason, and if I should feel suicidal, I will (a) talk to a staff member, or (b) talk to my therapist." (If accepted procedure at your institution.)
- List support people and agencies to use as outpatient and crisis hotline numbers for clients/family/friends.

Risk for Self-Directed Violence

Behaviors in which an individual demonstrates that he or she can be physically, emotionally, and/or sexually harmful to self

Related To (Etiology)

◆ Age 15–19; age over 45; marital status (single, widowed, divorced)
◆ Manic excitement/panic states/cognitive disorders
◆ Spouse/child abuse
◆ History of multiple suicide attempts
◆ Rage reaction/anger/hostility
◆ Recent loss(es) (e.g., job, home, relationship, death, divorce, health)
◆ Severe depression/psychosis/severe personality disorder, substance abuse
● Hopelessness, helplessness, anhedonia
● Loneliness
● Panic attacks

As Evidenced By (Assessment Findings/Diagnostic Cues)

◆ Suicidal behavior (attempt, talk, ideation, plan, available means)
◆ Suicide plan (clear and specific, lethal method and available means)
● Suicidal cues
  • **Overt**—"No one will miss me"; "Nothing left to live for"; "I'd be better off dead"
  • **Covert**—Making out a will, giving valuables away, writing forlorn love notes, taking out large life insurance policy
● Statements of despair, hopelessness, helplessness, and nothing left to live for

Outcome Criteria

Clients will:

• State they want to live
• Name two people they can call if thoughts of suicide reoccur
• Name at least one acceptable alternative to their situation

Short-Term Goals

Client will:

• Remain safe while in the hospital with aid of nursing intervention and support (if in the hospital)

◆ NANDA accepted; ● In addition to NANDA.

- Make a no-suicide contract with the nurse covering the next 24 hours, then renegotiate the terms at that time (if in hospital and accepted at your institution)
- Stay with a friend or family if person still has potential for suicide (if in the community)
- Keep an appointment for the next day with a crisis counselor (if in the community)
- Join family in crisis family counseling
- Have links to self-help groups in the community, as will family

Interventions and Rationales

IN THE HOSPITAL

Intervention	**Rationale**
1. During the crisis period, health care workers will continue to emphasize the following four points: a. The crisis is temporary. b. Unbearable pain can be survived. c. Help is available. d. You are not alone.	1. Because of "tunnel vision" clients do not have perspective on their lives. These statements give perspective to the client and helps offer hope for the future.
2. **Follow unit protocol** for suicide regarding creating a safe environment (taking away potential weapons—belts, sharps, ties, glass items, etc. (See Box 13–1 for ensuring hospital safety.)	2. Provide safe environment during time client is actively suicidal and impulsive; self-destructive acts are perceived as the only way out of an intolerable situation.
3. Put on either *suicide precaution* (one-to-one monitoring at one arm's length away) or *suicide observation* (15-minute visual check of mood, behavior, and verbatim statements), depending on level of suicide potential.	3. Protection of client's life at all costs during crisis is part of medical and nursing staff responsibility to preserve life. **Follow hospital protocol.**
4. Keep accurate and timely records, document client's activity usually every 15 minutes (what client is	4. Accurate documentation is vital. Chart is a legal document as to client's "ongoing status" and

---

❖ B O X   1 3 – 1   ❖

Guidelines for a Safe Hospital Environment

1. Use plastic utensils.
2. Do not allow clients to spend too much time alone in their rooms. Do not assign to a private room.
3. Jump-proof and hang-proof the bathrooms by installing break-away shower rods and recessed shower nozzles.
4. Keep electrical cords to minimal length.
5. Install unbreakable glass in windows. Install tamper-proof screens or partitions too small to pass through. Keep all windows locked.
6. Lock all utility rooms, kitchens, adjacent stairwells, and offices. All nonclinical staff (e.g., housekeepers and maintenance workers) should receive instructions to keep doors locked.
7. Take all potentially harmful gifts (e.g., flowers in glass vases) from visitors before allowing them to see clients.
8. Go through client's belongings with client and remove all potentially harmful objects (e.g., belts, shoelaces, metal nail files, tweezers, matches, and razors).
9. Take care that client doesn't hoard medical supplies (e.g., IV tubing) or, if on an IV, client is carefully observed.
10. Ensure that visitors do not leave potentially harmful objects in client's room (e.g., matches and nail files).
11. Search clients for harmful objects (e.g., drugs, sharp objects, and cords) on return from pass.

Data from Schultz, B.M. (1982). Legal Liability in Psychotherapy. San Francisco: Jossey-Bass Publishing.

---

doing, whom with, etc.).
Follow unit protocols.

5. Construct a *no suicide contract* between the suicidal client and nurse. Use clear, simple language. When contract is up, it is renegotiated. (If accepted procedure at your institution.)

6. Encourage clients to talk about their feelings and problem solve alternatives.

interventions taken and by whom.

5. The no suicide contract helps clients know what to do when they begin to feel overwhelmed by pain (e.g., "I will speak to my nurse/counselor/support group/family member when I first begin to feel the wish to harm myself.").

6. Talking about feelings and looking at alternatives can minimize suicidal acting out.

INTERVENTION IN THE COMMUNITY

Intervention	Rationale
1. Arrange for client to stay with family or friends. If no one is available and the person is highly suicidal, hospitalization must be considered.	1. Relieve isolation and provide safety and comfort.
2. Weapons and pills are removed by friends, relatives, or the nurse.	2. To help ensure safety.
3. Encourage clients to talk freely about feelings (anger, disappointments) and help plan alternative ways of handling anger and frustration.	3. Gives clients alternative ways of dealing with overwhelming emotions and gaining a sense of control over their life.
4. Encourage client to avoid decisions until alternatives can be considered during the time of crisis.	4. During crisis situations, people are unable to think clearly or evaluate their options.
5. Contact family members, arrange for individual and/or family crisis counseling. Activate links to self-help groups.	5. Re-establishes social ties. Diminishes sense of isolation, and provides contact from individuals who care about the suicidal person.
6. If anxiety is extremely high, or client has not slept in days, a tranquilizer may be prescribed. **ONLY a 1- to 3-day supply of medication should be given. Family member or significant other could monitor pills for safety.**	6. Relief of anxiety and restoration of sleep loss can help the client think more clearly and may help restore some sense of well-being.

Hopelessness

A subjective state in which an individual sees limited or no alternatives or personal choices available and is unable to mobilize energy on own behalf

Related To (Etiology)

- ◆ Failing or deteriorating physiological conditions (AIDS, cancer)
- ◆ Prolonged isolation
- ◆ Long-term stress
- ◆ Abandonment
- ◆ Lost belief in transcendent values/God
- ● Chronic pain
- ● Perceived helplessness, powerlessness
- ● Loss of significant support system(s)
- ● Severe stressful event(s) (financial reversals, relationship turmoil, loss of job)
- ● Perceiving the future as bleak and wasted

As Evidenced By (Assessment Findings/Diagnostic Cues)

- ◆ Passivity, decreased verbalization
- ◆ Decreased affect
- ◆ Verbal cues (despondent content: "I can't"; "Life is hopeless"; "What's the use?"; "There is no way out")
- ◆ Lack of involvement in care
- ◆ Turning away from speaker
- ◆ Lack of initiative
- ● Decreased judgment
- ● Decreased problem solving
- ● Lack of motivation
- ● Loss of interest in life
- ● Impaired decision making

Outcome Criteria

Client will:

- State three optimistic expectations for the future by (date)
- Demonstrate reframing skills when viewing aspects of client's life that appear all negative by (date)
- Demonstrate two new problem-solving skills that client finds effective in making life decisions by (date)
- Describe and plan for at least two future-orientated goals by (date)

Short-Term Goals

Client will:

- Identify two alternatives for one life problem area by (date)
- Identify three things that they are doing right by (date)

◆ NANDA accepted; ● In addition to NANDA.

- Reframe two problem areas in their life that encourage problem-solving alternative solutions
- Make two decisions related to their care by (date)
- Name one community resource (support group, counseling, social service, family counseling) that they have attended at least twice

Interventions and Rationales

Intervention	Rationale
1. Teach client steps in the problem-solving process.	1. Stress that it is not so much *people* who are ineffective, but rather it's often the coping strategies they are using that are not effective.
2. Encourage clients to look into their negative thinking, and reframe negative thinking into neutral objective thinking.	2. Cognitive reframing helps people look at situations in ways that allow for alternative approaches.
3. Point out unrealistic and perfectionistic thinking.	3. Constructive interpretations of events and behavior open up more realistic and satisfying options for the future.
4. Work with client to identify strengths.	4. When people are feeling overwhelmed, they no longer view their lives or behavior objectively.
5. Spend time discussing client's dreams and wishes for the future. Identify short-term goals they can set for the future.	5. Renewing realistic dreams and hopes can give promise to the future and meaning to life.
6. Identify things that gave meaning and joy to life. Discuss how these things can be reincorporated into their present lifestyle (e.g., religious or spiritual beliefs, group activities, creative endeavors).	6. Reawakens in client abilities and experiences that tapped areas of strength and creativity. Creative activities give people intrinsic pleasure and joy, and a great deal of life satisfaction.

> # Ineffective Individual Coping
>
> Inability to form a valid appraisal of the stressors, inadequate choices of practical responses, and/or inability to use available resources

Related To (Etiology)

- ◆ Situational or maturational crises
- ◆ Disturbance in pattern of tension release
- ◆ Inadequate opportunity to prepare for stressor
- ◆ Inadequate resources available
- ◆ Inadequate social support created by characteristics of relationship
- ● Inadequate coping skills
- ● Poorly developed social skills
- ● Personal loss or threat of rejection
- ● Impulsive use of extreme solutions

As Evidenced By (Assessment Findings/Diagnostic Cues)

- ◆ Lack of goal-directed behavior
- ◆ Verbalization of inability to cope or inability to ask for help
- ◆ Abuse of chemical agents
- ◆ Inability to meet basic needs
- ◆ Decreased use of social supports
- ◆ Inability to problem solve
- ◆ Poor problem solving
- ◆ Destructive behavior toward self or others
- ◆ Inability to meet role expectations
- ◆ Use of forms of coping that might impede adaptive behavior
- ◆ Change in usual communication pattern
- ◆ Expression of anxiety, depression, fear, impatience, frustration, and/or discouragement

Outcome Criteria

Clients will:

- • Demonstrate an absence of self-destructive behaviors
- • Demonstrate adaptive behaviors in dealing with emotional pain

---

◆ NANDA accepted; ● In addition to NANDA.

- Name two persons to whom they can talk if suicidal thoughts recur in the future
- State that they believe their life has value and that they have an important role to play (mother, son, husband, father, provider, friend, job-related position, etc.)

Short-Term Goals

Clients will:

- Discuss with the nurse/counselor at least three situations that trigger suicidal thoughts, and feelings about these situations by (date)
- Name two effective ways to handle difficult situations in the future by (date)
- State that they feel comfortable with one new coping technique after three sessions of role playing by (date)

Interventions and Rationales

Intervention	Rationale
1. Identify situations that trigger suicidal thoughts.	1. Identify targets for learning more adaptive coping skills.
2. Assess client's strengths and positive coping skills (talking to others, creative outlets, social activities, problem-solving abilities).	2. Use these to build upon and draw from in planning alternatives to self-defeating behaviors.
3. Assess client's coping behaviors that are not effective and that result in negative emotional sequelae: drinking, angry outbursts, withdrawal, denial, procrastination.	3. Identify areas to target for teaching and planning strategies for supplanting more effective and self-enhancing behaviors.
4. Role play with client adaptive coping strategies that client can use when situations that lead to suicidal thinking begin to emerge.	4. Not all new coping strategies may be effective. *The idea is that the nurse and client work together to find what does work, and that there is no ONE RIGHT way to behave.*
5. Assess need for assertiveness training. Assertive-	5. When people have difficulty getting their needs

ness skills can help client develop a sense of control and balance.

met or asking for what they need, frustration and anger can build up, leading to, in some cases, ineffective outlets for stress.

6. Clarify those things that are not under the person's control. One *cannot* control another's actions, likes, choices, or health status.

6. Recognizing one's limitations in controlling others is, paradoxically, a beginning to finding one's strength.

7. Assess client's social supports.

7. Have client experiment with attending at least two chosen possibilities.

◆ CLIENT AND FAMILY RESOURCES—SUICIDE

Associations

American Foundation for Suicide Prevention
120 Wall Street, 22nd Floor
New York, NY 10005
1-888-333-2377; 1-212-363-3500
http://www.afsp.org

American Suicide Foundation
1045 Park Avenue, Suite 3C
New York, NY 10028
1-800-ASF-4042; 1-212-410-1111
(Provides referrals to national support groups for suicide survivors)

American Association of Suicidology
4201 Connecticut Avenue NW, Suite #310
Washington, DC 20008
1-202-237-2280

Friends for Survival
P.O. Box 214463
Sacramento, CA 95821
1-916-392-0664; 1-800-646-7322
(For family, friends, and professionals after a suicide death)

Ray of Hope
P.O. Box 2323
Iowa City, IA 52244
1-319-337-9890

SOSAD (Save Our Sons and Daughters)
1-313-361-5200
(For family and friends of survivors of homicide and suicide)

Internet Sites

Suicide Awareness Voices of Education
http://www.save.org

The Samaritans
http://www.samaritans.org.uk/

(If You Are Thinking About) Suicide . . . Read This First
http://www.metanoia.org/suicide/

Suicide@rochford.org
http://www.rochford.org/suicide

C H A P T E R   1 4

Anger and Aggression

People who are prone to acting out anger and assaultive behavior are becoming an increasing public health concern. An increase in such behaviors has become a national concern, and anger is now being recognized as a crucial problem area. Severe angry episodes are experienced by as much as 20% of the population (Suinn, 1998). One example is the phenomenon of "road rage." Another example is the need to develop programs to train flight attendants to deal with aggression and assaultive behavior by passengers in flight. Child/family abuse, community property damage, dysfunctional work performance, and physical or verbal assaults are the result of inappropriate and destructive acting out of anger.

Anger is a universal emotion, perhaps one of the most difficult for people to deal with, whether it is one's own or someone else's angry or aggressive impulses. Anger and aggression are the last stages of a response that begins with feelings of vulnerability and then uneasiness (Alvarez, 1998). Ideally, the most useful nursing interventions would be instituted during these **initial phases**, before a client's anger starts to escalate out of control. An understanding of the kinds of situations and client attributes that may make a client predisposed to angry and aggressive behaviors is important for nurses. Assessment skills guiding the nurse to signals of escalating anger and aggression are vital. Accurate assessment and intervention during the early stages of escalating anger are the best prevention of violent or aggressive behavior, which in most instances is the physical attempt to take control (Alverez, 1998).

However, there are times when anger has already escalated and the threat of violence is imminent. At this time, different intervention strategies are needed. Therefore, a whole different set of guidelines is needed when a client threatens to become physically violent.

Nurses encounter angry and aggressive clients in various settings. Clients in emergency rooms or medical units, in community health settings, and even during a home visit may feel anxious, overwhelmed, and/or threatened and lash out verbally or threaten aggressive physical behavior toward health care personnel. Some clients are more prone toward angry and aggressive behaviors than others. For example, clients who abuse substances have poor coping skills, are psychotic, have antisocial, borderline, or narcissistic traits, and have cognitive disorders, paranoia, or mania may at times be at risk for violent behaviors.

No nurse need ever accept or tolerate anger or aggression. Preventative measures are required for the safety of the nurse as well as the client's safety.

The following sections offer nursing guidelines for assessing anger and potential aggression for when a client is angry and verbally abusive, and interventions for when a client's anger has escalated to physical abuse.

In the hospital, specific protocols that follow legal and ethical guidelines need to be followed when restraining or secluding clients.

There are psychopharmacological agents that have been found useful for angry and aggressive clients as well. Guidelines for working with angry and aggressive clients follow the least restrictive means of helping a client in gaining control. Least restrictive usually starts with verbal restraints, then chemical restraints, and finally physical restraints/seclusion.

◆ ASSESSING POTENTIAL FOR VIOLENCE

History

1. Any past history of violence **(The best predictor of future behavior is past behavior.)**
2. Paranoia
3. Alcohol/drug ingestion
4. Certain clients with mania or agitated depression
5. Personality disorder clients prone to rage, violence, or impulse dyscontrol (antisocial, borderline, and narcissistic)
6. Oppositional defiant disorder or conduct disorder
7. Clients experiencing command hallucinations
8. Any client with psychotic features (hallucinations, delusions, illusions)
9. Clients with a cognitive disorder (e.g., dementia or delirium)

10. Clients known to have intermittent explosive disorder (e.g., domestic violence)
11. Certain medical conditions (e.g., chronic illness or loss of body function) may strain a person's coping abilities and lead to uncharacteristic anger

Presenting Signs and Symptoms

1. Violence is usually (BUT NOT ALWAYS) preceded by:
   a. Hyperactivity: most important predictor of imminent violence (e.g., pacing, restlessness)
   b. Increasing anxiety and tension: clenched jaw or fist, rigid posture, fixed or tense facial expression, mumbling to self (Client may have shortness of breath, sweating, and rapid pulse.)
   c. Verbal abuse: profanity, argumentativness
   d. Loud voice, change of pitch or very soft voice forcing others to strain to hear
   e. Intense eye contact or avoidance of eye contact
2. Recent acts of violence, including property violence
3. Stone silence
4. Alcohol or drug intoxication
5. Carrying a weapon or object that may be used as a weapon (e.g., fork, knife, rock)
6. Milieu conducive to violence:
   a. Overcrowding
   b. Staff inexperience
   c. Staff provocative/controlling
   d. Poor limit setting
   e. Arbitrarily taking away privileges

Sample Questions

The nurse uses a variety of therapeutic techniques to obtain the answers to the following questions. Use your discretion and decide which questions are appropriate to complete your assessment.

1. "Tell me about a time you felt compelled or driven to do things you didn't want to do."
2. "Have you ever been fired/evicted/arrested? Describe the circumstances."
3. "Tell me about a time you lost control." (e.g., thrown/broken things)
4. "Have you ever hit/attacked anyone?" (Ask for examples.)

5. "Have you ever or do you now hear voices telling to do things to hurt other people? Tell me about one time."
6. "What do you do when you get very upset?"

Assessment Guide

Box 14–1 presents an overt aggression scale.

☰	ASSESSMENT ALERTS
	1. History of violence is the single best predictor of violence.
	2. *Assess client for risk of violence*:
	• Has violent wish or intention to harm another?
	• Has a plan?
	• Has availability or means to carry out plan?
	• Consider demographics: sex (male), age (14 to 24), socioeconomic status (low), and support system (few).
	3. Assess situational characteristics (Box 14–2).
	4. Assess self for defensive response or taking client's anger personally, which may accelerate the anger cycle. For example, are you:
	• Responding aggressively toward client?
	• Avoiding client?
	• Suppressing or denying either your own or client's anger?
	5. Assess your level of comfort in the situation and the prudence of enlisting other staff to work with you to deal with a potentially explosive situation.

◆ NURSING DIAGNOSES WITH INTERVENTIONS

People who commit acts of violence often lack conflict resolution skills, and resort to more primitive and physical ways of acting and responding. Many believe that a lack of assertiveness or problem-solving skills is an area of dysfunction in violent people (Maiuro, 1997). Therefore, teaching clients new coping skills and effective behavioral alternatives to manage their anger is helpful for many clients and is a primary prevention intervention. Many practitioners use psychoeducational and cognitive-behavioral approaches for people with anger, violence, and abuse control problems. Some of the focus in therapy is directed toward (Maiuro, 1997):

❖   B O X   1 4 – 1   ❖
Overt Aggression Scale

Verbal Aggression

_____   Makes loud noises, shouts angrily

_____   Yells mild personal insults (e.g., "You're stupid.")

_____   Curses viciously, uses foul language in anger, makes moderate threats to others or self

_____   Makes clear threats of violence towards others or self ("I'm gonna kill you.") or requests help to control self

Physical Aggression Against Objects

_____   Slams doors, scatters clothing, makes a mess

_____   Throws objects down, kicks furniture without breaking it, marks the wall

_____   Breaks objects, smashes window

_____   Sets fires, throws objects dangerously

Physical Aggression Against Self

_____   Picks or scratches skin, hits self, pulls hair (with no or minor injury only)

_____   Bangs head, hits fist into objects, throws self onto floor or onto objects (hurts self without serious injury)

_____   Small cuts or bruises, minor burns

_____   Mutilates self; causes deep cuts, bites that bleed, internal injury, fracture, loss of consciousness, loss of teeth

Physical Aggression Against Other People

_____   Makes threatening gesture, swings at people, grabs at clothes

_____   Strikes, kicks, pushes, pulls hair (without injury to them)

_____   Attacks others, causing mild-moderate physical injury (bruises, sprain, welts)

_____   Attacks others, causing severe physical injury (broken bones, deep lacerations, internal injury)

From Yudofsky, S.C., Silver, J.M., Jackson, W., et al. (1986). The Overt Aggression Scale for the objective rating of verbal and physical aggression. American Journal of Psychiatry 143:35–39; reprinted with permission. Copyright 1986 American Psychiatric Association.

❖   B O X   1 4 – 2   ❖

Assessing Situational Characteristics for Violence

- **Availability of Potential Victim(s):** most violent crimes occur between people who know each other.
- **Access to Weapons:** People with martial arts training or combat experience and those who possess great physical strength are capable of inflicting great harm.
- **Substance Use**
- Stressors: Daily stressor such as relationship and financial problems can reduce a person's frustration tolerance.

Data from Vandercreek, L. (1998). Models for clinical decision making with dangerous patients. In Koocher, G.P., Norcross, S.C., and Hill, S.S. (eds.), Psychologists' Desk Reference. New York: Oxford University Press, pp. 496–499.

---

1. Increasing client's awareness, appreciation, and accountability for his or her acts
2. Enhancing the client's ability to identify and manage the attitudes and emotions that are associated with violent behaviors
3. Decreasing social isolation and providing a supportive milieu for change
4. Decreasing hostile-dependent relationships when they exist
5. Developing nonviolent and constructive conflict resolution skills

Ineffective Individual Coping is an appropriate nursing diagnosis for clients who have angry and aggressive responses to stressful, frustrating, or threatening situations. When a client's anxiety and anger escalate to levels where there is a threat of harm to self or others, then **Risk for Violence: Directed at Others** is more appropriate and necessitates a whole different set of interventions. During this time, talking-down skills are employed. If psychopharmacology or chemical restraints are not effective, restraint or seclusion of an aggressive client may be warranted.

Nurses are better prepared when they are familiar with the medications that can be effective during an episode of acute aggression or violence. Again, the least restrictive intervention is usually used first: (1) interpersonal (verbal), then (2) chemical (psychopharmacology), and finally, (3) physical restraint or seclusion.

OVERALL GUIDELINES FOR NURSING INTERVENTION

1. Always minimize personal risks—stay at least one arm's length away from client. Give client lots of space.
2. Set limits at the outset:
   - Use *DIRECT APPROACH* (e.g., "Violence is unacceptable."). Describe the consequences (restraints, seclusion). Best for confused or psychotic clients.
   - Use *INDIRECT APPROACH* if client is **not** confused or psychotic (e.g., "You have a choice. You can take this medication and go into the interview room [or hallway] and talk, or you can sit in the seclusion room until you feel less anxious.").
3. Follow guidelines for setting limits as identified in Box 14–3.

❖   B O X   1 4 – 3   ❖
Setting Limits

1. Set limits only in those areas in which a clear need to protect the client or others exists.
2. Establish realistic and enforceable consequences of exceeding limits.
3. Make the client aware of the limits and the consequences of not adhering to the limits before incidents occur. The client should be told in a clear, polite, and firm manner what the limits and consequences are and should be given the opportunity to discuss any feelings or reactions to them.
4. All limits should be supported by the entire staff. The limits should be written in the care plan, if the client is hospitalized, and should also be communicated verbally to all those involved.
5. When the limits are consistently adhered to, a decision to discontinue the limits should be made by the staff and should be noted on the nursing care plan. The decision should be based on consistent behavior, not on promises or sporadic efforts.
6. The staff should formulate a plan to address their own difficulty in maintaining consistent limits.

From Chitty, K.K., and Maynard, C.K. (1986). Managing manipulation. Journal of Psychosocial Nursing and Mental Health Services 24(6):9; reprinted with permission.

The following text discusses two nursing diagnoses, one for intervention with clients who are angry and hostile, and a second for intervention with those whose anger has escalated to threat of violence toward self or others. Guidelines are given for restraint procedure, and appropriate pharmacological agents for acute anger and aggression are noted.

Ineffective Individual Coping

Inability to form a valid appraisal of the stressors, inadequate choices of practical responses, and/or inability to use available resources

Related To (Etiology)

◆ Inadequate level of perception of control
◆ High degree of threat
◆ Disturbance in pattern of tension release
◆ Inadequate opportunity to prepare for stressors
◆ Disturbance in pattern of appraisal of threat
● Ineffective problem-solving strategies/skills
● Inappropriate/ineffective use of defense mechanisms
● Personal vulnerability
● Knowledge deficit
● Overwhelming crisis situations
● Impaired reality testing
● Excessive anxiety
● Intoxication or withdrawal of substances of chemical abuse
● Chemical or biological brain changes

As Evidenced By (Assessment Findings/Diagnostic Cues)

◆ Inappropriate/ineffective use of defense mechanisms
◆ Inability to meet role expectations
◆ Use of forms of coping that impede adaptive behavior
◆ Abuse of chemical agents
◆ Destructive behavior toward self and others
◆ Change in usual communication patterns
● Verbal manipulations
● Expressed inability to cope
● Perceptual distortions

◆ NANDA accepted; ● In addition to NANDA.

- Aggressive rather than assertive behaviors
- Immature maladaptive behaviors
- Reports feeling anxious, apprehensive, fearful and/or depressed, angry

Outcome Criteria

Client will:

- Identify two new safe and appropriate behaviors that will reduce anxiety, frustration, and anger by (date)
- Discuss alternative ways of meeting demands of current situation by (date)
- Recognize when anger and aggressive tendencies begin to escalate and employ tension-reducing behaviors at that time (time outs, deep breathing, talk to a previously designated person, employ an exercise such as jogging) by (date)
- Verbalize an understanding of aggressive behavior, associated disorders, and medications, if any by (date)
- Identify own strengths and skills to cope with problems, and work with nurse to build upon these skills (e.g., problem solving) (ongoing)
- Practice stress-management techniques (exercising, talking, relaxation, journal writing) as evidenced by staff observations and family report (ongoing)

Short-Term Goals

Client will:

- Refrain from harming others or destroying property
- Be free of self-inflicted harm
- Be rule-compliant during hospitalization
- Begin to implement at least two new coping techniques when angry and aggressive feelings begin to escalate
- Experience a decrease of anxiety, anger using a self-reported scale of 1 to 10 (1 feeling least anger and 10 feeling the most anger) after trying new coping techniques

Interventions and Rationales

Intervention	Rationale
1. Assess your own feelings in the situation, guard against taking client's abusive	1. Although clients are often skillful at making personal and pointed statements,

◆ NANDA accepted; ● In addition to NANDA.

Intervention	**Rationale**
statements personally or becoming defensive.	they do not know nurses personally, and have no basis on which they can make accurate judgments.
2. Refrain from responding with sarcasm or ridicule, no matter how threatened or angry you feel.	2. An angry or sarcastic remark by an authority figure will serve as an attack on the client's self-esteem, and encourage more defensive behaviors (e.g., increased hostility).
3. Pay attention to angry and aggressive behavior; do not minimize such behavior in the hope that it will go away.	3. *Minimization of angry behaviors* and *ineffective limit setting* are the **most frequent factors contributing to the escalation of violence**.
4. Set clear, consistent, and enforceable limits on behavior (see Box 14–3 for guidelines).	4. Clear limits give client understanding of expectations for acceptable behaviors and stress the consequences of not adhering to those behaviors.
5. Emphasize to clients that they are responsible for all consequences of their aggressive behavior, including legal charges.	5. Focusing on the "here and now" rules, and that client is responsible for the consequences of any and all aggressive behaviors, can help decrease the chronically angry client's need to "test limits."
6. Emphasize to the client that you are setting limits on specific behaviors, not feelings (e.g., "It is OK to be angry at Tom, but it is not OK to threaten him or verbally abuse him.").	6. Underlines that behavioral limits are not punitive while communicating expectation for positive behaviors.
7. Use a matter-of-fact, neutral approach. Remain calm and use a moderate,	7. Fear, indignation, and arguing are gratifying to many verbally abusive

firm voice and calming hand gestures.

clients. A matter-of-fact approach can help interrupt the cycle of escalating anger.

8. When a client starts to become abusive, and anger threatens to escalate, inform the client that the nurse will leave the room for a period of time (20 minutes) and will be back when the situation is calmer. Return when time is up.

8. When this response is given in a neutral, matter-of-fact manner, the client's abusive behavior does not get rewarded. Always returns in the time specified, and focus communication on neutral topics.

9. Attend positively to non-abusive communication, such as non–illness-related topics, by responding to requests and by providing emotional support.

9. Reinforces appropriate communication and behaviors. This gives the client and nurse time to share healthier communication and build up a sounder working relationship.

10. Avoid power struggles and control battles.

10. Power struggles and control battles are perceived as a challenge, and generally lead to escalation of the conflict.

11. Respond to client anxiety or anger with active listening and validation of client distress. Apologize when appropriate.

11. Allows the client to feel heard and understood; builds trust.

12. Work with client to identify the internal and interpersonal factors that provoke violence or that strengthen a relationship against anger and aggression.

12. Helps both nurse and client identify triggers for aggression, and factors that can mitigate or reduce the escalation of anger and aggression. **This is the first step in a structured violence prevention strategy** (Goodwin, 1985).

Intervention

13. Identify serious risk factors for further violence (family chaos, other mental or environmental risk factors).

14. Work with client to identify what supports are lacking, and problem solve ways to achieve needed support.

15. Teach the client (and family) the steps in the problem-solving process.

16. Role play alternative behaviors with clients that they can use in stressful and overwhelming situations when anger threatens.

17. Work with clients to set goals for their behavior. Give positive feedback when clients reach their goals.

18. Provide the client with other outlets for stress and anxiety (exercising, listening to music, reading, talking to a friend, support groups, participation in a sport).

Rationale

13. Whenever possible, reduce the possibility of continued violence by treating the risk factors (e.g., getting family counseling, finding job). **This is the second step in a structured violence prevention strategy** (Goodwin, 1985).

14. Advocacy with support is **the third step in intervention for violence** (Goodwin, 1985).

15. Many people have never learned a systematic and effective approach to dealing with and mastering tough life situations/problems.

16. Role playing allows client to rehearse alternative ways of handling stressful and angry feelings in a safe environment.

17. Gives client a sense of control while learning goal-setting skills. Achieving self-set goals may enhance a person's sense of self, and can foster new and more effective approaches to frustrating feelings.

18. Alternative means of channeling aggression and angry feelings can help clients decrease their anxiety and stress, and allow for more cognitive approaches to their situa-

19. Provide the client and family with community resources that teach assertiveness training, anger management, and stress reduction techniques. These may take a while to master, but give client more satisfying experiences in life.

19. When clients are motivated, there are a number of techniques they can learn that can aid in helping them get what they want through acceptable and rewarding means (e.g., using a problem-solving approach).

Risk for Violence: Directed at Others

Behaviors in which an individual demonstrates that he or she can be physically, emotionally, and/or sexually harmful to others

---

Related To (Etiology)

◆ History of violent antisocial behavior
◆ History of violence against others (hitting, biting, kicking, spitting, rape, etc.)
◆ Panic states
◆ Stamping feet, running in corridors
◆ Rage reactions
◆ Neurological impairment (positive EEG, computed tomography scan, or magnetic resonance image; head trauma, positive neurological findings, seizure disorders)
◆ Manic excitement
◆ Cognitive impairment
◆ Substance abuse or withdrawal
◆ Psychotic symptoms (auditory, visual, common hallucinations, paranoid delusions, illogical thought processes)
◆ Poor impulse control

As Evidenced By (Assessment Findings/Diagnostic Cues)

◆ Increased motor activity, pacing, excitement, irritability, agitation
◆ Provocative behavior (argumentative, overactive, complaining, demanding behaviors)

◆ NANDA accepted; ● In addition to NANDA.

◆ Hostile, threatening verbalizations (loud, threatening, profane speech)
◆ Overt and aggressive acts; goal-directed destruction of objects in the environment
◆ Possession of destructive means (gun, knife, other weapon)
◆ Verbal threats against property/person, threatening notes/letters
◆ Body language: angry facial expressions, rigid posture, clenched fists, threatening posture
◆ History of assaultive behavior

Outcome Criteria

Client will:

• Display nonviolent behaviors toward self and others
• Demonstrate three new ways to deal with tension and aggression in a nondestructive manner
• Make plans to continue with long-term therapy (individual, family, group) to work on violence prevention strategies and increasing coping skills

Short-Term Goals

• Client's behavior will not escalate to aggressive acts toward self, others, or property while in hospital.
• Client will demonstrate increased self-control while in hospital.
• Client will participate in time outs, moving to a less stimulating environment, and verbal limits set by staff during hospital stay.
• Client will refrain from hurting self or others with the aid of verbal, chemical, or physical restraints.

Interventions and Rationales

Intervention	Rationale
1. Keep environmental stimulation at a minimum (e.g., lower lights, keep stereos down, ask clients and visitors to leave the area or have staff take client to another area).	1. Increased stimulation may increase client's anxiety level, leading to increased agitation or aggressive behaviors.
2. Keep voice calm, speak in a low tone.	2. High-pitched rapid voice can increase anxiety levels in others; the opposite is

---

◆ NANDA accepted; ● In addition to NANDA.

true when the tone of voice is low and calm, and the words are spoken slowly.

3. Call client by name, introduce yourself, orient the client when necessary, tell the client beforehand what you are going to do.

3. Calling client by name helps to establish contact. Orienting and giving information can minimize misrepresentation of nurses' intentions.

4. Always use personal safety precautions:
   a. Either leave the door open in the interview room or use a hallway.
   b. If you feel uncertain of client's potential for violence, other staff should be nearby.
   c. Never turn your back on an angry client.
   d. Have a quick exit available.
   e. If on home visit, go with a colleague if there is concern regarding aggression.

   Leave the home immediately if there are any signs that the client's behavior is escalating out of control.

4. *Your safety is first always.* Always call in colleagues or other staff if you feel threatened or in physical danger. Nursing and security staff should have received frequent training in dealing with angry and hostile clients, including frequent training in steps in anger de-escalation and seclusion and restraint procedures. Ask for training, and learn from more experienced colleagues about unit precautions for staff as well as client safety.

5. When interventions are needed to reduce escalating anger, always use the least restrictive first:
   a. Interpersonal—verbal interventions
   b. Chemical—appropriate medications
   c. Physical—restraints or seclusion

5. Seclusion or restraints should never be used as punishment or substitute for staffing. Restraints should be used only when there is no less restrictive alternative.

Intervention	Rationale
6. *Verbal Interventions:* Encourage the client to talk about angry feelings and find ways to tolerate or reduce angry and aggressive feelings.	6. When client feels heard and understood and has help with problem-solving alternative options, de-escalation of anger and aggression is often possible.
7. Use empathetic *verbal interventions* (e.g., "It must be frightening to be here and to be feeling out of control.").	7. Empathetic verbal intervention is the most effective method of calming an agitated, fearful, panicky client.
8. When interpersonal interventions fail to decrease the client's anger, consider the need for *chemical* or *physical restraints*. (See Table 14–1 in next section for medications used for clients with acute anger.)	8. Often psychopharmacological interventions can help clients gain control of their behavior, and prevent continued escalation of anger and hostile impulses.
9. Alert hospital security and other staff in a quiet and unobtrusive manner *before* violent behavior escalates so that they are prepared to intervene in a safe and knowledgeable manner if needed.	9. **Hospital staff and security should have frequent training in restraining or secluding clients.** Alerting staff and security beforehand best ensures that the restraint or seclusion process will be handled safely for client, staff, and other clients on the unit.
10. When interpersonal and pharmacological interventions fail to control the angry client, *physical intervention (restraints or seclusion)* is the final resort. **Always follow hospital protocols.** Refer to Box 14–4 for some guidelines for use of restraints.	10. Hospital protocols that are clear and well written tell staff when to restrain, how to restrain, how long before a physician's order is needed, nursing interventions for client during period of restraint or seclusion, how often to check restraints or client in seclusion, whom to

---

❖   B O X   1 4 – 4   ❖
Guidelines for Restraining a Client

---

1. The specific indications should be clearly documented.
2. Anyone impaired enough to require restraints should have continuous staff observation.
3. Restraints are used when there is **NOT** a less restrictive alternative left.
4. Restraints should be properly used and designed.
5. Five staff are necessary to restrain a resistant client.
6. Security should be called to assist.
7. During the procedure, the client should be told in calm, simple terms, what is happening.
   "You are in a hospital . . . these people are nurses and security staff . . . no one is going to hurt you . . . we are trying to make things safe for you."
8. Nursing and security staff should receive training in this procedure on a regular basis.

From Goldberg, R.J. (1995). Practical Guide to the Care of the Psychiatric Patient. St. Louis: Mosby, p. 168; reprinted with permission.

11. Specific interventions should be documented, including times, types of intervention, and behavioral responses before restraints/seclusion was employed.

12. If restraints or seclusion has been used, check on client every 15 minutes, check restraints and circulation (color, temperature, pulses on extremities), need for toileting, nutrition, and hydration. **Use unit protocol as a guide.**

call, how often the need for restraints/seclusion needs to be re-evaluated by physician.

11. Record what works with client, so that how to intervene with client in the future can be gleaned from careful documentation.

12. Client safety is an important part of our care. Checking client frequently helps ensure client safety **(use unit protocol as a guide)**, and written records are kept in client's permanent record.

◆ PSYCHOPHARMACOLOGY FOR ACUTE AGGRESSION

Medications are often needed to help clients maintain control and prevent harm to self or others. Table 14–1 helps identify some medications useful for acute aggression.

Table 14–1 ◆ Medication Useful for Acute Aggression

Haloperidol (Haldol)	• Should be limited to psychosis-induced violence. • Not to be used for aggression alone for more than 6 weeks.
Lorazepam (Ativan)	• Initially 1–2 mg orally or intramuscularly every hour until calm. Taper at 10% per day from highest dose to avoid withdrawal symptoms unless drug is used less than 1 week. • Not to be used for aggression alone for more than 6 weeks.
Trazodone (Desyrel)	Acutely lowers aggression and agitation in demented or mentally retarded clients without impairing cognition. Doses up to 500 mg have been used.

C H A P T E R   1 5

Crisis Intervention and Rehabilitation

A**crisis** is an acute, time-limited phenomenon experienced as an overwhelming emotional reaction to a:

- stressful situational event,
- developmental event,
- societal event, or
- cultural event, or to the perception of that event.

A crisis is not a pathological state, and being in crisis is not pathological. It is a struggle for equilibrium and adjustment when problems are perceived as insolvable.

Nurses intervene through a variety of crisis intervention modalities, such as disaster nursing, mobile crisis units, group work, health education and crisis prevention, victim outreach programs, and telephone hot lines.

It is important to keep in mind that, in crisis work, particularly, the client may be an individual, group, or community:

- **Individual client** (as in physical abuse)
- **Group** (as in students in a classmate's suicide event or shootings)
- **Community** (as in disaster nursing—tornadoes, shootings, airplane crashes)

It is difficult to predict what one person may perceive as a disastrous event constituting a crisis. A pregnancy, a breakup of a relationship, failing a test, or being given an adverse medical diagnosis may be catastrophic for one person but not to another. Some crises are more universal, such as the death of a child or spouse; these events are experienced as crises to most everyone.

Crisis by definition is self-limiting and is resolved within 4 to 6 weeks. The goal of crisis intervention is to maintain the precrisis level of functioning. However, a person may emerge from the crisis at a higher level of functioning, at the same level, or at a lower level of functioning. Crisis intervention deals with the present (here-and-now) only, and nurses take a much more active and directive role with their clients in crisis.

◆ TYPES OF CRISES

There are basically three types of crises: maturational, situational, and adventitious crises.

Maturational

Erikson identified eight stages of growth and development that must be completed in order to reach maturity. Each stage identifies a specific task that must be successfully mastered in order to progress through the growth process. When a person arrives at a new stage, former coping styles may no longer be age appropriate, and new coping mechanisms have yet to be developed. During this period of transition, psychological disequilibrium may be present. This temporary disequilibrium may affect interpersonal relationship, body image, and social and work roles (Hoff, 1995).

Situational

A situational crisis arises from an external rather than an internal source. Examples of internal situations that could precipitate a crisis include loss of a job, the death of a loved one, witnessing a crime, abortion, a change of job, a change in financial status, "coming out" as to homosexual orientation, divorce, and school problems. These external situations are often referred to as "life events" or "crucial life problems" because most people encounter some of these problems during the course of their lives.

Adventitious

An adventitious crisis is a crisis of disaster, and is not a part of everyday life; it is unplanned and accidental. Adventitious crises can be divided into three subcategories:

1. Natural disaster (floods, earthquakes, fires, tornadoes)
2. National disasters (wars, riots, airplane crashes)
3. Crimes of violence (assault or murder in the workplace, bombing in crowded places, spousal or child abuse)

◆ PHASES OF CRISIS

1. A problem arises that contributes to increase in anxiety levels. The anxiety stimulates the use of usual problem-solving techniques.
2. If the usual problem-solving techniques don't work, anxiety continues to rise and trial-and-error attempts at restoring balance are tried.
3. If trial-and-error attempts fail, anxiety escalates to severe or panic levels and the person adopts automatic relief behaviors.
4. If these measures do not reduce anxiety, anxiety can overwhelm the person and lead to serious personality disorganization, which signals the person is in crisis.

◆ LEVELS OF CRISIS INTERVENTION

There are three levels of crisis intervention: (1) preventive, (2) crisis intervention, and (3) rehabilitation. Psychotherapeutic nursing interventions are directed toward these three levels of care.

Preventive (Primary Care)

Primary preventions are interventions that promote mental health and reduce the incidence of mental illness in an individual, group, or community. Interventions are aimed at altering causative factors before they can do harm—for example, anticipating and preparing people for stressful events such as parenting classes, premarital counseling, preoperative teaching, respite care, or childbirth classes. Environmental manipulation may also help allay a crisis by providing support or removing the client from the stressor. Examples include finding shelter for an abused woman and her children, offering sick leave to an individual, or obtaining shelter for a homeless individual.

Crisis Intervention (Secondary Care)

Intervention during an acute crisis aims to prevent prolonged anxiety from diminishing personal effectiveness and personality organization.

Rehabilitation (Tertiary Care)

Rehabilitation provides support for those who have experienced and are now recovered from a disabling mental state and are as a result psychologically disabled. There are notably different aspects of response between a mentally healthy person and a severe and persistently mentally ill person in crisis. The mentally healthy person can make good use of crisis intervention (secondary care). The severely mentally ill or psychologically disabled person, in contrast, will fare much better with rehabilitation (tertiary care). Table 15–1 gives the reader an idea of some of the basic differences.

◆ ASSESSMENT

History

A positive history for potential crises might include:

1. Overwhelming life event (situational, maturational, or adventitious)
2. A history of violent behavior
3. A history of suicidal behavior
4. A history of a psychiatric disorder (e.g., depression, personality disorder, bipolar disorder, schizophrenia, or an anxiety disorder)
5. A history of or concurrent serious medical condition (cancer, ongoing cardiac problems, uncontrolled diabetes, lupus, multiple sclerosis)
6. Religious or cultural beliefs that may affect the way the person experiences the crisis event

Table 15–1 ◆ Mentally Healthy Versus Severe and Persistently Mentally Ill Person in Crisis

MENTALLY HEALTHY PERSON	LONG-TERM MENTALLY ILL PERSON
1. Has realistic perception of potential crisis event.	1. Because of severe biologically based mental illness or psychologically disabling illness, potential crisis event is usually distorted by minimizing or maximizing the event.
2. Has healthy sense of self, place, and purpose in life. Good problem-solving abilities.	2. Inadequate sense of self and purpose or abilities. Inadequate problem-solving abilities. Nurse becomes more active in assisting the person in crisis.
3. Usually has adequate situational supports.	3. Person often has no family or friends and may be living an isolated existence, or even homeless.
4. Usually has adequate coping skills. Has a number of techniques that can be used to lower anxiety and adapt to the situation.	4. Because coping ability for the severely and persistently mentally ill is poor, coping mechanisms are usually inadequate or poorly utilized.

Presenting Symptoms

People in crisis may present with a variety of behaviors. For example, some behaviors may include:

- Confusion/disorganized thinking
- Immobilization/social withdrawal
- Violence against others/suicidal thoughts or attempts
- Running about aimlessly/agitated increased psychomotor activity
- Crying/ adness
- Flashbacks/intrusive thoughts/nightmares
- Forgetfulness/poor concentration

Sample Questions

The nurse uses a variety of therapeutic techniques to obtain the answers to the following questions. Use your discretion and decide which questions are appropriate to complete your assessment.

The nurse assesses three main areas during a crisis: (1) the meaning of the precipitating event, (2) support system, and (3) coping skills.

Determine the Meaning of the Precipitating Event

1. "What has happened in your life before you started to feel this way?"
2. If this is an ongoing problem, ask the person, "What is different today than yesterday about the problem? Be specific."
3. "What does this event/problem mean to you?"
4. "How does this event/problem affect your life?"
5. "How do you see this event/problem as affecting your future?"

Evaluate the Client's Support System

1. "To whom do you talk when you feel overwhelmed?"
2. "Whom can you trust?"
3. "Who is available to help you?"
4. "Are these people available now?"
5. "Where do you worship (talk to God)? Go to school? Are there community-based activities that you are involved in?"

Identify Personal Coping Skills

1. "What do you usually do when you feel stressed or overwhelmed?"
2. "What has helped you get through difficult times in the past?"

3. "When these things haven't helped, why do you think your previous coping skills aren't working now?"
4. "What have you done so far to cope with this situation?"
5. "Have you thought of killing yourself or someone else?"

Assessment Guide

There are many factors than can influence how a person responds to a potential crisis situation. Some factors that can limit a person's ability to cope with stressful life events are:

- The number of other stressful life events with which the person is currently coping
- The presence of other unresolved losses the person may be dealing with
- The presence of concurrent medical problems
- Experiencing excessive fatigue or pain

Assessing for stressful life events can be a very useful tool (see Table 15–2).

ASSESSMENT ALERTS

1. Identify if the client's response to the crisis warrants psychiatric treatment or hospitalization to minimize decompensation (suicidal behavior, psychotic thinking, violent behavior).
2. Do the nurse and client have a clear understanding of the *precipitating event*?
3. Assess client's understanding of his or her present *situational supports.*
4. What *coping styles* does the client usually use? What coping mechanisms may help the situation in the present?
5. Are there certain religious or cultural beliefs that need to be considered in assessing and intervening in this person's crisis?
6. Is this situation one in which the client needs primary (education, environmental manipulation, or new coping skills), secondary (crisis intervention), or tertiary (rehabilitation) intervention?

◆ NURSING DIAGNOSES WITH INTERVENTIONS

During a crisis, a person may exhibit a variety of behaviors that indicate a number of human problems. When anxiety levels escalate to high-moderate, severe, or panic levels, the ability to prob-

Table 15–2 ◆ Life-Changing Event Questionnaire

SOCIAL AREA	LIFE CHANGES	LCU VALUE*
Family	Death of spouse	105
	Marital separation	65
	Death of a close family member	65
	Divorce	62
	Pregnancy	60
	Change in health of family member	52
	Marriage	50
	Gain of new family member	50
	Marital reconciliation	42
	Spouse begins or stops work	37
	Son or daughter leaving home	29
	In-law trouble	29
	Change in number of family get-togethers	26
Personal	Jail term	56
	Sex difficulties	49
	Death of a close friend	46
	Personal injury or illness	42
	Change in living conditions	39
	Outstanding personal achievement	33
	Change in residence	33
	Minor violations of the law	32
	Begin or end school	32
	Change in sleeping habits	31
	Revision of personal habits	31
	Change in eating habits	29
	Change in church activities	29
	Vacation	29
	Change in school	28
	Change in recreation	28
	Christmas	26
Work	Fired at work	64
	Retirement from work	49
	Trouble with boss	39
	Business readjustment	38
	Change to different line of work	38
	Change in work responsibilities	33
	Change in work hours or conditions	30
Financial	Foreclosure of mortgage or loan	57
	Change in financial state	43
	Mortgage (home, car, etc.)	39
	Mortgage or loan less than $10,000 (stereo, etc.)	26

Directions: Sum the LCUs for your life change events during the past 12 months. 250–400 LCUs per year: minor life crisis; 400 and over LCUs per year: major life crisis

*LCU, life change unit. The number of LCUs reflects the average degree or intensity of the life change.
Adapted from Rahe, R. (1990). Psychosocial stressors and adjustment disorder: Van Gogh's life chart illustrates stress and disease. Journal of Clinical Psychiatry 51(11, Suppl.):15; reprinted with permission.

lem solve is impaired, if present at all. **Ineffective Individual Coping** may be evidenced by inability to meet basic needs, use of inappropriate defense mechanisms, and/or alteration in social participation.

Anxiety (moderate, severe, panic) is always present, and lowering of anxiety so that clients are able to start problem solving on their own is key in crisis management.

Altered Family Coping may be related to a situational or maturational event within the family, or two or more events going on simultaneously. Family members may have difficulty responding to each other in a helping manner. Communications may become confused, and inability to express feelings may be evident.

The following sections thread Ineffective Individual Coping through:

1. **CRISIS INTERVENTION**
2. **REHABILITATION**

Ineffective Individual Coping

Inability to form a valid appraisal of the stressors, inadequate choices of practiced responses, and/or inability to use available resources

---

Related To (Etiology)

◆ Inadequate level of confidence in ability to cope
◆ Inadequate social support created by characteristics of relationships
◆ Inadequate level of perception of control
◆ Inadequate resources available
◆ High degree of threat; situational or maturational crises
◆ Inadequate opportunity to prepare for stressors
◆ Disturbance in pattern of appraisal of threat
◆ Disturbance in pattern of tension release
● Mass disaster (bombing, tornado, flood, hostage situation)
● Crime of violence (rape, witnessing robbery or murder, spouse/child abuse)

As Evidenced By (Assessment Findings/Diagnostic Cues)

◆ Inability to meet basic needs
◆ Destructive behavior toward self or others

◆ NANDA accepted; ● In addition to NANDA.

◆ Inability to meet role expectations
◆ Use of forms of coping that impede adaptive behavior
◆ Abuse of chemical agents
◆ Change in usual communication patterns
◆ Risk taking
◆ Decreased use of social support
◆ Inadequate problem solving
◆ Verbalization of inability to cope or inability to ask for help

Crisis Intervention

Outcome Criteria

Clients will:

• Return to precrisis level of functioning within 4 to 6 weeks
• Identify skills and information that can help prevent future crises
• State that they have learned more adaptive ways to cope with stress
• State that they have a stronger existing support system

Short-Term Goals

• Client's anxiety level will go from severe to moderate or moderate to mild by end of first encounter (a person in mild to moderate levels of anxiety can still problem solve).
• Client and nurse will clarify the problem in solvable terms by end of first session.
• Client and nurse will identify existing supports and identify other needed supports by end of first session.
• Client and nurse will set realistic goals to deal with problem situations by end of first session.
• Client and nurse will identify a clear step-by-step plan of action by end of first session, revised throughout.
• Client will remain safe throughout crisis situation.

Interventions and Rationales

Intervention	Rationale
1. Provide liaison to social agencies to take care of emergency needs.	1. Physical needs such as shelter, food, protection from abuser need to be handled immediately.
2. Make appointments for needed medical care	2. For example, child or elder may have acute

◆ NANDA accepted; ● In addition to NANDA.

Intervention	Rationale
or other health care providers. Write out time of appointment and directions for client.	physical problems that might need emergency attention.
3. Assess for client's safety, for example: Are there suicidal thoughts? Is there child or spouse abuse? Are there unsafe living conditions?	3. Client safety is first consideration.
4. Identify client's perception of the event. Reframe perception of the event if event is seen as overwhelming or hopeless, and/or client views self as helpless.	4. Distorted perception raises anxiety. Help client experience event as a problem that can be solved.
5. Assess stressors and precipitating cause of the crisis.	5. Identify areas for change and intervention.
6. Identify client's current skills, resources, and knowledge to deal with problems.	6. Encourage client to use strengths and usual coping skills.
7. Identify other skills client may need to develop (e.g., decision-making skills, problem-solving skills, communication skills, relaxation techniques).	7. Additional skills can help minimize crisis situations in the future and help clients regain more control over their present situation.
8. Assess client's support systems. Rally existing supports *(with client's permission)* if client is overwhelmed at present.	8. Client may be initially immobilized. Nurses often need to take an active role during crisis intervention.
9. Identify and arrange for extra supports if current support system is either not available or insufficient.	9. Client may have lost important supports (death, divorce, distance) or may not have sufficient supports in place.

10. Nurse often needs to take an active role in crisis intervention (e.g., make telephone calls; arrange temporary child care; arrange for shelters, emergency food, first aid, etc.).

10. Clients in crisis are often temporarily immobilized by anxiety and unable to problem solve. Nurse organizes situation so it is seen as solvable and controllable.

11. Give only small amounts of information at a time.

11. Only small pieces of information can be understood when a person's anxiety level is high.

12. Encourage client to stay in the "here-and-now" to deal with the immediate situation only.

12. Crisis intervention deals with the immediate problem disrupting client's present situation.

13. Listen to client's story. Refrain from interrupting.

13. Telling of the story can in itself be healing.

14. Help client to set achievable goals.

14. Working in small achievable steps helps client gain sense of control and mastery.

15. Work with client on devising a plan to meet goals.

15. A realistic and specific plan helps decrease anxiety and promotes hopefulness.

16. Identify and contact other members of the health team who can work with client to solve crisis event.

16. Provides a broad base of support to intervene with problem and enlarges client's network for future problems.

17. In some situations, **DEBRIEFING** is a valuable technique for use with a group of people. Examples of debriefing: with staff on a unit when a client suicides; in a disaster situation (e.g., plane crashes, bombings, natural disasters).

17. Survivors, family members, and staff all need to discuss the impact of a disaster, and debriefing provides a structure in which to do so (Weeks, 1999).

Rehabilitation

Outcome Criteria

Client will:

- Maintain optimum level of functioning in:
  - Work
  - Home
  - Community
- Function in the community with minimal use of inpatient services
- Increase life skills and available supports to use during times of stress
- Maintain stable functioning between episodes of exacerbation

Short-Term Goals

Client will:

- Retain positive coping strategies during times of stress with aid of nurse/family/friends
- Work with nurse to find needed supports, for example:
  - Residential
  - Financial
  - Employment/education
  - Medical
  - Social
  - Recreational

Interventions and Rationales

Intervention	Rationale
1. Nurse works with client and family to assess the variety of needs that clients may have.	1. Client with psychiatric disabilities has a wide range of needs.
2. Identify client's highest level of functioning in terms of: a. Living skills b. Learning skills c. Working skills See Table 15–3.	2. Identifies client's potential and so arrangements can be made to support client's potential.
3. Identify the social supports available to the family: a. Education about the disease, treatment, prognosis, and medications	3. Family members need a variety of supports to prevent family deterioration.

Table 15–3 ♦ Living, Learning, and Working
Skills for Psychiatrically Disabled Clients

Potential skilled activities needed to achieve goal of psychiatric rehabilitation:

PHYSICAL	EMOTIONAL	INTELLECTUAL
Living Skills		
Personal hygiene	Human relations	Money management
Physical fitness	Self-control	Use of community
Use of public	Selective reward	resources
transportation	Stigma reduction	Goal setting
Cooking	Problem solving	Problem development
Shopping	Conversational	
Cleaning	skills	
Sports participation		
Using recreational		
facilities		
Learning Skills		
Being quiet	Speech making	Reading
Paying attention	Question asking	Writing
Staying in seating	Volunteering answers	Arithmetic
Observing	Following directions	Study skills
Punctuality	Asking for directions	Hobby activities
	Listening	Typing
Working Skills		
Punctuality	Job interviewing	Job qualifying
Use of job tools	Job decision making	Job seeking
Job strength	Human relations	Specific job tasks
Job transportation	Self-control	
Specific job tasks	Job keeping	
	Specific job tasks	

Data from Anthony, W.A. (1980). Principles of Psychiatric Rehabilitation.
Baltimore: University Park Press; reprinted.

    b. Community supports
       to help client function
       optimally
    c. Community supports
       that offer family support/
       groups/ongoing psycho-
       education
4. Identify specific community
   supports that can provide
   client and family with
   continuity of care, for
   example (Public Policy
   Committee, 1999):

4. NAMI (Public Policy Committee, 1999) contends that
   a comprehensive array
   of community support
   services must be available
   for individuals to help

Intervention	**Rationale**
a. Residential support services	people function at optimum level and slow down relapse rate.
b. Transportation support services	
c. Intensive case management	
d. Psychosocial rehabilitation	
e. Peer support	
f. Consumer-run services	
g. Round-the-clock crisis services	
h. Outpatient services with mobile capabilities.	
5. Provide *social skills training*, especially if client is living with family.	5. Some studies have shown that social skills training did lower relapse over time, especially for those living with families (Public Policy Committee, 1999).
6. Work with family and client to identify client's prodromal (early) signs of impending relapse.	6. Client and family can secure medical help before exacerbation of illness occurs.
7. Work with client and family to identify an appropriate vocational rehabilitation service for client. Box 15–1 describes types of vocational rehabilitation services available.	7. Employment makes a significant contribution to relapse prevention, improved clinical outcomes, and improved self-image (Palmer-Erbs and Manos, 1998).
8. Teach client and family about psychoactive medications:	8. Medication teaching can do a lot to reduce relapse rate and prolong time between relapses.
a. Side effects	
b. Toxic effects	
c. What medication can do	
d. What medication can't do	
e. Whom/where to call for questions, for emergencies	

❖   B O X   1 5 – 1   ❖
Some Vocational Rehabilitation Models

Supported Employment Programs (SE)

This model has proven to be most successful in assisting persons with the most serious disabilities to attain and maintain an attachment to the work force. It is individualized and provides on-site, one-on-one supports and job coaching services, and occurs in competitive, "real work" settings; job coach services are gradually faded and removed.

Transitional Employment Programs (TE)

This model offers a temporary work experience to individuals offering the same supports and services as SE. TE positions are contracted to a service program that fills openings and staffs positions to meet contractual obligations. No individual participants receive permanent TE positions: they must move on to competitive employment within an agreed-upon length of time. Staff often cover contract positions, working in the job for a day in cases of illness or with changes in participants' schedules.

Clubhouses

Programs are "member directed," with members defined as individuals with serious mental illness. Clubhouse services and supports are provided to members according to the structure of the "work-ordered day." Members have individual daily responsibilities and schedules to fulfill as preparation for entry or re-entry into the world of work. Membership in a clubhouse is lifelong, and members provide each other ongoing support.

Job Clubs

There are two main types: in-house clubs and postprogram graduate clubs. Members discuss issues, uncertainties, and problems that they may face while seeking employment or maintaining employment gains. In-house clubs can provide practical guidelines in resumé writing, guidelines for work exploration, opportunities to practice interviewing skills, and, in some cases, vocational assessment and interest identification. Postprogram graduate clubs provide essential off-site support services, such as working with new co-workers, adjusting to job requirements, handling issues of stigma and disclosure, and feelings of isolation.

Peer and Natural Supports

These circles of support are central to the continued success of individuals with serious psychiatric conditions who are attaining and maintaining employment. Circles expand connections beyond the usual family and friends to include wider community

Continued

links to religious organizations, recreational/activity groups, public libraries, volunteer activities, peer support activities (such as job clubs, support groups that meet regularly, one-on-one relationships, "warm lines" for crisis intervention and supports, and Internet chat rooms).

Adapted from Donegan, K.R., and Palmer-Erbs, V.K. (1998). Promoting the importance of work for persons with psychiatric disabilities. Journal of Psychosocial Nursing 36(4):13–23; reprinted with permission.

◆ NURSE, CLIENT, AND FAMILY RESOURCES—CRISIS INTERVENTION

Associations

Emotions Anonymous
P.O. Box 4245
St. Paul, MN 55104-0245
1-612-647-9712
(12-step program of recovery from emotional difficulties)

Workaholics Anonymous
P.O. Box 289
Menlo Park, CA 94026-0289
1-510-273-9253
(12-step program of recovery from compulsive overworking)

Red Cross Disaster Mental Health Services (DMHS)
Contact local Red Cross for information

Internet Sites

Alliance for Psychosocial Nursing
http://www.psychnurse.org

NAMI (National Alliance for the Mentally Ill)
http://www.nami.org

Mental Health Net
http://mentalhelp.net

CHAPTER 16

Family Violence and Sexual Assault

Physical and psychological trauma causes long-lasting and devastating damage to people's lives, their children's lives, and lives of generations to come. Violence has moved from the home into schools, the workplace, and neighborhoods, onto the road, and into the air, and touches every corner of community life. This chapter deals with child, spouse, and elder abuse and rape. **Part I covers child, spouse, and elder abuse; Part II covers sexual assault (rape).**

◆ PART I: CHILD, SPOUSE, AND ELDER ABUSE

One of the most disturbing aspects of family violence or victimization is the horrifying legacy of violence:

> I and the public know what all school children learn
> Those to whom evil is done do evil in return (Auden, 1939)

Victims of abuse are often debilitated when their ability to cope is overwhelmed. Zerbe (1999) states that, during a course of a lifetime, few escape traumatic events, but the victims are often left to deal with the devastating consequences by themselves.

The nurse is often the first point of contact for people experiencing family violence, and is in the ideal position to contribute to prevention, detection, and effective intervention. All forms of interpersonal abuse can be devastating. Abuse can take the form of emotional, physical, and/or sexual abuse and neglect. Emotional abuse kills the spirit and the ability to succeed later in life, to feel deeply, or to make emotional contact with others. Physical abuse includes emotional abuse in addition to the potential for long-term physical deformity, internal damage, and acute painful tissue damage, bone damage, and/or in some cases death. The consequences of being sexually abused as a child are devastating and often never-ending. Survivors of sexual abuse experience low self-esteem, self-hatred, affective instability, poor control of aggressive impulses, and disturbed interpersonal relationships compounded by an inability to trust and difficulty in protecting themselves. Sexual abuse occurs all too often in conjunction with spouse abuse and elder abuse.

Assessing for Family Violence

Sensitivity is required on the part of the nurse who may suspect family violence. Interview guidelines are suggested in Box 16–1. A person who feels judged or accused of wrongdoing is most likely to become defensive, and any attempts at changing coping strategies in the family will be thwarted. It is better for the nurse to ask about ways of solving disagreements or methods of disciplining children, rather than use the word *abuse* or *violence*, which appear judgmental and thus are threatening to the family (Smith-DiJulio, 1998).

❖   B O X   1 6 – 1   ❖
Interview Guidelines

DOs
- Conduct the interview in private
- Be direct, honest, and professional
- Use language the client understands
- Ask client to clarify words not understood
- Be understanding
- Be attentive
- Inform the client if you must make a referral to child/adult protective services and explain the process
- Assess safety and help reduce danger (at discharge)

DON'Ts
- Do *not* try to "prove" abuse by accusations or demands
- Do *not* display horror, anger, shock, or disapproval of the perpetrator or situation
- Do *not* place blame or make judgments
- Do *not* allow the client to feel "at fault" or "in trouble"
- Do *not* probe or press for responses or answers the client is not willing to give
- Do *not* conduct the interview with a group of interviewers
- Do *not* force a child to remove clothing

History

1. **Child:** Is there a history of unexplained "accidents" and physical injuries?
2. **Child:** Does the child appear well nourished, appropriately dressed, clean, and appropriately groomed?
3. **Adult Woman:** Does she have a history of abuse as a child?
4. **Adult Man:** Does he have a history of abuse as a child?
5. **Elder:** Is there a history of unexplained "accidents" or physical injuries?
6. **Elder:** Does the elder have a history of being abused as a child, or abusing his or her children?
7. Does there seem to be a history of drug or alcohol abuse within the family system?
8. Does the client re-experience the abuse through flashbacks, dreams or nightmares, or intrusive thoughts?
9. Does the client or other family member state that he or she has had suicidal or homicidal thoughts in the past?

Presenting Signs and Symptoms

1. Feelings of helplessness or powerlessness
2. Repeated emergency room or hospital visits
3. Vague complaints, including insomnia, abdominal pain, hyperventilation, headache, or menstrual problems
4. Poorly explained bruises in various stages of healing
5. Injuries (bruises, fractures, scrapes, lacerations) that do not seem to fit the description of the "accident"
6. Frightened, withdrawn, depressed, and/or despondent appearance

Sample Questions

The nurse uses a variety of therapeutic techniques to obtain the answers to the following questions. Use your discretion and decide which questions are appropriate to complete your assessment.

FOR ALL CLIENTS

1. "Tell me about what happened to you?"
2. "Who takes care of you?" (for children or dependent elderly)
3. "What happens when you do something wrong?" (for children)
4. "How do you and your partner/caregiver resolve disagreements?" (for women and elderly)
5. "What do you do for fun?"
6. "Who helps you with your child(ren)? Parents?"
7. "What time do you have for yourself?"

FOR SPOUSE (Feldhaus et al., 1997)

1. "Have you been hit, kicked, or otherwise hurt by someone in the past year? By whom?"
2. "Do you feel safe in your current relationship?"
3. "Is there a partner from a previous relationship who is making you feel unsafe now?"

FOR PARENTS

1. "What arrangement do you make when you have to leave your child alone?"
2. "How do you discipline your child?"
3. "When your infant cries for a long time, how do you get him or her to stop?"
4. "What about your child's behavior bothers you the most?"

Assessment Guidelines

Box 16–2 is an Abuse Assessment Screen developed by the Nursing Research Consortium on Violence and Abuse and is a helpful tool for nurses in the clinical area.

ASSESSMENT ALERTS
During your assessment and counseling, maintain an interested and empathetic manner. Refrain from displaying horror, anger, shock or disapproval of the perpetrator or the situation. Assess for: 1. Presenting signs and symptoms of victims of family violence   2. Potential problem in vulnerable families. For example, some indicators of vulnerable parents who might benefit from education and effective coping techniques are listed in Box 16–3.   3. Physical, sexual, and/or emotional abuse and neglect and economic maltreatment in the case of elders   4. Family coping patterns   5. Client's support system   6. Drug or alcohol use   7. Suicidal or homicidal ideas   8. Post-trauma syndrome   9. If the client is a child or an elder, identify the protection agency in your state that will have to be notified.

❖   B O X   1 6 – 2   ❖
Abuse Assessment Screen

1. Have you ever been emotionally or physically abused by
   your partner or someone important to you?
   Yes _____ No _____
   If yes, by whom? _____
   Number of times _____
2. Within the past year, have you been hit, slapped, kicked, or
   otherwise physically hurt by someone?
   Yes _____ No _____
   If yes, by whom? _____
   Number of times _____
3. Since you have been pregnant, have you been hit, slapped,
   kicked, or otherwise physically hurt by someone?
   Yes _____ No _____
   If yes, by whom? _____
   Number of times _____
4. Within the past year, has anyone forced you to have sexual
   activities?
   Yes _____ No _____
   If yes, by whom? _____
   Number of times _____
5. Are you afraid of your partner or anyone listed above?
   Yes_____ No _____

The Abuse Assessment Screen was developed by the Nursing Research
Consortium on Violence and Abuse (1989). Its reproduction and use
is encouraged. Used with permission of Peace at Home, Boston,
Massachusetts.

◆ NURSING DIAGNOSES WITH INTERVENTION

Violence brings with it pain, psychological and physical injury and
anguish, the potential for disfigurement, and the potential for
death. Therefore, **Risk for Injury** is a major concern for nurses
and other members of the health care team.

Within all families where violence occurs, severe communication problems are evident. Coping skills are not adequate to handle
the emotional and environmental events that trigger the crisis situation. Inadequate coping skills among family members result in
family members not getting their needs met, including the need for
safety, security, and sense of self. Therefore, there exists **Altered
Role Performance** within the family.

There are many other nursing diagnoses that the nurse may use in caring for children and adults who are suffering from abuse at the hands of others. Some include **Anxiety, Fear, Ineffective Family Coping, Post-Trauma Syndrome, Powerlessness, Caregiver Role Strain, Body Image Disturbance, Self-Esteem Disturbance, Altered Parenting,** and **Pain.**

This chapter discusses Risk for Injury for the child, adult, and elder and Altered Role Performance geared toward the abuser.

OVERALL GUIDELINES FOR NURSING INTERVENTIONS

1. Establish rapport before focusing in on the details of the violent experience.
2. Reassure client that he or she did nothing wrong.
3. Allow client to tell his or her story without interruptions.
4. If clients is an **adult**, assure client of confidentiality, and that any changes are his or hers to make.
5. If client is a **child**, report abuse to appropriate authorities designated in your state.
6. If client is an **elder**, check with state laws for reporting information.
7. Establish a safety plan in situations of **spouse abuse**. (See Box 16–5 for a full personalized plan.)
8. **Keep your charting detailed, accurate, and up-to-date.**
   - Verbatim statements of who caused the injury and when it occurred
   - A body map to indicate size, color, shape, areas, and types of injuries with explanation
   - Physical evidence, when possible, of sexual abuse
   - Ask for permission to take photos.
9. Be aware of your own feelings of anger, frustration, and need to rescue.
10. Use peer supervision for validation, support, and guidance.

Risk for Injury

A state in which an individual is at risk of injury as a result of environmental conditions interacting with the individual's adaptive and defensive resources

---

❖   B O X   1 6 – 3   ❖
Assessing Parents Vulnerable
for Child Abuse

---

1. New parents whose behavior toward the infant is rejecting, hostile, or indifferent
2. Teenage parents, most of whom are children themselves, require special help and guidance in handling the baby and discussing their expectations of the baby and their support systems.
3. Retarded parents, for whom careful, explicit, and repeated instructions on caring for the child and recognizing the infant's needs are indicated
4. People who grew up watching their mother being beaten. This is the biggest risk factor for perpetuation of family violence.

Related To (Etiology): Perpetrator's

- Rage reaction (parents, partner, caregiver)
- Poor coping skills
- History of violence, neglect, or emotional deprivation as a child
- History of drug or alcohol abuse
- Poor impulse control
- Decline in mental status or has a mental illness
- Pathological family dynamics

As Evidenced By (Assessment Findings/Diagnostic Cues): Victim's

- Recurrent emergency department (ED) visits for injuries attributed to being "accident prone"
- Presenting problems reflecting signs of high anxiety and chronic stress:
  - Hyperventilation
  - Panic attacks
  - Gastrointestinal disturbances
  - Hypertension
  - Physical injuries
- Depression
- Stress related conditions:
  - Insomnia

◆ NANDA accepted; ● In addition to NANDA.

- • Violent nightmares
- • Anxiety
- • Extreme fatigue
- • Eczema, loss of hair
- ● Inability to concentrate as seen in poor school or work performance
- ● Poor hygiene and disheveled appearance at school or work or in the home
- ● Bruises of various ages and specific shapes (fingers, belts)

Child Abuse Client

Outcome Criteria

Child will:

- • Know what plans are made for the child's protection and state them to nurse after decision is made by health care team
- • Demonstrate renewed confidence and feelings of safety during follow-up visits

Short-Term Goals

Child will:

- • Be safe until adequate home and family assessment is made by (date)
- • Be treated by nurse practitioner or physician and receive medical care for injuries within 1 hour
- • Participate with therapists (nurse, social worker, counselor) for purpose of ongoing therapy and emotional support (art, play, group, or other) within 24 to 48 hours

Interventions and Rationales

Intervention	Rationale
1. Adopt a non-threatening, nonjudgmental relationship with the parent(s).	1. If the parent(s) feel judged or blamed or become defensive, they may take the child and either seek help elsewhere or seek no help at all.
2. Understand that children do not want to betray their parent(s).	2. Even in an intolerable situation, the parent(s) are the only security that child knows.

◆ NANDA accepted; ● In addition to NANDA.

3. Provide (or have physician provide) a complete physical assessment of child.

3. Provide competent care and to substantiate reporting to child welfare agency if required.

4. Use of dolls may help child tell his or her story of how "accident" happened.

4. Child may not know how to articulate what happened or may be afraid of punishment. Dolls may be an easier way for child to act out what happened.

5. **Be aware of your agency's and state's policy on reporting child abuse.** Contact supervisor and/or social worker to implement appropriate reporting (Gorman et al., 1996).

5. Health care workers are mandated to report any cases of "suspected" or actual child abuse.

6. Ensure that proper procedures are followed, and evidence is collected.

6. If child is temporarily taken to a safe environment, appropriate evidence helps protect the child's future welfare.

7. Keep accurate and detailed records of incident:
   • Verbatim statements of who caused the injury and when it occurred
   • A body map to indicate size, color, shape, areas, and types of injuries with explanation
   • Physical evidence, when possible, of sexual abuse
   • Use of photos can be helpful. Check hospital policy.

7. Accurate records could help ensure child's future safety.

Spouse Abuse Client

Outcome Criteria

Clients will:

• Within 3 weeks, state that they believe that they do not deserve to be beaten
• Within 3 weeks, state they have joined a support group or are receiving counseling (families, couples, individual)

- State that their living conditions are now safe from spouse abuse or potential abuse; *or*
- Within 2 months, state that they have found safe housing for self and children

Short-Term Goals

Clients will:

- Have timely access to medical care for fractures, wounds, burns, and other injuries
- After initial interview, name four community resources they can contact (hotlines, shelters, support groups, neighbor, crisis center, or spiritual advisors who do not support violence)
- After initial interview, describe a safety plan to be used in future violent situations
- State their right to live in a safe environment by (date)

Interventions and Rationales

Intervention	**Rationale**
1. Ensure that medical attention is provided to client. Ask permission to take photos.	1. If client wants to file charges, photos boost victim's confidence to press charges now or in the future.
2. Set up interview in private and ensure confidentiality.	2. Client may be terrified of retribution and further attacks from partner if she "tells."
3. Assess in a nonthreatening manner information concerning: a. Sexual abuse b. Chemical abuse c. Thoughts of suicide or homicide	3. These are all vital issues in determining appropriate interventions: a. Increases risk for Posttrauma syndrome. b. Many victims self-medicate. c. May seem the only way out of an intolerable, catastrophic situation.
4. Encourage client to talk about the battering incident without interruptions.	4. When you ask clients to share their story, you understand that you are there to listen.
5. Assess for level of violence in the home (refer to Box 16–4).	5. Each cycle of violence can become more intense. Danger for life of victim

6. Ask how client is faring with the children in the home.

7. Assess if clients have a safe place to go when violence is escalating. If NO, include a list of shelters or safe houses with other written information.

8. Identity if client is interested in pressing charges. If yes, give information on:
   a. Local attorneys who handle spouse abuse cases
   b. Legal clinics
   c. Battered women's advocates

9. **Know the requirement in your state about reporting suspected spouse abuse.**

10. Discuss with client an escape plan during

and children increases during escalation.

6. In homes where the mother is abused, children also tend to be abused.

7. When abused clients are ready to go, they will need to go quickly.

8. Often clients are afraid of spouse or partner retaliation, but when they are ready to seek legal advice, appropriate list of lawyers well trained in this area are needed.

9. Many states have or are developing laws and/or guidelines for protecting battered women.

10. Write out plan and put in shelter and referral

❖   B O X   1 6 – 4   ❖

Spouse Abuse—Assessing Level of Violence in the Home

1. Does the client feel safe?
2. Has there been a recent increase in violence?
3. Has the client been choked?
4. Is there a weapon in the house?
5. Has the abuser used/threatened to use a weapon?
6. Has the abuser threatened to harm the children?
7. Has the abuser threatened to kill the client?

Adapted from Jezierski, M. (1994). Abuse of women by male partners: Basic knowledge for emergency nurses. Journal of Emergency Nursing 20(5):361; reprinted with permission.

Intervention	**Rationale**
escalation of anxiety, before actual violence erupts. (Box 16–5 is an example of a personalized safety plan.)	numbers. This can prevent further abuse to children and client.
11. Throughout work with battered spouses emphasize: a. "**No one** deserves to be beaten" b. "You **cannot make anyone hurt you.** It is **not** your fault."	11. When self-esteem is eroded, people often buy into the myth that they deserved the beatings because they did something "wrong," and if they hadn't done x, then it wouldn't have happened.
12. Encourage clients to reach out to family and friends they may have been avoiding.	12. Old friends and relatives can make helpful allies and validate that client doesn't deserve to be beaten.
13. Know the psychotherapists in your community who have experience working with battered spouses/partners.	13. Psychotherapy with victims of trauma requires *special skills* on the part of even an experienced therapist.
14. If client is not ready to take action at this time, give her a list of community resources available: a. Hotlines b. Shelters c. Battered women's groups d. Battered women's advocates e. Social services f. Medical assistance/ Aid to Families with Dependent Children (AFDC)	14. It may take time for clients to make decisions to change their life situation. People need appropriate information.

Box 16–5 provides a personalized safety plan for when the client is in the relationship and when the relationship is over.

❖   B O X   1 6 – 5   ❖
Personalized Safety Plan

Suggestions for Increasing Safety—in the Relationship

- I will have important phone numbers available to my children and myself.
- I can tell _____ and _____ about the violence and ask them to call the police if they hear suspicious noises coming from my home.
- If I leave my home, I can go (list four places) _____, _____, _____, or _____.
- I can leave extra money, car keys, clothes, and copies of documents with _____.
- If I leave, I will bring _____ (see checklist next page).
- To ensure safety and independence, I can: keep change for phone calls with me at all times; open my own savings account; rehearse my escape route with a support person; and review safety plan on _____ (date).

Suggestions for Increasing Safety—When the Relationship Is Over

- I can: change the locks; install steel/metal doors, a security system, smoke detectors, and an outside lighting system.
- I will inform _____ and _____ that my partner no longer lives with me and ask them to call the police if he or she is observed near my home or my children.
- I will tell people who take care of my children the names of those who have permission to pick them up. The people who have permission are: _____, _____, and _____.
- I can tell _____ at work about my situation and ask _____ to screen my calls.
- I can avoid stores, banks, and _____ that I used when living with my battering partner.
- I can obtain a protective order from _____. I can keep it on or near me at all times as well as have a copy with _____.
- If I feel down and ready to return to a potentially abusive situation, I can call _____ for support or attend workshops and support groups to gain support and strengthen my relationships with other people.

Continued

Important Phone Numbers

Police _____
Hotline _____
Friends _____
Shelter _____

Items To Take Checklist

Identification
Birth certificates for me and my children
Social Security cards
School and medical records
Money, bankbooks, credit cards
Keys—house/car/office
Driver's license and registration
Medications
Change of clothes
Welfare identification
Passport(s), Green Cards, work permits
Divorce papers
Lease/rental agreement, house deed
Mortgage payment book, current unpaid bills
Insurance papers
Address book
Pictures, jewelry, items of sentimental value
Children's favorite toys and/or blankets

❖   B O X   1 6 – 6   ❖
Home Assessment—Elder Abuse/Neglect

Environmental Conditions

- House in poor repair
- Inadequate heat, lighting, furniture, cooking utensils
- Presence of garbage or vermin
- Old food in kitchen
- Lack of assistive devices
- Locks on refrigerator
- Blocked stairways
- Victim lying in urine, feces, or food
- Unpleasant odors

Medication

- Medication not being taken as prescribed

Elder Abuse Client

Outcome Criteria

Client will:

- State that caregiver has provided adequate food, clothing, housing, and medical care by (date)
- Be free of physical signs of abuse by (date)

Short-Term Goals

Clients will:

- State that they feel safer and more comfortable by (date) using a scale of 1–5 (1 being the safest); *or*
- Ask to be removed from violent situation by (date)
- Name two people who can be called for help by (date)

Interventions and Rationales

Intervention	Rationale
1. Assess severity of signs and symptoms of abuse and potential for further abuse on a weekly level.	1. Determines need for further intervention.
2. Assess environmental conditions as factors in abuse or neglect (refer to Box 16–6).	2. Identifies areas in need of intervention and degree of abuse or neglect.
3. If abuse is suspected, talk with client and caregiver separately.	3. Helps attain a better understanding of what is happening, and to minimize friction between the two.
4. Discuss with client factors leading to abuse.	4. Identifies triggers to abusive behaviors and areas for teaching for abuser.
5. Stress concern for physical safety.	5 Validates situation is serious.
6. Know your state laws regarding elder abuse. Notify supervisor, physicians, and social services when a suspected abuse is reported.	6. Keeps channels of communications open. Emphasizes the need for accurate and detailed records.

Intervention	**Rationale**
7. Stress that no one has the right to abuse another person.	7. Often people who have been abused begin to believe that they "deserve" the abuse.
8. Discuss with client: a. Hotlines b. Crisis units c. Emergency numbers	8. Maximizes client safety through use of support systems.
9. Explore with client ways to make changes.	9. Directs assessment to positive areas.
10. Assist client in making decisions for future action.	10. Helps lower feelings of helplessness and identifies realistic options to an abusive situation.
11. Involve community supports to help monitor and support elder.	11. Involve as many agencies as can take a legitimate role in maintaining client safety.

Altered Role Performance

The pattern of behavior and self-expression do not match the environmental context, norms, and expectations

---

Related To (Etiology)

◆ Domestic violence
◆ Inadequate support system
◆ Family conflict
◆ Young age, developmental level
◆ Low socioeconomic status
◆ Substance abuse
◆ Mental health disorder
◆ Lack of resources
◆ Lack of knowledge about role skills

As Evidenced By (Assessment Findings/Diagnostic Cues)

◆ Inadequate external support for role enactment
◆ System conflict

◆ NANDA accepted; ● In addition to NANDA.

- ◆ Change in usual patterns of responsibility
- ◆ Domestic violence
- ◆ Inadequate role competency and skills
- ◆ Role overload
- ◆ Inadequate coping
- ● Anxiety or depression

Parents of Abused Child

Outcome Criteria

Parent(s) will:

- State that group meetings with other parents who have battered are useful
- Demonstrate at least four new parenting skills that they find effective
- Share in two planned pleasurable activities twice a day with child when child returns home
- Attend workshops/group classes for effective parenting on an ongoing basis
- Attend an anger management training (AMT) course within 2 weeks

Short-Term Goals

Parent(s) will:

- Be able to name and call three agencies that can help financially during the crisis within 24 hours
- Name two places they can contact to discuss feeling of rage and helplessness by end of first interview
- Be able to name three alternative actions to take when feelings of helplessness and rage start to surface within 1 week

Interventions and Rationales

Intervention	Rationale

1. Identify if the child needs:
  a. Hospitalization for treatment and observation, *and/or*
  b. Referral to child protective services
	1. Immediate safety of the child is foremost. Temporary removal of the child in volatile situations gives the nurse/ counselor time to assess

---

◆ NANDA accepted; ● In addition to NANDA.

Intervention	**Rationale**
	the family situation, and coping skills and rally community resources to lower family stress.
2. Discuss with parent(s) stresses the family unit is currently facing. Contact appropriate agencies to help reduce stress: *Economic* a. Job opportunities b. Social services c. Family service agencies *Social supports* a. Public health nurse b. Day care teacher c. Schoolteacher d. Social worker e. Respite worker f. AMT Encourage and provide family therapy.	2. Lower family stress can lead to improved ability to problem solve with help of outside resources.
3. Reinforce parent(s) strengths and acknowledge the importance of continued medical care for the child (Gorman et al., 1996).	3. Gives parent(s) credit and reinforce positive parenting skills.
4. Work with parent(s) to try out safe and effective methods to discipline the child.	4. Gives parent(s) alternatives and can help minimize feelings of frustration and helplessness.
5. Strongly encourage parent(s) to join a self-help group (e.g., Parents Anonymous, family counseling, group counseling).	5. Learning new ways of dealing with stress takes time, and support from others acts as an important incentive to change.
6. Provide written information on hotlines, community supports, and agencies.	6. Have resources available for immediate use.

Perpetrator and Client in Spouse Abuse

Outcome Criteria

Abuser will:

- State he must change in order to stay with family
- Join and attend a group for spouses who batter
- Recognize inner states of anger
- Attend a structured AMT program
- Demonstrate at least four alternative ways to deal with anger and frustration
- Within 6 months, couple will state that violence has ceased altogether

Short-Term Goals

Clients will:

- State that they are interested in knowing about family treatment modalities
- State that they no longer choose to live in a situation with violence
- Name three places they can call to receive counseling for self and family
- Obtain a restraining order
- Have information on safe houses or name people they can stay with

Interventions and Rationales—Spouse Abuser

Intervention	Rationale
1. If abuser is motivated, make arrangements for abuser to participate in an AMT program.	1. Empirical results show a 6- to 8-week structural program trains clients to deactivate angry emotional state (Suinn, 1998).
2. Work with abuser to recognize signs of escalating anger.	2. Often abuser is unaware of process of what leads up to rage reaction.
3. Work with abuser to learn ways of channeling anger nonviolently.	3. Violence is often a learned coping skill. Adaptive skills for dealing with anger need to be learned.
4. Encourages abuser to discuss thoughts and feelings with others who have similar problems.	4. Minimizes isolation and encourages problem solving.

Intervention	Rationale
5. Refer to self-help groups in the community for abusive men, such as Batterers Anonymous.	5. Self-help groups help clients look at own behaviors among those who have similar problems.

Perpetrator and Client of Elder Abuse

Outcome Criteria

- Client will state the abuse has stopped, or state that he or she is now in a safe place.
- Family members will state that they will meet the nurse/counselor on a weekly basis for counseling starting by (date).
- Abuser will meet with other family members and discuss feelings on care of elderly by (date).
- Family members will meet together and discuss alternatives for care of elder by (date).
- Client and family will meet together and discuss resources and supports they feel are important to them by (date).
- Abuser will demonstrate, instead of violence, two appropriate methods of dealing with frustration by date.

Short-Term Goals

- Family members will meet together with nurse/counselor and discuss alternative approaches toward their elderly family member within 1 week.
- Family members will role play two strategies for avoiding physical or emotional violence toward elder (relaxation, assertive behaviors, anger management techniques) by (date).
- Family members will demonstrate two safe alternative methods of dealing with their emotions in "hot" situations by date.
- Family members will name two support services to whom they can turn for help within 2 days.
- One other family member or support person will spend time with elder and relieve abuser of caregiving duties for stated periods of time within 1 week.

Interventions and Rationals—Elder Abuser

Intervention	Rationale
1. Check your state for laws regarding elder abuse.	1. Many states have adopted laws to help protect elders and support their needs for safety.

2. Encourage abuser to verbalize feelings about elder and the abusive situation.

2. It may be that the abuser feels overwhelmed, isolated, and unsupported.

3. Encourage problem-solving approach when identifying stressful areas.

3. Assesses abuser's problem-solving skills and explores alternatives.

4. Meet with entire family and identify stressors and problem areas.

4. Other family members may not be aware of the strain the abuser is under or the lack of safety to the abused family member.

5. If there are no other family members, notify other community agencies that might help abuser and elder stabilize situation, for example:
   a. Support group for elder
   b. Support group for abuser
   c. Meals on Wheels
   d. Day care for seniors
   e. Respite services
   f. Visiting nurse service

5. Minimizes family stress and isolation, and increases safety.

6. Initiate referrals for available support services.

6. Rallies needed support for abusive situation.

7. Encourage abuser's use of counseling.

7. Increases coping skills and social supports.

8. Suggest that family members meet together on a regular basis for problem solving and support.

8. Encourages family to learn to solve problems together.

9. Act as a facilitator in the beginning to assess and teach problem-solving skills and offer referral information.

9. Families increase their communication skills, effectiveness in interactions, and self-esteem.

◆ PART II: SEXUAL ASSAULT

Rape is an act of violence, and sex is the weapon used by the perpetrator. **Rape is a nonconsensual vaginal, anal, or oral penetration, obtained by force or threat of bodily harm, or when a person is incapable of giving consent**. It is usually men who rape, and most of those raped are women. A male who is raped is more likely to have physical trauma and to have been victimized by several assailants than is a female (Smith-DiJulio, 1998). The male experiences the same devastating severe and long-lasting trauma as do females. Long-term psychological effects of sexual assault may include the development of depression, dysfunction, and somatic complaints in many survivors. Incest victims may experience a negative self-image, self-destructive behavior, and substance abuse. All catastrophic events may result in a post-trauma syndrome. The **Rape-Trauma Syndrome** is a variant of PTSD and consists of two phases: (1) the acute phase, and (2) the long-term reorganization phase. Nurses may encounter clients right after the sexual assault or weeks, months, or even years after the sexual assault. In either case, the individual will benefit from compassionate and effective nursing interventions.

Assessment for Sexual Assault

History

A positive history includes:

1. A history of a previous sexual assault
2. A history of incest within the family
3. The individual suffers from any of the signs and symptoms of PTSD

Presenting Signs and Symptoms

ACUTE PHASE OF RAPE-TRAUMA SYNDROME
(0 TO 2 WEEKS AFTER THE RAPE)

Typical reactions to crisis reflecting cognitive, affective, and behavioral disruptions:

1. Shock, numbness, and disbelief.
2. May appear calm and self-contained.
3. May appear hysterical, restless.
4. May cry a lot; *or*
5. May smile or laugh a lot.
6. Complains of disorganization in his or her life.
7. Complains of somatic symptoms.

LONG-TERM REORGANIZATION PHASE (2 WEEKS OR MORE)

1. Intrusive thought of the rape throughout day and night
2. Flashbacks of the incident (re-experiencing the traumatic event)
3. Dreams with violent content
4. Insomnia

5. Increased motor activity (moving, taking trips, changing phone numbers, staying with friends)
6. Mood swings, crying spells, depression
7. Fears and phobias may develop:
   a. Fear of indoors (if rape occurred indoors)
   b. Fear of outdoors (if rape occurred outdoors)
   c. Fear of being alone
   d. Fear of crowds
   e. Fear of sexual encounters

Sample Questions

Questioning should be done in a very nonthreatening manner using open-ended types of questions (e.g., "It must have been very frightening to know you had no control of what was happening.").

☰	ASSESSMENT ALERTS
	1. Assess physical trauma—use a body map and ask permission to take photos.
	2. Assess psychological trauma—write down verbatim statements of client.
	3. Assess available support system. Often partners or family members don't understand about rape, and may not be the best supports to rally at this time.
	4. Assess level of anxiety. If clients are in severe to panic levels of anxiety, they will not be able to problem solve or process information.
	5. Identify community supports (e.g., attorneys, support groups, therapist) that work in the area of sexual assault.
	6. Encourage clients to tell their story. **Do not** press them to.

Nursing Diagnoses with Interventions

Rape-Trauma Syndrome is the nursing diagnosis that applies to the physical and psychological effects resulting from a sexual assault. The diagnosis includes the acute phase of disorganization of the survivor's lifestyle and the long-term phase reorganization.

Rape-Trauma Syndrome: Compound Reaction includes the above diagnosis with:

• Reliance on alcohol or other drugs
• Reactivated symptoms of previous conditions, such as physical or psychiatric illness

Rape-Trauma Syndrome: Silent Reaction is a complex stress reaction to rape. The individual is usually unable to describe or discuss the rape. Some of the symptoms are:

- Abrupt changes in relationships with men
- Nightmares
- Increasing anxiety during the interview, silence, blocking, stuttering
- Marked change in sexual behavior
- Sudden onset of phobic reactions
- No verbalization of the occurrence of rape

Each ED or crisis center needs to have its own rape protocol. Most EDs and crisis centers also have rape kits that facilitate collection of specimens.

OVERALL GUIDELINES FOR NURSING INTERVENTION

1. Follow your institution's protocol for sexual assault.
2. Do not leave the person alone.
3. Maintain a nonjudgmental attitude.
4. Ensure confidentiality.
5. Encourage the person to talk; listen empathetically.
6. Emphasize that the person did the right thing to save his or her life.
7. Keep accurate records:
   - Physical trauma—size, color, distribution of trauma with a body map.
   - Ask permission to take photos.
   - Take verbatim statements as to client's reaction to rape.
   - Document emotional status.
8. Explain everything that you are going to do beforehand.
9. Obtain medicolegal specimens with client's written permission.
10. Alert client as to what he or she may experience during the long-term reorganization phase.
11. Arrange for support follow-up, for example:
    - Support groups
    - Group therapy
    - Individual therapy
    - Crisis counseling

Rape-Trauma Syndrome

Sustained maladaptive response to a forced, violent, sexual penetration against the victim's will and consent

---

Related To (Etiology)

◆ Rape

As Evidenced By (Assessment Findings/Diagnostic Cues)

◆ Disorganization
◆ Change in relationships
◆ Physical trauma (bruising, tissue irritation)
◆ Suicide attempts
◆ Denial
◆ Guilt, humiliation, embarrassment
◆ Aggression; muscle tension
◆ Mood swings
◆ Nightmare and sleep disturbances
◆ Sexual dysfunction
◆ Feelings for revenge
◆ Phobias
◆ Loss of self-esteem
◆ Inability to make decisions
◆ Vulnerability, helplessness
◆ Substance abuse
◆ Depression, anxiety
◆ Shame, shock, fear
◆ Self-blame
◆ Dissociative disorders
◆ Hyperalertness

Outcome Criteria

The survivor will:

• Discuss the need for follow-up crisis counseling and other supports by (date)
• State that the acuteness of the memory of the rape subsides over time and is less vivid and less frightening within 3 to 5 months

---

◆ NANDA accepted; ● In addition to NANDA.

- State that the physical symptoms (e.g., sleep disturbances, poor appetite, and physical trauma) have subsided within 3 to 5 months

Short-Term Goals

The survivor will:

- Begin to express reactions and feelings about the assault before leaving the ED or crisis center
- Have a short-term plan for handling immediate situational needs before leaving the ED or crisis center
- List common physical, social, and emotional reactions that often follow a sexual assault before leaving the ED or crisis center
- Speak to a community-based rape victim advocate in the ED or crisis center
- State the results of the physical examination completed in the ED or crisis center

Interventions and Rationales

Intervention	Rationale
1. Have someone stay with the client (friend, neighbor, or staff member) while he or she is waiting to be treated in ED.	1. People in high levels of anxiety need someone with them until anxiety level is down to moderate.
2. **Very Important:** Approach client in a nonjudgmental manner.	2. Nurses' attitudes can have an important therapeutic impact. Displays of shock, horror, disgust, or disbelief are not appropriate.
3. Confidentiality is crucial.	3. The client's situation is not to be discussed with **anyone** other than medical personnel involved unless client gives their consent.
4. Explain to client the signs and symptoms that many people experience during the long-term phase, for example: a. Nightmares b. Phobias c. Anxiety, depression d. Insomnia e. Somatic symptoms	4. Many individuals think they are going crazy as time goes on and are not aware that this is a process that many people in their situation have experienced.

5. Listen and let the client talk. **Do not** press client to talk.

5. When people feel understood, they feel more in control of their situation.

6. Stress that they did the right thing to save their life.

6. Rape victims may feel guilt or shame. Reinforcing that they did what they had to do to stay alive can reduce guilt and maintain self-esteem.

7. Assess the signs and symptoms of physical trauma.

7. Most common injuries are to face, head, neck, extremities.

8. Make a body map to identify size, color, and location of injuries. Ask permission to take photos.

8. Accurate records and photos can be used as medicolegal evidence for the future.

9. Carefully explain all procedures before doing them (e.g., "We would like to do a vaginal exam and do a swab. Have you had a vaginal exam before?" [rectal exam in case of raped male]).

9. The individual is experiencing high levels of anxiety. Matter-of-factly explaining what you plan to do and why can help reduce fear and anxiety.

10. Explain the evidence you plan to collect; inform client that it can be used for identification and prosecution of the rapist, for example:
    a. Combing pubic hairs
    b. Skin from underneath nails
    c. Semen samples

10. Collecting body fluids and swabs is essential (DNA) for identifying the rapist.

11. Explain to the client that many medical facilities automatically treat for sexually transmitted diseases.

11. Many survivors are lost to follow-up after being seen in the ED or crisis center and won't otherwise get protection.

12. Many clinics offer prophylaxis to pregnancy with norgestrel (Ovral).

12. About 3% to 5% of women who are raped become pregnant.

Intervention	**Rationale**

13. All data must be carefully documented:
    a. Verbatim statements
    b. Detailed observations of physical trauma
    c. Detailed observations of emotional status
    d. Results from the physical examination
    e. All lab tests should be noted.

13. Accurate and detailed documentation is crucial legal evidence.

14. Arrange for support follow-up:
    a. Rape counselor
    b. Support group
    c. Group therapy
    d. Individual therapy
    e. Crisis counseling

14. Many individuals carry with them constant emotional trauma. Depression and suicidal ideation are frequent sequelae of rape. The sooner the intervention, the less complicated the recovery may be.

◆ NURSE, CLIENT, AND FAMILY RESOURCES— FAMILY VIOLENCE AND SEXUAL ASSAULT

Associations

Family Violence Sexual Assault Institute (FUSAI)
1300 Clinic Drive
Tyler, TX 75701
1-903-595-6600 (voice); 1-904-595-6799 (Fax)

National Domestic Violence Hotline (NDV Hotline)
3616 Far West Boulevard, Suite 101-297
Austin, TX 78731-3074
1-800-799-SAFE (Hotline)

Rape, Abuse, Incest National Network (RAINN)
1-800-656-HOPE
http://www.feminist.com/rainn.htm

Batterers Anonymous
8485 Tamarinal #D
Fontana, CA 92335
1-909-355-1100
(For men who wish to control their anger and eliminate their abusive behavior)

Sexual Abuse Survivors Anonymous (SASA)
P.O. Box 241046
Detroit, MI 48224
(12-step program for survivors of rape, incest, or sexual abuse)

Survivors of Incest Anonymous (SIA)
P.O. Box 26870
Baltimore, MD 21212
1-410-282-3400
(12-step program for survivors of incest)

Child Abuse Prevention—Kids Peace
1-800-257-3223

Child Help USA Hotline
1-800-422-4453 (24 hours)

Youth Crisis Hotline
1-800-HIT-HOME

Runaway Hotline
1-800-231-6946

Internet Sites

National Coalition Against Domestic Violence
http://www.ncadv.org

National Clearinghouse Child Abuse and Neglect Information
1-800-394-3366
http://www.calib.com/nccanch

Prevent Child Abuse America Home Page
http://www.childabuse.org

Child Abuse Prevention Network
http://child.cornell.edu

Victim Services Domestic Violence Shelter Tour
http://www.dvsheltertour.org

David Baldwin's Trauma Information Page
http://www.trauma-pages.com/
Site focuses on emotional trauma and traumatic stress

Especially for Men

Men Who Have Experienced Sexual Abuse (NOMSV)
http://www.malesurvivor.org/

Men's Rape Prevention Project
http://www.mrpp.org
(Helping men who rape)

CHAPTER 17

Manipulation

Healthy manipulation is essentially purposeful behavior directed at getting needs met. It (1) is goal oriented and used only when appropriate, (2) considers others' needs, and (3) is only one of several coping mechanisms used.

Individuals manipulate events every day to manage their lives (e.g., carry out financial obligations, optimize social activities, ensure the welfare of their families), and to keep their lives and the lives of those they care about as secure and stable as possible. Most nurses are good at organizing their daily schedules to provide the optimum care to their clients. This may include consults with other health care professionals, changing time schedules, organizing care into priorities, and countless other ways to ensure quality care. These are all healthy uses of manipulation. Nurses manipulate situations and events not just to complete their assignment, but to best serve their clients.

Manipulation is maladaptive when (Chitty and Maynard, 1986):

- It is the primary method used for getting needs met.
- The needs, goals, and feelings of others are disregarded.
- Others are treated as objects in order to fulfill the needs of the manipulator.

Manipulation is in effect a matter of gaining a sense of control. When manipulation is used in a maladaptive manner, individuals will say or do most anything to get what they want, even if it is at the expense of others.

Maladaptive manipulation in the health care system may present a real challenge to staff. Staff are most effective when they are working together on intervention for manipulation. One way staff members can be alert to being manipulated is when each staff member views and experiences the client in extremely different ways. This inevitably results in staff confusion and disagreements. Infighting may result when discussing caring for the client. Varia-

434

tions in experiences can occur between nurses and physicians, between shifts, between individuals on the nursing staff, and/or between administrators and staff (Gorman et al., 1996).

Potential for staff manipulation is particularly high among individuals who:

- Have personality disorders (especially borderline and antisocial PDs)
- Abuse substances
- Are in the manic phase of bipolar disorder
- Have long histories of physical complaints without physical cause
- Are children or adolescents who have the diagnosis of conduct disorder

People who manipulate may be trying to gain a variety of different things, although a need for control is usually the underlying force. For example, people may manipulate to get nurturance, power over a situation or person, possessions, or some other material gratification.

Clients may manipulate by the use of pitting one person or group against another person or group:

"Nurse X really understands my situation, she lets me take my own medications (etc.) Why can't you? Please don't tell anyone I told on nurse X. I don't want her to get into trouble."

Or, when talking to a member of the day staff, a manipulative client might say something like:

"The night staff are awful, they just sit around and drink coffee, yell at the patients when they ring their bells, and really say some nasty stuff about you day people."

Once staff is all stirred up and angry with each other, the client is better able to get what he or she wants without interference. Staff splitting is a real challenge in the health care setting. Clients also manipulate when they flatter and behave in such a way as to give the impression of sincerity, caring, and appreciation when their only goal is to get their own needs met in any manner possible:

"You are the kindest nurse on the unit, and the only one here who cares enough to understand me. You know how much I need to go out on pass even if I did come in late yesterday. I know I'm not supposed to but please trust me just this once. I promise I will be on time. "

Clients with *substance abuse* problems are used to soothing anxiety and denying or postponing unattractive realities through use of their substance. Clients learn to manipulate others through anger, threatening, swindling, cajoling, instilling guilt, flattering, or any other method in order to get their drugs. For most people dependent upon a drug(s), the drug is the only thing in the world they care about.

Another form of manipulation is seen in clients who are profane, fault finding, and adept at exploring others' vulnerabilities. They constantly push limits. Their manipulative behaviors often alienate family, friends, employers, health care providers, and others.

◆ ASSESSING FOR MANIPULATON

History

A positive history may include some of the following:

1. A history of a PD (borderline, antisocial, passive-aggressive)
2. A history of mania
3. A history of substance abuse
4. A history of unreliable or immature behaviors marked by instability, frequent changes in jobs, relationships, and physicians
5. A long history of unsubstantiated physical complaints

Presenting Symptoms

1. Manipulation of staff, family, and others
2. Playing one person against another (nurse against nurse, family member against staff, therapist against family member)
3. Attempts to get special treatment or privileges
4. Attention-seeking behaviors
5. Use of somatic complaints to get out of doing things
6. Lacks insight
7. Denies problems
8. Focuses on other people's problems (clients, staff, unit dynamics)
9. May use intimidation to control or feel superior
10. Demanding (the more staff try to cater to client's demands, the more they escalate)
11. Frustration causes more intense manipulative behavior
12. Lies, cheats, steals
13. Exploitive with little concern for others
14. Quick to recognize vulnerability in others
15. Devalues others to feel good about self

Assessing Risk for Manipulation

1. Client has low frustration tolerance.
2. Client resists limits set on negative behaviors.

3. Staff confusion and upset related to client pitting staff against staff.
4. Client seeks out one staff member as "the one who really under-stands me . . . is the nicest . . . etc."
5. Client doesn't take responsibility for his or her actions in family, staff, or unit altercations.

Sample Questions

The nurse uses a variety of therapeutic techniques to obtain the an-swers to the following questions. Use your discretion and decide which questions are appropriate to complete your assessment.

1. "How do you feel when you don't get your way?"
2. "What do you do when you don't get your way?"
3. "Whom do you trust?"
4. "When do you feel the safest?"
5. "In what situations do you feel the most vulnerable?"

ASSESSMENT ALERTS

1. Assess for history of physical or psychosocial problems.
2. Identify client's usual coping responses.
3. Assess medications client is taking.
4. Assess for a history of substance abuse, spouse abuse, legal difficulties, violent behavior.
5. Assess client's strengths as well as weaknesses.
6. Is the client at risk for suicide? Homicide?
7. Is the client abusing others? Child? Spouse? Elder? Other?

◆ NURSING DIAGNOSES WITH INTERVENTIONS

Clients who employ manipulation as a primary means of getting their needs met often have no motivation to change, as long as they can get what they want when they want it, even if it is at the ex-pense of others. **Impaired Social Interaction** is most always pre-sent because the individual's actions usually impact negatively on others. People who employ maladaptive manipulation in their rela-tionships with others usually present with a history of interpersonal difficulties and unstable relationships. The manipulative individual may feel no compunction about lying, stealing, cheating, threaten-ing, tormenting, devaluing, demeaning, or swindling to get what he or she wants.

Staff working with manipulative clients are best prepared when they establish firm rules that are rigidly interpreted and consistently enforced among all members of the health care team. Frequent discussions regarding the client's progress can help reduce staff frustration and isolation, and minimize the client's attempts at staff splitting. Smith (1994) identifies important guidelines when intervening with manipulative behaviors:

- Ignoring manipulative behaviors won't make them go away; they get worse when ignored.
- Interventions such as employing limit-setting techniques help reduce stress and hostility for both client and staff.
- To successfully limit problem behavior, limits must be consistent and reinforced by everyone, including all health care personnel as well as family.

Therefore, **confronting** unacceptable, inappropriate, or harmful behavior needs to be done immediately, and **setting limits** on client behaviors is the pivotal intervention when working with manipulative clients. Clear, enforceable consequences of continuing unacceptable behaviors need to be clearly spelled out and consistently and matter-of-factly enforced by all staff involved in the client's care.

Schultz and Videbeck (1998) point out that it is not the nurse's purpose to be a friend to the client, nor the client a friend to the nurse. The most effective approach with the client is to maintain a professional therapeutic relationship with clear boundaries. A professional relationship is based upon the client's therapeutic needs, not on being liked or the nurse's personal feelings. People who manipulate others need clear and firm boundaries with clear and firm consequences identified for overstepping those boundaries.

Manipulative clients often have great difficulty with impulse control, and become inappropriately angry and may even become aggressive with little or no provocation when they can't get their own way. Therefore, anger management is often useful and important for nurses to learn and employ. **Chapter 14 identifies some useful guidelines for dealing with anger and aggression.**

OVERALL GUIDELINES FOR NURSING INTERVENTIONS

1. Anger is a natural response to being manipulated. Deal with your own feelings of anger toward client. Peer supervision can be useful.
2. Assess your feelings toward clients that use manipulation, and work on being assertive in stating limits. Workshops in assertiveness can be very helpful for nurses.

Continued

3. State limits and the behavior you expect from the client in a matter-of-fact, nonthreatening tone.
4. Be sure the limits are:
   • Appropriate, not punitive
   • Enforceable
   • Stated in a nonpersonal way (e.g., "Alcohol is not allowed," **not** "I don't want you to drink alcohol on the unit.")
5. State the consequences if behaviors are not forthcoming. Written limits and consequences can be useful (one copy for client and one for staff).
6. Be sure all staff understand the expectations, limits, and consequences discussed with the client to provide consistency. A written copy should be in Kardex or client folder.
7. Follow through with the consequences.
8. Enforce all unit, hospital, group, or community center policies. State reasons for not bending the rules.
9. Be direct and assertive if necessary in a neutral, factual manner, not out of anger.
10. Do **not:**
    • Discuss yourself or other staff members with the client
    • Promise to keep a secret for the client
    • Accept gifts from the client
    • Attempt to be liked, "the favorite," or popular with the client
11. Withdraw your attention when client's behavior is inappropriate.
12. Give attention and support when client's behavior is appropriate and positive.
13. Emphasize the client's feelings, not his or her rationalizations or intellectualizations.
14. Encourage the expression of feelings.
15. Set limits on frequency and time of interactions with the client, especially those that involve therapists significant to the client.
16. Encourage identification of feelings or situations that trigger manipulative behaviors.
17. Role play situations so that client may practice more direct and appropriate ways of relating.
18. Provide positive feedback when client interacts without use of manipulation.
19. Where appropriate, see that client and family have names and numbers of appropriate community resources (e.g., Alanon, Alcoholics Anonymous, Parents Anonymous, Tough Love).

Continued

20. Keep detailed records in client's chart as to client's responses to limit setting and any increase or decrease in undesirable, unacceptable, maladaptive manipulative behavior. Identify what seems to work and what doesn't seem to work. Share information with all staff.

Impaired Social Interaction

The state in which an individual participates in an insufficient or excessive quantity or ineffective quality of social exchange

---

Related To (Etiology)

- Longstanding patterns of maladaptive behaviors
- Biochemical/neurological imbalances
- Impulsive and chronic need for immediate gratification without regard to consequences to others
- Inability or unwillingness to respect the rights and wishes of others

As Evidenced By (Assessment Findings/Diagnostic Cues)

- ◆ Observed use of unsuccessful social interactions
- ◆ Dysfunctional interaction with peers, family, and/or others
- ● Use of forms of coping that impede adaptive behavior
- ● Destructive behavior toward self or others
- ● Inability to meet role expectations
- ● Inability to take responsibility for own actions
- ● Lack of remorse when actions hurt or hinder others

Outcome Criteria

Client will:

- Respond in a positive manner to confrontation and limit setting
- Learn and master at least three skills that facilitate adaptive behaviors (particularly anger management)
- Demonstrate an increase in responsible behavior in dealing with others as witnessed by staff and stated by others (clients/family/acquaintances)
- Use acceptable methods of getting needs met

◆ NANDA accepted; ● In addition to NANDA.

- Participate in ongoing management of anger, impulsivity, control issues, and the like
- Demonstrate a decrease in manipulative, attention-seeking, or passive-aggressive behaviors as reported by staff, family, and peers

Short-Term Goals

Clients will:

- Participate in treatment program, activities, responsibilities, and the like within 1 to 3 days
- State they understand the unit (community center/rehabilitation program, etc.) rules and understands the consequences of breaking them by first day
- Sign and discuss the content of a contract defining staff and client expectations by first day
- Participate in articulating a contract to modify specific inappropriate and unacceptable behaviors that spells out the consequences of continuing behaviors by first or second day (a copy goes to the client and the Kardex/community center/rehabilitation counselor, etc.)
- Target two inappropriate behaviors to work on learning alternative ways of behaving within 2 to 3 days
- Role play with nurse new skills in dealing with targeted behaviors (ongoing)

Interventions and Rationales

Interventions	Rationales
1. Assess your own reactions toward client. If you feel angry, discuss with peer(s) ways to reframe your thinking to defray feelings of anger.	1. Anger is a natural response to being manipulated. It is also a block to effective nurse-client interaction.
2. Assess client's interactions over a short period before labeling them manipulative.	2. A client may just be responding to one particular high-stress situation with maladaptive behaviors, but use appropriate behaviors in other situations.
3. Approach client in calm, neutral manner when confronting client with unacceptable behavior. Focus on	3. Focusing on behavior (drinking) is less accusing than personalizing the behavior (your drinking).

Interventions	**Rationales**
the behavior, not the client (e.g., "Drinking alcohol is not allowed here," *not* "I don't want you to drink alcohol on this unit.").	
4. State clearly the limits and behavior the staff expects of client.	4. Client needs to be aware of specific expectations and boundaries.

5. Limits are:
  a. Appropriate—not punitive
  b. Enforceable
  c. Stated in a nonpunitive manner
  d. Written with consequences of nonadherence clearly stated.
Make one copy for client, and one copy for client's record (e.g., Kardex).
	5. Clear, enforceable limits give client specific boundaries of expected behavior(s).

6. Meet with client to formulate a written contract detailing specific undesirable behaviors that are to be changed, alternatives to those behaviors, and specific consequence(s) of nonadherence.	6. Encouraging clients to participate in contract drafting may encourage compliance.
7. Both nurse and client sign the contract; one copy goes to client and another copy goes to nurse (Kardex).	7. Validates that the contract is a serious document and will be a guideline for all staff, and a reminder for the client.
8. Communicate frequently to all staff about specific limits and consequences set for clients. Post copy on Kardex.	8. Limits and consequences have to be adhered to by all of the staff in order to be effective means for modifying behavior.
9. Follow through with consequences in a nonpunitive manner (e.g., "The unit rules we went over together when you arrived, Mr. Miller, clearly stated	9. Clients begin to understand that they will be taking responsibility for their behavior. In this example, the client chose to drink on the

that clients were not to have alcohol on the unit or their weekend passes were to be cancelled. Because you brought alcohol to the unit, your weekend pass is canceled.").

unit, but by doing so, he has also chosen to forgo his weekend pass.

10. Discuss with clients their thoughts and feelings right before the undesirable behavior.

10. Identifies specific thoughts and feelings that can be discussed and dealt with in alternative ways.

11. Discuss with clients alternative behaviors they could use to effectively deal with these kinds of thoughts, feelings, or situation in the future.

11. Clients may not be aware of what they are feeling (anger, anxiety, and sadness) or the thinking that triggers specific maladaptive behaviors.

12. Teach or refer client to appropriate place to learn needed coping skill (e.g., anger management, assertiveness training).

12. If clients are NOT TO DO a specific maladaptive behavior, they need to learn WHAT TO DO to deal with intense thoughts/feelings and impulsive behaviors.

13. Role play situations so that client can practice the use of new behaviors.

13. Gives client chances to practice more direct and appropriate ways of relating and getting needs met.

14. Be vigilant; **AVOID:**
    a. Discussing yourself or other staff members with client
    b. Promising to keep a secret for the client
    c. Accepting gifts from the client
    d. Doing special favors for the client

14. Client can use this kind of information to manipulate you and/or split staff. Decline all invitations in a firm, but matter-of-fact manner, for example:
    a. "I cannot keep secrets from other staff. If you tell me something I may have to share it."
    b. " If you want to know about Ms. Williams, you will have to ask her."
    c. "I am here to focus on you."

Interventions	**Rationales**
	d. "You are to return to the unit by 4 PM on Sunday, period."
15. Meet frequently with staff to discuss client's care plan and progress. Revise care plan as a team.	15. Helps ensure consistency of enforcing limits, and minimize staff splitting.
16. Give client attention and support when behavior is appropriate and positive.	16. Reinforces appropriate behaviors.
17. Withdraw attention when client's behavior is inappropriate (unless there is a need to enforce consequences).	17. Client learns that inappropriate behavior will not be rewarded by attention he or she may be seeking.
18. Maintain a neutral manner at all times. Avoid power struggles or trying to outmanipulate client.	18. You cannot win a power struggle or outmanipulate a manipulative client. In any case, this isn't a game.
19. Provide positive feedback when client interacts without use of manipulation.	19. Encourages and reinforces appropriate behaviors.
20. Keep detailed and accurate notes on: a. Client's behaviors b. Frequency of behaviors c. Limits set d. Consequences enforced	20. Helps staff identify what is working and not working. Can minimize manipulation of staff.
21. Include family in client education.	21. The same skills used when working with the client may be useful for the family (Gorman et al., 1996).

# CHAPTER 18

Nonadherence to Medications or Treatment

Nonadherence to prescribed health care is thought to be a frequent phenomenon. In fact, it is estimated that up to 50% of clients may fail to adhere to their prescribed health care regimen (Postrado and Lehman, 1995).

When clients do not follow medication and treatment plans, they are often labeled as **"noncompliant."** The term *noncompliant* applied to clients often brings with it negative connotations. The term *compliance* refers to the extent to which a client obediently and faithfully follows health care providers' instructions. "That client is noncompliant" often translates into he or she is "bad" or "lazy." The "noncompliant" client is then open to blame and criticism. The situation often results in a power struggle between the health care worker and client that can leave both frustrated and angry. Clients who are labeled as noncompliant are often seen as "deviant," and the term is invariably judgmental.

By contrast, the term *adherence* implies a more active, voluntary, and collaborative involvement of the client in a mutually acceptable course of behavior (Meichenbaum and Turk, 1987). Lerner (1997) suggests that, rather than seeing the health care worker's role as trying to "get a noncompliant client to comply," we should emphasize the importance of negotiation and accommodation within the client–health care worker relationship. Therefore, the term *nonadherence* has less of a negative connotation, and frames the behavior more as a problem to be solved, not so much willful negative behavior. For that reason, the term *nonadherence* is used here.

The reasons clients do not adhere to their treatment of care, even though they may fully understand their health care regimen, are many and complex. Nonadherence to medications and treatment by itself is not the problem. Nonadherence is usually a *symptom* of

445

more complex underlying problems. Although inadequate client education is a common reason for nonadherence to a medical regimen, it is by no means the only reason.

A number of complex issues may complicate a person's willingness to follow a path leading to increased health or health maintenance. These issues, once addressed, can increase a person's adherence toward their health care regimen. Table 18–1 presents some factors that will need to be uncovered and dealt with before medical compliance can be a reality.

◆ ASSESSING FOR NONADHERENCE TO MEDICATIONS OR TREATMENT

History

A positive history includes:

1. A history of not keeping appointments
2. A history of not taking medications
3. Escalation of signs and symptoms despite the availability of appropriate medication
4. A history of emergency visits that are effectively treated with prescribed medication or treatment
5. Religious or cultural beliefs that contradict medical/psychological health care regimen
6. A poor outcome from past medical/psychological treatments
7. A history of poor relationships with past health care providers
8. A history of leaving the hospital against medical advice (AMA)

Presenting Signs and Symptoms

1. Objective tests (e.g., blood and urine) are inconsistent with reported medication intake (e.g., low lithium levels, low neuroleptic blood levels, high sugar levels).
2. Family members or friends state that client is not adhering to prescribed regimen.
3. Progression of disease/behaviors despite appropriate medication/treatment ordered.
4. Fails to follow through with referrals.
5. Fails to keep appointments.
6. Denies the need for medication or treatment.

Sample Questions

The nurse uses a variety of therapeutic techniques to gain the answers to the following questions. Use your discretion and decide which questions are appropriate to complete your assessment.

Table 18–1 ◆ Selected Factors That Contribute
to Nonadherence

FACTOR	SUGGESTED INTERVENTIONS
Use of power struggles to gain a sense of control	Devise ways to give client more control over regimen by giving alternate effective treatment options.
Reluctance to give up a behavior that is a usual coping mechanism (e.g., smoking, diet, drugs/alcohol)	Teach client alternative coping strategies (relaxation, exercise, creative pursuits) and role play ceasing the one and employing another.
Secondary gains from the "sick" role	Teach family and staff to give positive reinforcement for healthy behavior and use of healthy coping skills, and draw away from giving attention to problem behavior.
Self-destructive behavior (suicide, anorexia, bulimia, drugs)	Perform good nursing assessment and work or refer client to competent specially trained clinician.
Negative family influence related to denial, lack of understanding, or need for client to maintain sick role	Family teaching and possibly family therapy to clarify issues, identify long-range consequences of nonadherence, and involve them in treatment plan.
Lack of economic resources (can't afford medications or time off to keep appointments)	Refer to social services; identify community resources that may be helpful.
Lack of transportation	Refer to social services.
Unsatisfactory relationships with health care personnel	Work to establish a partnership with client showing concern and interest; avoid power struggles.
Cultural and/or religious beliefs	Identify specific concerns. Emphasize what can happen when regimen is not followed. Attempt to engage client, family/friends to problem solve alternative solutions.
Language problems, inability to read or understand instructions	Obtain an interpreter, and involve other members of the family who may have more facility with English. Have written instructions in client's primary language.
Uncomfortable side effects	Encourage client and family to share untoward reactions to drug so adjustments can be made before client stops taking medication or treatment.
Lack of skills to adhere to treatment regimen	Assess and identify needed skills. Some of these skills include decision-making skills, relaxation skills, assertiveness training skills, relapse prevention techniques.

(Table continued on following page)

Table 18–1 ♦ Selected Factors That Contribute to Nonadherence (*Continued*)

FACTOR	SUGGESTED INTERVENTIONS
Conflict with self-image, especially children and adolescents (e.g., taking medication or imposing limits on activity)	Refer and encourage client to join a group with others grappling with similar issues.
Confusion about (1) taking the medication, (2) when to take, or (3) if he or she has already taken medication	Set up concrete system for taking medications (cross-off chart, pillbox with separate compartments). Try to enlist help from family or others if available.

Data from Gorman et al. (1996, pp. 243–245) and Schultz and Videbeck (1998).

1. "What, if any, religious or cultural beliefs go against taking this medication/treatment? Please tell me about them."
2. "Does taking this medication/treatment pose any large financial problems for your family? In what way?"
3. "What questions haven't been answered regarding how the medications/treatments work, the side effects, or how the medications are to be taken? Please go over them with me."
4. "Would it help if we could put the instructions for taking the medications/treatment in another language?"
5. "What would you want us to be able to change about how the medications/treatments affect you?" (Erectile dysfunction in men is a common side effect with a number of medications. Gaining weight is an unwanted side effect that affects many women.)
6. "What are your thoughts about these medications/treatment? Do you believe they are necessary or helpful to you? Give me an example."
7. "Do you find taking so many medications/treatments a bit confusing? Would it help if we could figure out some ways to make remembering all this information easier?"
8. "What is the most difficult part for you about taking the medications/treatment?"

ASSESSMENT ALERTS

1. Do self-assessment (e.g., personal feelings of anger, feeling responsible for noncompliance, critical and judgmental feelings toward client).
2. Identify any ethnic and/or cultural beliefs that may conflict with the client adhering to medical management.

Continued

3. Evaluate age-related issues interfering with adherence to medication/treatment protocols (see above).
4. Assess presence of side effects of medications/treatments and how they affect client's lifestyle.
5. Does client believe that the medications/treatments are really necessary?
6. Assess client's thoughts and feelings toward health care personnel.
7. What does client identify as being the most difficult aspect of following through with medication/treatment regimen?

◆ NURSING DIAGNOSES WITH INTERVENTIONS

Nonadherence to medications or treatment can be voluntary, or a result of a variety of factors that make adherence difficult if not impossible. The nursing diagnosis of **Noncompliance** coincides with the *active decision of an individual or family to fully or partially nonadhere to an agreed upon medication/treatment regimen.* In contrast, **Ineffective Management of Therapeutic Regimen: Individual** refers to the *difficulty or inability to regulate or integrate a medication/treatment plan into daily life.* A distinction between the two is important in obtaining desired results.

The position taken in this chapter is that Noncompliance is used to identify **voluntary nonadherence** to a medical/psychiatric/treatment regimen, and Ineffective Management of Therapeutic Regimen refers to those situations in which the client **may be willing to comply, but is having difficulty** integrating the therapeutic regimen into his or her life or lifestyle.

Noncompliance

The extent to which a person's and/or caregiver's behavior coincides or fails to coincide with a health-promoting or therapeutic plan agreed upon by the person (and/or family, and/or community) and health care professional. In the presence of an agreed-upon health-promoting or therapeutic plan, person's or caregiver's behavior may be fully, partially, or nonadherent and may lead to clinically effective, partially effective, or ineffective outcomes.

Related To (Etiology)

◆ Health care plan
   * Duration
   * Significant others
   * Cost
   * Intensity
   * Complexity
◆ Individual factors
   * Personal and developmental abilities
   * Health beliefs and cultural influences
   * Spiritual values
   * Individual value system
   * Knowledge and skill relevant to the regimen behavior
   * Motivational forces
◆ Health System
   * Satisfaction with care
   * Credibility of provider
   * Access and convenience of care
   * Financial flexibility of plan
   * Client-provider relationships
   * Provider reimbursement of teaching and follow-up
   * Provider continuity and regular follow-up
   * Individual health coverage
   * Communication and teaching skills of the provider
◆ Network
   * Involvement of members in health plan
   * Social value regarding plan
   * Perceived beliefs of significant others

As Evidenced By (Assessment Findings/Diagnostic Cues)

◆ Behavior indicative of failure to adhere (by direct observation or by statements of patient or significant others)
◆ Evidence of development of complications
◆ Evidence of exacerbation of symptoms
◆ Failure to keep appointments
◆ Failure to progress
◆ Objective tests (blood, urine, physiological markers)

Outcome Criteria

Clients will:

• State correct information about their condition, benefits of treatment, risks of treatment, and treatment options each time changes are made to their treatment plan

---

◆ NANDA accepted; ● In addition to NANDA.

- Participate in decision making concerning treatment plan on an ongoing basis
- Demonstrate adherence to the treatment plan
- Follow behavioral contract in assuming his or her responsibility for self-care on an ongoing basis

Short-Term Goals

Client will:

- Discuss the impact of illness on lifestyle (ongoing)
- Discuss fears, concerns, and beliefs that influence noncompliance (ongoing)
- Identify one barrier to compliance (by end of session)
- With family, problem solve ways to minimize or erase barrier (within 1 week)
- With family, discuss with nurse the potential undesirable consequences of nonadherence to therapeutic regimen (within 1 week)
- Negotiate acceptable changes in the treatment plan that client is willing to follow (ongoing)
- Participate in one decision regarding their treatment plan (by end of first session)
- Sign a behavioral contract defining their mutual participation and responsibility for care (at end of session and review/update frequently)

Interventions and Rationales

Intervention	Rationale
1. Explore with clients their feelings about the illness/ disorder and the need for ongoing treatments (medications).	1. Setting up a rapport with clients who believe you are interested in them encourages understanding of client's perspective.
2. Use therapeutic nursing techniques to encourage client to share feelings in an atmosphere of acceptance.	2. When clients feel understood, they are less likely to feel defensive and more likely to be open to suggestions and information regarding optimizing their health.
3. Identify communication barriers that may impede client's (family's) comprehension. Identify need for: a. Interpreters	3. When we make assumptions going by what we teach clients, and not what they might or might not understand,

Intervention	**Rationale**
b. Use of nontechnical language	a great potential for miscommunication is present.
c. Need for written material	
d. Understanding religious barriers	
e. Attitudes toward health care system	
4. Assess clients' (family's) understanding about the illness/disorder, treatment options, how they work, and side and toxic effects.	4. Client (family) misperceptions about disease/disorder or treatments result in faulty decision making.
5. Assess how the client's disease/disorder and subsequent treatments/medications impact upon client's (and family's) lifestyle.	5. Age, religion, cultural beliefs, expectations of others all impact on our value system and factor into how we make decisions.
6. Ask clients to share their rationale for nonadherence to medical/psychosocial regimen.	6. Identifies areas of misunderstanding.
7. **Do not** argue with clients about the value of their beliefs; **rather**, point out the negative outcomes these beliefs may cause.	7. Arguing or getting into power struggles with clients makes them defensive and not open to alternative actions.
8. Engage family, friends, caregivers to explain negative actions of nonadherence to treatment regimen.	8. Those whom client trusts, and from similar background, culture, and the like, may inspire trust and open the way for negotiation.
9. Encourage clients to participate in decision-making process regarding their plan of care.	9. Can give clients a sense of control, and give them the opportunity to choose those interventions they might decide to try.
10. Give the client a range of assignments from which to choose.	10. Giving client choices in making a decision increases client involvement in treatment planning.

11. Negotiate with clients one or two areas they will comply with, if client refuses the whole treatment plan outright.

11. Clients may "try" one or two items from the treatment regimen to comply with at first. Hopefully this can form a base for further adherence.

12. Negotiate a behavioral contract with client, and review it periodically. Give a written copy to client and file one in client's chart.

12. Contracts have been found to enhance adherence in both adult and child populations (Kobayashi et al., 1998).

13. Reduce the complexity of the treatment plan (prioritize, facilitate schedules, fits lifestyle).

13. The more complicated a treatment plan, the more likely nonadherence.

14. When appropriate, encourage support groups.

14. While giving support, groups also share information, and encourage healthy choices.

15. Determine if a different medication or a different type of therapy might be acceptable to the client.

15. Client may engage in treatment if alternative but equally effective treatment options are available.

16. Recognize that it might not be possible to alter strong cultural or religious beliefs.

16. Ultimately, the final choice is with the client. Our job is to provide information and effective treatment options that best suit the client's lifestyle.

MEDICATION NONADHERENCE

Intervention

Rationale

1. Assess if clients believe they need the medication. Identify need for teaching.

1. If client denies need for medication, motivation for adherence is lacking.

2. Use a variety of teaching strategies for client and family member(s) (e.g., pamphlets, videotapes, role playing, group teaching with others in

2. Knowledge and understanding can increase adherence to treatment regimen.

Intervention	Rationale
similar circumstances, support groups).	
3. If clients stops taking medication when they feel "better," more client and family teaching is needed.	3. People need to know that, in most instances, medications can't cure them, but they can help stabilize their symptoms over time.
4. Encourage reporting side effects (e.g., "Do these medications affect your ability to function sexually? They affect **many** people that way.").	4. Physician may lower dose, or give client an alternative medication, when side effects are affecting adherence.
5. Encourage client to report any disturbing side effects right away, rather than stopping medication.	5. Some side effects can be minimized through simple actions.

Ineffective Management of Therapeutic Regimen

A pattern of regulating and integrating into daily living a program for treatment of illness and the sequelae of illness that is satisfactory for meeting specific health goals

---

Related To (Etiology)

◆ Perceived barriers
◆ Social support deficits
◆ Mistrust of regimen and/or health care personnel
◆ Knowledge deficits
◆ Family patterns of health care
◆ Economic difficulties
◆ Complexity of therapeutic regimen
◆ Inadequate number and types of cues to action

As Evidenced By (Assessment Findings/Diagnostic Cues)

◆ Choices of daily living ineffective for meeting the goals of a treatment or prevention program

---

◆ NANDA accepted; ● In addition to NANDA.

◆ Verbalized that they did not take action to reduce risk factors for progression of illness and sequelae
◆ Verbalized difficulty with regulation/integration of one or more prescribed regimens for treatment
◆ Acceleration of illness symptoms
◆ Verbalized that they did not take action to include treatment regimens in daily routines

Outcome Criteria

Client will:

• Demonstrate adherence to treatment regimen
• Verbalize acceptance and adherence to the treatment plan
• Keep follow-up appointments
• Demonstrate skills or knowledge needed for adherence
• Establish a network of referrals to call upon if and when difficulties with carrying out treatment regimen arise
• Participate in adjunctive services when appropriate

Short-Term Goals

Client will:

• Establish a supportive therapeutic partnership with health care worker(s)
• Identify obstacles that interfere with carrying out treatment plan
• Identify resources needed to ensure compliance
• Negotiate acceptable changes in the treatment plan that he or she is willing to follow

Interventions and Rationales

Intervention	Rationale
1. Establish an open and supportive partnership with client.	1. Adherence is positively correlated with client's perception of health care personnel's caring and interest (DiMatteo and DiNicola, 1982).
2. Identify areas in the treatment regimen that interfere with adherence: a. Economic b. Transportation	2. Targets areas for interventions.

◆ NANDA accepted; ● In addition to NANDA.

Intervention	Rationale
c. Knowledge barrier d. Language barrier e. Lack of or negative family involvement f. Lack of appropriate skills	

3. Involve adjunctive services when appropriate, for example:
  a. Social services for financial or transportation problems
  b. Interpreters if language difficulties
  c. Family teaching and or alternative teaching strategies if knowledge deficit
  d. Skills training
	3. Nonadherence is often a symptom of an underlying problem. That problem has to be identified.

4. Teach needed skills (e.g., problem-solving skills, assertiveness skills, relaxation skills, decision-making skills).	4. Skills training can help foster adherence to health care regimen.
5. Keep the treatment plan as clear and simple as possible.	5. The easier the regimen is to follow, the greater the likelihood of compliance.
6. Evaluate client comprehension by having client repeat or demonstrate what is to be done.	6. Clarifies misunderstandings and reinforces learning.

7. Use behavioral reminders for follow-up:
  a. Calendars
  b. Linking appointments
  c. Written reminders on refrigerators
  d. Sending reminder postcards
	7. Behavioral reminders have shown to be successful for long-term adherence (Kobayashi et al., 1998).

8. Facilitate short-term goal setting with client (explicitly defined, achievable goals).	8. Clients who use short-term goals rather than long-term goals are most successful at maintenance (Meichenbaum and Turk, 1987).

9. Provide feedback on client's progress and develop positive reinforcers for self-regulation.

9. Encouragement and recognition by clinician as to progress of goals can act as a motivator for positive change.

10. Tailor treatment plan to be congruent with client's social, cultural, and environmental milieus.

10. Optimizes client feeling comfortable with adhering to medications/treatments.

11. Teach relapse prevention skills.

11. Helps clients learn behavioral cues to potential relapse and how to cope with relapse.

12. Repeat everything.

12. Information that is repeated is more likely to be retained than information that is not repeated.

CHAPTER 19

Grieving and
Dysfunctional Grieving

L oss is part of the human experience, and grief is the normal
response to loss. Loss may be of a relationship (divorce,
separation, death, abortion), of health (a body function or
part, mental or physical capacity), of status or prestige, of security
(occupational, financial, social), of self-confidence, of self-concept,
or of a dream, or loss can be of a symbolic nature.

Even though grief and loss are universal experiences, loss
through death is a major life crisis for most of us. Grief is not a
mood disorder, although a depressive syndrome is often part of the
grieving process (see Chapter 8).

Grief is the characteristic painful feelings precipitated by the
death of a loved one or by some other significant loss. **Bereavement** is the state of being deprived of a loved one by death.
Mourning is the processes (grief work) by which the grief is resolved, and includes various phenomena identified subsequently.

Although grief is a normal phenomenon, it may at times be the
focus of treatment. Most bereaved persons resolve their loss with
help and support from family and friends. However, more than
30% may require professional support (Lloyd-Williams, 1995).
Unresolved grief reactions may account for many of the physical
symptoms seen in medical clinics and hospital units. Suicide is
higher among people who have had a significant loss, especially if
losses are multiple and grieving mechanisms are limited (Gregory,
1994). Deaths of children and multiple deaths are regarded as the
most severe types of loss. We as nurses are not immune to grief reactions. As health care workers, as nurses, as friends, as people
who will experience grief and loss throughout our own lifetimes, it
is helpful to know what happens during the process of mourning,
what might help others through this process, and how to identify a

person who is having difficulty resolving his or her pain and sorrow (dysfunctional grieving).

Most nurses and clinicians are familiar with Kubler-Ross's (1969) classic review of the stages of death and dying (denial, isolation, anger, bargaining, depression, and acceptance).

The resolution of the loss usually occurs through these stages, and a person may demonstrate a different clinical picture at each stage of mourning. Each stage has its own characteristics, and the duration and form of each stage may vary considerably from person to person. People react within their own cultural patterns and their own value and personality structure, as well as within their own social environment. Most of us are programmed in our response to death. Distinct characteristics, however, can be identified throughout the grieving process. It is important to keep in mind that these stages do not necessarily progress in an orderly fashion, and may overlap during the grief process.

What we are not often taught is what to say or do to facilitate the healing of those who must learn to live with their anguish.

Normal grief reaction includes depressed mood, insomnia, anxiety, poor appetite, loss of interest, guilt feelings, dreams about the deceased, and poor concentration. Psychological states include shock, denial, and yearning and searching for the deceased. The acute grief reaction lasts from 4 to 8 weeks, the active symptoms of grief usually last from 3 to 6 months, and the complete work of mourning may take from 1 to 2 years or more to complete. However, acute grief can be a time of exacerbation of any medical or psychiatric problems. A history of depression, substance abuse, or PTSD can complicate grief and certainly deserves specific treatment (Prigerson et al., 1995).

Nurses have a wonderful opportunity to care for the bereaved through listening, assisting in communication, teaching families about the process of dying, or facilitating bereavement with opportunities to prevent ill health and to help families find new directions for growth.

◆ ASSESSING FOR GRIEF AND POTENTIAL DYSFUNCTIONAL GRIEF REACTIONS

History

1. Does the bereaved exhibit some of the factors that can complicate the successful completion of mourning?
   a. Was the bereaved heavily dependent on the deceased?

    b. Were there persistent unresolved conflicts with the deceased?
    c. Was the deceased a child (often the most profound loss)?
    d. Does the bereaved have a meaningful relationship/support system?
    e. Has the bereaved experienced a number of previous losses?
    f. Does the bereaved person have sound coping skills?

2. Was the deceased's death associated with a cultural stigma (e.g., AIDS, suicide)?
3. Was the death unexpected or associated with violence (murder, suicide)?
4. Has the bereaved had difficulty resolving past significant losses?
5. Does the bereaved have a history of depression, drug or alcohol abuse, or other psychiatric illness?
6. If the bereaved is young, are there indications for special interventions?

Presenting Symptoms of Dysfunctional Grief

1. Prolonged severe symptoms lasting over 2 or more months
2. Limited response to support
3. Profound and persistent feelings of hopelessness
4. Completely withdrawn, or fear of being alone
5. Inability to work, to create, to feel emotion or positive states of mind
6. Maladaptive behaviors in response to the death, for example:
    a. Drug or alcohol abuse
    b. Promiscuity
    c. Fugue states
    d. Feeling dead or unreal
    e. Suicidal ideation
    f. Aggressive behaviors
    g. Compulsive spending
7. Recurrent nightmares, night terrors, compulsive re-enactments
8. Exhaustion from lack of sleep and hyperarousal

Sample Questions

The nurse uses a variety of therapeutic techniques to obtain the answers to the following questions. Use your discretion and decide which questions are appropriate to complete your assessment.

Many of these questions, if asked in the early phases of mourning (3 to 6 months), would not be significant in detecting a dysfunctional reactions. However, **if after 3 to 6 months, a person's life** is negatively altered because of any of the following problems, then professional assistance to complete the task of mourning might be indicated.

1. "Since the death, what alterations have you experienced as to concentration, or ability to perform simple tasks?"
2. "Describe any disturbing emotions you've experienced since the death." (extreme guilt, anxiety, anger)
3. "Compared with your relationships before the death, describe any difficulty at your job, in your personal life, or socializing with your friends since the loss."
4. "Tell me about any recurrent nightmares/night terrors/compulsive re-enactments of the loss you may have had since the death."
5. "Sometimes people have unusual experiences as if the loved one is still there. Tell me about the times you've had visions or heard voices (hallucinations), or have had dreams that beckon you to reunite with the person you lost."
6. "How would you describe any changes in your patterns of weight, eating, sleeping, or bowel function since the loss?"

Assessment Guide

Table 19–1 presents a comparison of the symptoms seen in a "normal" mourning process contrasting those seen in a dysfunctional grief reaction. This may be used as a helpful guide in your assessment.

☰	ASSESSMENT ALERTS
	1. Identify if the individual is at risk for complicated dysfunctional grieving (see History).
	2. Evaluate for psychotic symptoms, agitation, increased activity, alcohol/drug abuse, and extreme vegetative symptoms (anorexia, weight loss, not sleeping).
	3. Do not overlook people who do not express significant grief in the context of a major loss. Those individuals may have an increased risk of subsequent complicated or unresolved grief reaction (Kaplan and Sadock, 1993).
	4. Complicated grief reactions require significant interventions. Suicidal or severely depressed people may require hospitalization. **Always assess for suicide** with signs of depression or other dysfunctional signs **(see Chapter 13)**.

Continued

5. Assess support systems. If support systems are limited, find bereavement groups in the bereaved's community.
6. When grieving is stalled or dysfunctional, a variety of therapeutic approaches have proved extremely beneficial (e.g., cognitive-behavioral interventions). Provide referrals.
7. Grieving can bring with it severe spiritual anguish. Would spiritual counseling or a specific counselor be useful for the bereaved at this time?

♦ NURSING DIAGNOSES WITH INTERVENTIONS

NANDA (1999) identifies two nursing diagnoses for nursing actions, **Dysfunctional Grieving** and **Anticipatory Grieving**. However, because nurses are in constant contact with people and their families experiencing painful losses, **Acute Grief Reaction** (not a NANDA nursing diagnosis) may also be the focus of treatment. During this time, the nurse may also have to intervene for **Ineffective Individual Coping** or **Ineffective Family Coping, Potential for** or **Spiritual Distress, Altered Thought Processes**, or other problems.

OVERALL GUIDELINES FOR NURSING INTERVENTION

1. Employ methods that can facilitate the grieving process and give support to a grieving person by (Robinson, 1997):
   • Being there for the bereaved, giving your full presence.
   • Offer physical touch suited to the moment and your relationship. **Do not** use touch if it will presume an intimacy that does not exist or as a tool to coerce a person to mourn.
   • Identify family or friends to assist with practical concerns.
   • Try to provide beauty or nourishment in some suitable form.
   • Encourage the individual and family to mourn on their own schedule.
2. Identify and treat/refer an individual with a pathological process.

Continued

Table 19–1 ◆ Common Experiences During Grief and Their Pathological Intensification

PHASE	TYPICAL RESPONSE	PATHOLOGICAL INTENSIFICATION
Dying	Emotional expression and immediate coping with the dying process.	Avoidant; overwhelmed; dazed, confused; self-punitive; inappropriately hostile.
Death and outcry	Outcry of emotions with news of the death and turning for help to others or isolating self with self-succoring.	Panic; dissociative reactions, reactive psychoses.
Warding off (denial)	Avoidance of reminders, social withdrawal, focusing elsewhere, emotional numbing, not thinking of implications to self or certain themes.	Maladaptive avoidances confronting the implications of death. Drug or alcohol abuse, counterphobic frenzy, promiscuity, fugue states, phobic avoidance, feeling dead or unreal.
Re-experience (intrusion)	Intrusive experiences, including recollections of negative relationship experiences with the deceased, bad dreams, reduced concentration, compulsive re-enactments.	Flooding with negative images and emotions, uncontrolled ideation, self-impairing compulsive re-enactments, night terrors, recurrent nightmares, distraught from intrusion of anger, anxiety, despair, shame, or guilt themes; physiological exhaustion from hyperarousal.
Working through	Recollection of the deceased and contemplation of self with reduced intrusiveness of memories and fantasies, increased rational acceptance, reduced numbness and avoidance, more "dosing" of recollections, and a sense of working it through.	Sense that one cannot integrate the death with a sense of self and continued life. Persistent warded off themes may manifest as anxious, depressed, enraged, shame-filled, or guilty moods, and psychophysiological syndromes.
Completion	Reduction in emotional swings with a sense of self-coherence and readiness for new relationships. Able to experience positive states of mind.	Failure to complete mourning may be associated with inability to work, create, to feel emotion or positive states of mind.

From Horowitz, M.J. (1990). A model of mourning: Change in schemas of self and others. Journal of the American Psychoanalytic Association 38:297–324; reprinted with permission.

3. Assess for suicide if there is persistent, severe depression and deep enduring feelings of hopelessness (**see Chapter 13**).
4. Know, share, and support with the bereaved the normal phenomena that occur during the normal mourning process, which may concern some people (intense anger at the deceased, guilt, symptoms the deceased had before death, unbidden flood of memories). Give bereaved a written handout to refer to.
5. Apply appropriate measures when the family member dies in the hospital that can help facilitate grieving for families (Table 19–2).

Remember, we each grieve differently depending upon age, culture, and spiritual levels. Make an effort to identify special/specific needs of the bereaved.

Acute Grief Reaction

Focuses on the devastating and often overwhelming pain people experience upon the death of someone they care about and who was an integral part of their lives. The acute phase lasts from 4 to 8 weeks after the death or a significant loss. (The *long-term phase* follows the acute phase and constitutes the main work of mourning, and may last from 1 to 2 years or more.)

Related To (Etiology)

● Recent loss of loved one (person, pet) or forced change (e.g., loss of job, home, disaster, divorce, body part)

As Evidenced By (Assessment Findings/Diagnostic Cues)

Signs of grief:

● Anguish and pain
● Anger at deceased or health care professionals
● Guilt
● Crying
● Vegetative signs (anorexia, insomnia, bowel dysfunction, immobility)
● Withdrawal from usual activities and preoccupation with the deceased

---

♦ NANDA accepted; ● In addition to NANDA.

Table 19–2 ◆ Nursing Interventions for Grieving Families

INTERVENTION	RATIONALE
1. At the death or imminent death of a family member:	
• Communicate the news to the family in an area of privacy.	• Family members can support each other in an atmosphere in which they can behave naturally.
• If only one family member is available, stay with that member until clergy, a family member, or a friend arrives.	• The presence and comfort of the nurse during the initial stage of shock can help minimize feelings of acute isolation and anxiety.
• If the nurse feels unable to handle the situation, the aid of another who can support the family should be enlisted.	• The individual or family will need support, answers to questions, and guidance as to immediate tasks and information.
2. If the family requests to see and take leave of the dying or dead person:	
• Grant this request.	• The need to take leave can be of overwhelming importance for some—to kiss good-bye, ask for forgiveness, or take a lock of hair. This helps people face the reality of death.
3. If angry family members accuse the nurse or doctor of abusing or mismanaging the care of the deceased:	
• Continue to provide the best care for the dying or final care to the dead. Avoid becoming involved in angry and painful arguments and power struggles.	• Complaints are not directed toward the nurse personally. The anger may serve the purpose of keeping grieving relatives from falling apart. Projected anger may be an attempt to deal with aggression and guilt toward the dying person.
4. If relatives behave in a grossly disturbed manner (e.g., refuse to acknowledge the truth, collapse, or lose control):	
• Show patience and tact, and offer sympathy and warmth.	• Shock and disbelief are the first responses to the news of death, and people need ways to protect themselves from the overwhelming reality of loss.
• Encourage the person to cry.	• Crying helps provide relief from feelings of acute pain and tension.
• Provide a place of privacy for grieving.	• Privacy facilitates the natural expression of grief.

(*Table continued on following page*)

Table 19–2 ◆ Nursing Interventions for Grieving Families (*Continued*)

INTERVENTION	RATIONALE
5. If the family requests specific religious, cultural, or social customs strange or unknown to the nurse: • Help facilitate steps necessary for the family to carry out the desired arrangements.	• Institutional mourning rituals of various cultures provide important external supports for the grief-stricken person.

Data from Engel, G.L. (1964). Grief and grieving. *American Journal of Nursing* 64(9):93.

Outcome Criteria

• The bereaved will seek support during the grieving process.
• The bereaved will demonstrate behaviors that signify the individual is completing the process of mourning (Box 19–1).
• In time, the family will engage in life and pursue other activities.

Short-Term Goals

• The bereaved will state the names of two support people he or she can share painful feelings and memories with.
• If the bereaved demonstrates signs of dysfunctional grief reaction, he or she will agree to seek support and treatment.

❖   B O X   1 9 – 1   ❖

Behaviors Signalling Successful Mourning

The person:
1. Can tolerate intense emotions.
2. Demonstrates increased periods of stability.
3. Takes on new roles and responsibilities.
4. Has energy to invest in new endeavors.
5. Remembers both positive and negative aspects of the deceased loved one.
6. Brief periods of intense emotions may occur at significant times, such as anniversaries and holidays.

Data from Gorman et al. (1996).

Interventions and Rationales: When Death Occurs in the Health Care Setting

Intervention	Rationale

1. Employ methods that can facilitate the grieving process (Robinson, 1997):

   a. Giving your full presence: use appropriate eye contact, attentive listening, and appropriate touch.

   a. Talking is one of the most important ways of dealing with acute grief. *Listening patiently* helps the bereaved express all feelings, even ones he or she thinks are negative. *Appropriate eye contact* helps to let him or her know you are there and sharing his or her sadness. *Suitable human touch* can express warmth and nurture healing. Inappropriate touch can leave a person confused and uncomfortable.

   b. Be patient with the bereaved in times of silence. Do not fill silence with empty chatter.

   b. Sharing painful feelings during periods of silence is healing and conveys your concern.

2. **Avoid** the use of euphemisms. We use euphemisms in the hope they will stave off or soften the intrusive vulgarity of the death (e.g., "passed away," "You lost your husband."). Instead say something like, "I am really sorry to hear that James died."

2. Euphemisms can do harm:

   a. May cause the bereaved to think we've not caught the gravity of the situation.

   b. Wanting at one level to deny what's happening, the bereaved may use euphemisms to help postpone facing the painful feelings they desperately needs to be working through.

Intervention	**Rationale**
3. **Avoid** banal advice and philosophical statements such as, "He's no longer suffering"; "You can always have another child"; or "It's better this way." It is *more helpful* to put into words acknowledgment of the bereaved's painful feelings, such as: a. "His death will be a terrible loss." b. "No one can replace her." c. "He will be missed for a long time."	3. Gives the bereaved the impression that their experience is not understood, and that you are minimizing the experience and pain. The fact that the deceased is no longer suffering doesn't mean that the bereaved isn't experiencing a devastating, painful loss, and may be feeling the pain during this time.
4. Encourage the support of family and friends. If no supports are available, refer the bereaved to a community bereavement group. (Bereavement groups are helpful even when a person has many friends and/or family support.)	4. There are routine matters that friends can help with, for example: a. Getting food to the house b. Making phone calls c. Driving to the mortuary d. Taking care of kids or other family members
5. Offer spiritual support and/or referrals when needed.	5. Dealing with an illness or catastrophic loss can cause the most profound spiritual anguish (Zerbe, 1999).
6. When intense emotions are in evidence, show understanding and support (see Box 19–2 for guidelines).	6. Empathetic words that reflect acceptance of a bereaved individual's feelings are always healing (Robinson, 1997).

Dysfunctional Grieving

Extended length or severity of grieving process (unresolved grieving) following an actual or perceived loss or change in pattern of relationships (includes people, possessions, job, status, home, ideals, and parts and processes of the body)

❖   B O X   1 9 – 2   ❖
Guidelines for What To Say

When you sense an overwhelming *sorrow*:	"This must hurt terribly."
When you hear *anger* in the bereaved's voice:	"I hear anger in your voice. Most people go through periods of anger when their loved one dies. Are you feeling anger now?"
If you discern *guilt*:	"Are you feeling guilty? This is a common reaction many people have. What are some of your thoughts about this?"
If you sense a *fear* of the future:	"It must be scary to go through this."
When the bereaved seems *confused*:	"This can be a bewildering time."
In almost any *painful situation*:	"This must be very difficult for you."

Adapted from Robinson, D. (1997). Good Intentions: The Nine Unconscious Mistakes of Nice People. New York: Warner Books, p. 249; reprinted by permission. Copyright © 1997 by Duke Robinson.

Related To (Etiology)

◆ Loss of support systems
◆ Loss or perceived loss/change (specific)
● Presence of factors identified in history (e.g., substance abuse, multiple losses, poor physical health, other mental health risks)

As Evidenced By (Assessment Findings/Diagnostic Cues)

◆ Verbal expression of distress or loss or denial of loss *and* one of the following:
    * Arrested grieving process before resolution
    * Prolonged grieving beyond expected time for cultural group
    * Emotional response more exaggerated than expected for cultural group (severity of reaction)
◆ Expression of unresolved issues
◆ Interference with life functioning
● Suicidal ideation

◆ NANDA accepted; ● In addition to NANDA.

- Prolonged panic attacks
- Prolonged depression
- Engagement in self-destructive activities
- Self-neglect
- Protracted social withdrawal

Outcome Criteria

Bereaved will:

- Resolve blocks to the grieving process (maladaptive avoidance, extreme prolonged denial), and the stages of mourning will be re-activated during grief counseling
- Demonstrate initial integration into their life within 6 months
- Demonstrate physical recuperation from the stress of loss and grieving within 6 months
- Demonstrate re-established relationships and social supports within 4 weeks

Short-Term Goals

Bereaved will:

- Be free of self-directed harm
- Demonstrate decreased suicidal, aggressive, depressive, or with-drawn behaviors within 2 weeks
- Express feelings, verbally and nonverbally
- Establish or maintain an adequate balance of rest, sleep, and activity with help from nurse and family
- Establish or maintain adequate nutrition, hydration, and elimination within 2 weeks

Interventions and Rationales

Intervention	Rationale
1. Always assess for presence of suicidal thoughts or ideation.	1. Severely depressed or suicidal individuals may require hospitalization and protection from self-harm and severe self-neglect.
2. Talk with the bereaved in realistic terms. Discuss concrete changes that have occurred in the person's life after the death and	2. Discussing the death and how it has and will continue to affect the person's life can help the death become more concrete

◆ NANDA accepted; ● In addition to NANDA.

how it might affect the person's future.

and real.

3. If the bereaved is not able to talk initially about the death, encourage other means of expression (e.g., keeping a journal, drawing, reading about the experience of grief).

3. Talking is usually the most important tool for resolving initial pain; however, any avenue for the expression of feelings can help the bereaved identify, accept and work through their feelings.

4. Stress that people often have strong feelings of anger (even hate) at the deceased, feel guilty, harbor strong feelings of resentment, and the like.

4. Understanding that strong "negative" feelings are in fact normal and experienced by most people can help allow these "negative" feelings to come more into awareness and then be worked through.

5. Encourage the person to recall memories (happy ones, sad ones, difficult ones), listen actively, and stay silent when appropriate.

5. Reviewing past memories is an important stage in mourning. Being with the bereaved and sharing painful feelings can be healing.

6. Encourage the person to talk to others individually, in small groups, or in community bereavement groups.

6. Talking and listening are the most important activities that can help resolve grief and reactivate the mourning process.

7. Carefully avoid false reassurances that everything will be okay as time passes.

7. For some, separation through death is never okay; even when the grieving process is complete, the person may be sorely missed.

8. Assess the need for psychotherapy "re-grief" work.

8. Many people find brief counseling (6 to 10 sessions) useful during the work of mourning.

9. Identify religious/spiritual background and if the bereaved would be receptive to a spiritual advisor.

9. For many people, spiritual needs and support are extremely comforting at this time, and sharing feelings with a trusted and empathetic religious figure may be of great comfort.

◆ GUIDELINES FOR COPING WITH GRIEF

Table 19–3 suggests guidelines that may help the bereaved through this period.

Table 19–3 ◆ Patient Guidelines for Coping with Catastrophic Loss

---

1. **Take the time you need to grieve.** The hard work of grief uses psychological energy. Resolution of the "numb state" that occurs after loss requires a few weeks at least. A minimum of 1 year, to cover all the birthdays, anniversaries, and other important dates without your loved one, is required before you can "learn to live" with your loss.

2. **Express your feelings.** Remember that anger, anxiety, loneliness, and even guilt are normal reactions and that everyone needs a safe place to express them. Tell your personal story of loss as many times as you need to—this repetition is a helpful and necessary part of the grieving process.

3. **Make a daily structure and stick to it.** Although it is hard to do, keeping to some semblance of structure makes the first few weeks after a loss easier. Getting through each day helps restore the confidence you need to accept the reality of loss.

4. **Don't feel that you have to answer all the questions asked of you.** Although most people try to be kind, they may be unaware of their insensitivity. Down the road, you may want to read books about how others have dealt with similar circumstances. They often have helpful suggestions for a person in your situation.

5. **As hard as it is, try to take good care of yourself.** Eat well, talk with friends, get plenty of rest. Be sure to let your primary care clinician know if you are having trouble eating or sleeping. Make use of exercise. It can help you let out pent-up frustrations. If you are losing weight, sleeping excessively or intermittently, or still experiencing deep depression after 3 months, be sure to seek professional assistance.

6. **Expect the unexpected.** You may begin to feel a bit better, only to have a brief "emotional collapse." These are expectable reactions. Moreover, you may find that you dream, visualize, think about, or search for your loved one. This, too, is a part of the grief process.

7. **Give yourself time.** Don't feel that you have to resume all of life's duties right away.

8. **Make use of rituals.** Those who take the time to "say good-bye" at a funeral or a viewing tend to find it helps the bereavement process.

9. **If you do not begin to feel better within a few weeks, at least for a few hours every day, be sure to tell your doctor.** If you have had an emotional problem in the past (e.g., depression, substance abuse), be sure to get the additional support you need. Losing a loved one puts you at higher risk for relapse of these disorders.

From Zerbe, K.J. (1999). Women's Mental Health in Primary Care. Philadelphia: W.B. Saunders Company, pp. 207–208; reprinted with permission.

◆ NURSE, BEREAVED, AND FAMILY RESOURCES—GRIEVING AND DYSFUNCTIONAL GRIEVING

Books

For People With a Terminally Ill Family Member

Callahan, M., and Kelley, P. (1997). Final Gifts: Understanding the Special Awareness, Needs and Communication of the Dying. New York: Poseidon.

For Survivors of Suicide

Chance, S. (1992). Stronger Than Death. New York: W.W. Norton.

For Widows

Brothers, J. (1990). Widowhood. New York: Ballantine Books.
Caine, L. (1988). Being a Widow. New York: Penguin Books.

For Bereaved Parents

Rosof, B.D. (1994). The Worst Loss: How Families Heal From the Death of a Child. New York: Henry Holt.

For Children

Lionni, L. (1995). Little Blue and Little Yellow. New York: Mulberry.

About Death

O'Gorman, S. (1998). Death and dying in contemporary society: An evaluation of current attitudes and rituals associated with death and dying and their relevance to recent understandings of health and healing. Journal of Advanced Nursing, 27:1127–1135.

Educational Resources

About Dying

National Hospice Organization
200 State Road
South Deerfield, MA 01373-0200
1-800-646-6460

Internet Sites

American Academy of Hospice and Palliative Medicine
http://www.aahpm.org

Approaching Death: Improving Care at the End of Life
http://books.nap.edu/html/approaching/
(online publication)

Webster's Death, Dying and Grief Guide
http://www.katsden.com/death/index.html

Hospice Foundation of America
http://www.hospicefoundation.org

National Institute of Aging
http://www.nih.gov/nia

APPENDICES

Appendix A

REFERENCES

Aguilera, D. (1994). Crisis Intervention: Theory and Methodology, 7th ed. St. Louis: Mosby.

Alvarez, C. (1998). Communication with angry and aggressive clients. In E.M. Varcarolis (ed.), Foundations of Psychiatric Nursing, 3rd ed. Philadelphia: W.B. Saunders Company.

American Nurses Association. (1994). Statement on Psychiatric–Mental Health Clinical Nursing Practice and Standards of Psychiatric–Mental Health Clinical Nursing Practice. Washington, DC: American Nurses Association.

American Psychiatric Association. (1987). Diagnostic and Statistical Manual of Mental Disorders, 3rd ed., rev. Washington, DC: American Psychiatric Press.

American Psychiatric Association. (1994). Diagnostic and Statistical Manual of Mental Disorders, 4th ed. Washington, DC: American Psychiatric Press.

Beeder, A.B., and Mellman, R.B. (1992). Treatment of patients with psychopathology and substance abuse. In J. Lowinson, P. Ruiz, R. Millman, and J. Langrod (eds.), Substance Abuse: A Comprehensive Textbook, 2nd ed. Baltimore: Williams & Wilkins.

Borson, S. (1997). Delirium and confusional states. In D.L. Dunner (ed.), Current Psychiatric Therapy, Vol 2. Philadlephia: W.B. Saunders Company.

Bullechek, G.M., and McCloskey, J.C. (1992). Nursing Interventions: Essential Nursing Treatments, 2nd ed. Philadelphia: W.B. Saunders Company.

Burnside, I. (1988). Nursing and the Aged, 3rd ed. New York: McGraw-Hill.

Chiles, J.A., and Strosahl, K. (1997). Assessment, crisis management, and treatment of the suicidal patient. In D.L. Dunner (ed.), Current Psychiatric Therapy, 2nd ed. Philadelphia: W.B. Saunders Company, pp. 547–551.

Chitty, K.K., and Maynard, C.K. (1986). Managing manipulation. Journal of Psycosocial and Mental Health Nursing Services 34(2):9.

Collins, M. (1993). Communication in Health Care. The Human Connection in the Life Cycle, 2nd ed. St. Louis: Mosby.

Dee, V. (1991). How can we become more aware of culturally specific body language and use this awareness therapeutically? Journal of Psychosocial Nursing and Mental Health Services 29(11):39–40.

Delaney, C. (1999). Reducing recidivism: Medication versus psychosocial rehabilitation. Journal of Psychosocial Nursing and Mental Health Services 36(11): 28–34.

DiMatteo, M.R., and DiNicola, D.D. (1982). Achieving Patient Compliance: The Psychology of the Medical Practitioner's Role. Elmsford, NY: Pergamon Press.

Dubin, W.R., and Weiss, K.J. (1991). Handbook of Psychiatric Emergencies. Springhouse, PA: Springhouse Corporation.

Dunner, D.L. (1997). Current Psychiatric Theory, 2nd ed. Philadelphia: W.B. Saunders Company.

Dunner, D.L., and Rosenbaum, J.F. (1999). The Psychiatric Clinics of North America Annual of Drug Therapy. Philadelphia: W.B. Saunders Company.

Eells, T. (1995). Relational therapy of grief disorders. In J.J.P. Barber and P. Crits-Christoph (eds.), Dynamic Therapies for Psychiatric Disorders (Axis 1). New York: Basic Books, pp. 86–419.

Egan, G. (1994). The Skilled Helper: A Problem-Management Approach, 5th ed. Pacific Grove, CA: Brooks/Cole.

Ekman, P. (1972). Darwin and Facial Expression: A Century of Research in Review. New York: Academic Press.

477

Feldhaus, K.L., Koziol-McLain, J., Amsbury, H.L., et al. (1997). Accuracy of three brief screening questions for detecting partner violence in the emergency department. JAMA, 227:1357–1361.

Finfgeld, D.L. (1999). Use of brief interventions to treat individuals with drinking problems. Journal of Psychosocial Nursing 37(4):23–30.

Goldberg, R.J. (1995). Practical Guide to the Care of the Psychiatric Patient. St. Louis: Mosby.

Goodwin, J. (1985). The Talk Book: The Intimate Science of Communicating in Close Relationships. New York: Ballantine.

Gorman, L.M., Sultan D.F., and Raines, M.L. (1996). Davis's Manual of Psychosocial Nursing for General Patient Care. Philadelphia: F.A. Davis Company.

Greden, J. (1995). Better outcomes with difficult cases. Presented at the U.S. Psychiatric and Mental Health Congress, New York, November 17, 1995.

Green, A.I., Mooney, J.J., Posner, J.A., and Schildkraut, J.J. (1995). Mood disorders: Biological aspects. In H.I. Kaplan and B.J. Sadock (eds.), Comprehensive Textbook of Psychiatry, 4th ed. Baltimore: Williams & Wilkins.

Gregory, R.J. (1994). Grief and loss among Eskimos attempting suicide in western Alaska. American Journal of Psychiatry 15(12):1815.

Hagerty, B.K. (1984). Psychiatric Mental Health Assessment. St. Louis: Mosby.

Hall, E.T. (1983). Excerpts from an interview conducted by Carol Travis. GEO 25(3):12.

Hall, E.T. (1997). Beyond Culture. Garden City, NJ: Anchor Press.

Harvard Mental Health Letter (August 1996). Alcohol Dependence: Treatment of Alcoholism. Boston: Harvard Medical School Publication Group.

Hill, S.S. (1998). Practice guidelines for major disorders. In G.P. Koocher, J.C. Norcross, and S.S. Hill (eds.), Psychologists' Desk Reference. New York: Oxford University Press.

Hodgson, B.B., and Kizior, R.J. (1999). Nurse's Drug Handbook 1999. Philadelphia: W.B. Saunders Company.

Hoff, L.A. (1995). People in Crisis: Understanding and Helping, 4th ed. San Francisco: Jossey–Bass.

Hoffman, L., and Halmi, K.A. (1997). Treatment of anorexia nervosa. In D.L. Dunner (ed.), Current Psychiatric Therapy, Vol. 2. Philadelphia: W.B. Saunders Company.

Hogarty, G.E. (1999). Schizophrenia and Modern Mental Health Services. National Alliance for the Mentally Ill: http://www/nami.org/research.

Hurt, R.D., Offord, K.P., Croghan, I.T., et al. (1996). Mortality following inpatient addictions treatment: Role of tobacco use in community-based cohort. JAMA, 275: 1097–1103.

Ibrahim, K. (1998). People with eating disorders. In E.M. Varcarolis (ed.), Foundations of Psychiatric Nursing, 3rd ed. Philadelphia: W.B. Saunders Company.

Ingram, C.A. (1991). How can we become more aware of culturally specific body language and use this awareness therapeutically? Journal of Psychosocial Nursing 29(11):39–40.

Kaplan, H.I., and Sadock, B.J. (1993). Pocket Handbook of Emergency Psychiatric Medicine. Baltimore: Williams & Wilkins.

Kaplan, H.I., and Sadock, B.J. (1996). Pocket Handbook of Clinical Psychiatry, 2nd. ed. Baltimore: Williams & Wilkins.

Keller, M. (1995). Depression in adults. Presented at the U.S. Psychiatric and Mental Health Congress, New York, November 18, 1995.

Kobayashi, M., Smith, T.P., and Norcross, J.C. (1998). Enhancing adherence. In G.P. Koocher, J.C. Norcross, and S.S. Hill (eds.), Psychologists' Desk Reference. New York: Oxford University Press.

Krupnick, S.L.W., and Wade, A.J. (1993). Psychiatric Care Planning. Springhouse, PA: Springhouse Corporation.

Kubler-Ross, E. (1969). On Death and Dying. New York: Macmillan.

Lazarus, R.S. (1993).Why we should think of stress as a subset of emotion. In L. Goldberger and S. Breznitz (eds.), Handbook of Stress: Theoretical and Clinical Aspects, 2nd ed. New York: The Free Press.

Lehne, R.A., Moore, L.A., Crosby, L.J., et al. (1998). Pharmacology for Nursing Care, 3rd ed. Philadelphia: W.B. Saunders Company.

Lerner, B.H. (1997). From careless consumptives to recalcitrant patients: The historical construction of *noncompliance*. Social Science and Medicine 45(9):1423–1431.

Lin, K., Anderson, D., and Poland, R.E. (1997). Ethnic and cultural considerations in psychopharmacotherapy. In D.L. Dunner (ed.), Current Psychiatric Therapy, 2nd ed. Philadelphia: W.B. Saunders Company.

Lloyd-Williams, M. (1995). Bereavement referrals to a psychiatric service: An audit. European Journal of Cancer Care 4(1):17.

Lyons, M.A. (1998). The phenomenon of compulsive overeating in a select group of professional women. Journal of Advanced Nursing 27(9):1158–1164.

Mairo, R.D. (1997). Anger and aggression. In D.L. Dunner (ed.), Current Psychiatric Therapy, 2nd ed. Philadelphia: W.B. Saunders Company.

Marris, P. (1975). Loss and Change. Garden City, NY: Anchor Books.

Maxmen, J.S., and Ward, N.G. (1995). Psychotropic Drugs Fast Facts, 2nd ed. New York: W.W. Norton.

McCloskey, J., and Bulechek, G.M. (1995). Nursing Interventions Classification (NIC). St. Louis: Mosby–Year Book.

McGee, D.E., and Linehan, M.M. (1997). Cluster B personality disorders. In D.L. Dunner (ed.), Current Psychiatric Therapy, 2nd ed. Philadelphia: W.B. Saunders Company, pp. 433–438.

Meichenbaum, D., and Turk, D.C. (1987). Facilitating Treatment Adherence: A Practitioner's Guidebook. New York: Plenum Press.

Meier, S.T., and Davis, S.R. (1989). The Elements of Counseling, 2nd ed. Pacific Grove, CA: Brooks/Cole.

Moore, J.M., and Heartman, C.R. (1988). Developing a therapeutic relationship. In C.K. Beck, R.P. Rawlins, and S.R. Williams (eds.), Mental Health Psychiatric Nursing. St. Louis: Mosby.

Moscato, B. (1998). The one-to-one relationship. In H.S. Wilson and C.S. Kneisel (eds.), Psychiatric Nursing, 3rd ed. Menlo Park, CA: Addison-Wesley.

National Alliance for the Mentally Ill. (1999). Senators Domenici and Wellstone Introduced Mental Health Equitable Treatment Act of 1999. NAMI E-News 99(116): April 16 (http://www.nami.org)

National Institute of Mental Health. (1995). Suicide. NIMH

North American Nursing Diagnosis Association. (1999). Nursing Diagnoses: Definition and Classification 1999–2000. Philadelphia: North American Nursing Diagnosis Association.

O'Malley, S.S., Jaffe, A.J., Chang, G., et al. (1992). Naltrexone and coping skills therapy for alcohol dependence. Archives of General Psychiatry 49:881–887.

O'Malley, S.S., Jaffe, A.J., Rode, S., et al. (1996). Experience of a "slip" among alcoholics treated with naltrexone or placebo. American Journal of Psychiatry 153: 281–283.

Pages, K.P. (1997). Bulimia nervosa. In D.L. Dunner (ed.), Current Psychiatric Therapy, Vol. 2. Philadelphia: W.B. Saunders Company.

Palmer-Erbs and Manos (1998). Are we there yet? When will we be there? Designing collaboration plans for future psychiatric nursing practice. Journal of Psychosocial Nursing and Mental Health Services 36(4):10–12.

Paquette, M., and Rodemich, C. (1997). Psychiatric Nursing Diagnosis Care Plans for DSM-IV. Sudbury, MA: Jones and Bartlett.

Parsons, R.D., and Wicks, R.J. (1994). Counseling Strategies and Intervention Techniques for Human Services, 4th ed. Needham Heights, MA: Allyn & Bacon.

Pascualy, M., and Raskind, M.A. (1997). Alzheimer's disease. In D.L. Dunner (ed.), Current Psychiatric Therapy, Vol. 2. Philadelphia: W.B. Saunders Company.

Patterson, W., et al. (1983). Evaluation of suicidal patients. The SAD PERSONS Scale. Psychosomatics, 24(4):343.

Peplau, H.E. (1952). Interpersonal Relations in Nursing. New York: G.P. Putnam & Sons.

Post, R.M. (1992). Anticonvulsants and novel drugs. In E.S. Paykel (ed.), Handbook of Affective Disorders, 2nd ed. New York: Guilford Press, pp. 387–418.

Postrado, L.T., and Lehman, A.F. (1995). Quality of life and clinical predictors of rehospitalization of persons with severe mental illness. Psychiatric Services 46(11): 1161–1165.

Prigerson, H.G., Franke, E., Kasl, S.V., et al. (1995). Complicated grief and bereavement-related depression as distinct disorders: Preliminary empirical validation in elderly bereaved spouses. American Journal of Psychiatry 152:22–30.

Profiri, F. (1998). Personality disorders. In E.M. Varcarolis (ed.), Foundations of Psychiatric Mental Health Nursing, 3rd. ed. Philadelphia: W.B. Saunders Company, pp. 507–537.

Public Policy Committee of the Board of Directors and the NAMI Department of Public Policy and Research. (1999). Public Policy Platform of The National Alliance for the Mentally Ill (NAMI), 3rd ed., Section 4: Services and Supports for Adults. (http://www.nami.org/update/platform/services.htm)

Ries, R.K., Sloan, K.L., and Miller, N.S. (1997). Concept, diagnosis, and treatment of dual diagnosis. In D.L. Dunner (ed.), Current Psychiatric Therapy, Vol. 2. Philadelphia: W.B. Saunders Company.

Roberts, J.K.A. (1984). Differential Diagnosis in Neuropsychiatry. New York: John Wiley, p. 26

Robers, L.J., and Marlatt, G.A. (1998). Guidelines for relapse prevention. In G.P. Koocher, J.C. Norcross, and S.S. Hill (eds.), Psychologists' Desk Reference. New York: Oxford University Press.

Robertson, R.G., and Paradiso, S. (1997). Treatment of psychiatric disorders, including dementia, associated with cerebrovascular disease. In D.L. Dunner (ed.), Current Psychiatric Therapy, Vol. 2. Philadelphia: W.B. Saunders Company.

Robinson, D. (1997). Good Intentions: The Nine Unconscious Mistakes of Nice People. New York: Warner Books

Rogers, S. (1998). To work or not to work: That is not the question. Journal of Psychosocial Nursing and Mental Health Services 36(4):42–46.

Salzman, C. (1997). Overview of the treatment of geriatric disorders. In D.L. Dunner (ed.), Current Psychiatric Therapy, Vol. 2. Philadelphia: W.B. Saunders Company.

Saxon, A.J. (1997). Treatment of opioid dependence. In D.L. Dunner (ed.), Current Psychiatric Therapy, Vol. 2. Philadelphia: W.B. Saunders Company.

Schatzberg, A.F., Cole, J.O., and DeBattista, C. (1997). Manual of Clinical Psychopharmacology, 3rd ed. Washington, DC: American Psychiatric Press.

Schofield, R. (1999). Empowerment education for individuals with serious mental illness. Journal of Psychosocial Nursing 36(11):35–42.

Schultz, J.M., and Dark, S.L. (1982). Manual of Psychiatric Nursing Care Plans. Boston: Little, Brown.

Schultz, J.M., and Videbeck, S.D. (1998). Lippincott's Manual of Psychiatric Nursing Care Plans. Philadelphia: J.B. Lippincott.

Shea, S.C. (1998). Psychiatric Interviewing: The Art of Understanding, 2nd ed. Philadelphia: W.B. Saunders Company.

Sieh, A., and Brentin, L.K. (1997). The Nurse Communicates. Philadelphia: W.B. Saunders Company.

Slaby, A.E. (1994). Handbook of Psychiatric Emergencies, 4th ed. Norwalk, CT: Appleton & Lange.

Smith, L.S. (1994). Coping with the "problem" resident. Nursing Care 43(1): 40–41.

Smith, S. (1992). Communications in Nursing. St. Louis: Mosby–Year Book.

Smith-Dijulio, K. (1998). Families in crisis: Family violence. In E.M. Varcarolis (ed.), Psychiatric Mental Health Nursing, 3rd. ed. Philadelphia: W.B. Saunders Company.

Stone, M.H. (1997). Cluster C personality disorders. In D.L. Dunner (ed.), Current Psychiatric Therapy, 2nd ed. Philadelphia: W.B. Saunders Company, pp. 439–445.

Stone, S. (1999). Refractory schizophrenia. Journal of Psychosocial Nursing 37(2): 19–23.

Stuart, G.W., and Laraia, M.T. (1998). Pocket Guide to Psychiatric Nursing, 4th ed. St. Louis: Mosby.

Suinn, R.M. (1998). Anxiety/anger management. In G.P. Koocher, J.C. Norcross, and S.S. Hill (eds.), Psychologists' Desk Reference. New York: Oxford University Press.

Vaillant, G.E. (1988). What can long-term follow-up teach us about relapse and prevention of relapse in addictions? British Journal of Addictions 83:1147–1157.

Varcarolis, E.M. (ed.). (1998). Psychiatric Mental Health Nursing, 3rd. ed. Philadelphia: W.B. Saunders Company.

Volpicelli, J.R., Alterman, A.I., Hayashida, M., et al. (1992). Naltrexone in the treatment of alcohol dependence. Archives of General Psychiatry 49:876–880.

Weeks, S. M. (1999). Disaster mental health services: A personal perspective. Journal of Psychosocial Nursing 37(2):14–18.

Weissman, M.M., et. al. (1989). Suicidal ideation and suicide attempts in panic disorder and attacks. New England Journal of Medicine 321:1209.

World Health Organization. (1992). International Statistical Classification of Diseases and Related Health Problems, 10th Revision. Geneva: World Health Organization.

Zajecka, J. (1995). Treatment strategies for depression complicated by anxiety disorder. Presented at the U.S. Psychiatric and Mental Health Congress, New York, November 16.

Zale, C.F., O'Brian, M.M., Trestman, R.L., and Siever, L.J. (1997). Cluster A personality disorders. In D.L. Dunner (ed.), Current Psychiatric Therapy, 2nd ed. Philadelphia: W.B. Saunders Company, pp. 427–432.

Zerbe, K.J. (1999). Women's Mental Health in Primary Care. Philadelphia: W.B. Saunders Company.

Zuckerman, E.L. (1995). Clinician's Thesaurus, 4th ed. New York: Guilford Press.

NANDA-APPROVED NURSING DIAGNOSES

This list represents the NANDA-approved nursing diagnoses for clinical use and testing.

Pattern 1: Exchanging

	1.1.2.1	Altered Nutrition: More Than Body Requirements
	1.1.2.2	Altered Nutrition: Less Than Body Requirements
	1.1.2.3	Altered Nutrition: Risk for More Than Body Requirements
	1.2.1.1	Risk for Infection
	1.2.2.1	Risk for Altered Body Temperature
	1.2.2.2	Hypothermia
	1.2.2.3	Hyperthermia
	1.2.2.4	Ineffective Thermoregulation
	1.2.3.1	Dysreflexia
*	1.2.3.2	Risk for Autonomic Dysreflexia
★	1.3.1.1	Constipation
	1.3.1.1.1	Perceived Constipation
	1.3.1.1.2	Colonic Constipation (deleted in 1998)
★	1.3.1.2	Diarrhea
★	1.3.1.3	Bowel Incontinence
*	1.3.1.4	Risk for Constipation
	1.3.2	Altered Urinary Elimination
	1.3.2.1.1	Stress Incontinence
★	1.3.2.1.2	Reflex Urinary Incontinence
	1.3.2.1.3	Urge Incontinence
★	1.3.2.1.4	Functional Urinary Incontinence
	1.3.2.1.5	Total Incontinence

---

*New diagnoses accepted in 1998.
★Revised diagnoses submitted and approved in 1998.
From North American Nursing Diagnosis Association. (1999). Nursing Diagnoses: Definitions and Classifications 1999–2000. Philadelphia: North American Nursing Diagnosis Association, pp. 1–7; reprinted with permission.

*	1.3.2.1.6	Risk for Urinary Urge Incontinence
	1.3.2.2	Urinary Retention
#	1.4.1.1	Altered Tissue Perfusion (specify type: Renal, Cerebral, Cardiopulmonary, Gastrointestinal, Peripheral)
*	1.4.1.2	Risk for Fluid Volume Imbalance
	1.4.1.2.1	Fluid Volume Excess
	1.4.1.2.2.1	Fluid Volume Deficit
	1.4.1.2.2.2	Risk for Fluid Volume Deficit
	1.4.2.1	Decreased Cardiac Output
★	1.5.1.1	Impaired Gas Exchange
★	1.5.1.2	Ineffective Airway Clearance
★	1.5.1.3	Ineffective Breathing Pattern
	1.5.1.3.1	Inability to Sustain Spontaneous Ventilation
	1.5.1.3.2	Dysfunctional Ventilatory Weaning Response
	1.6.1	Risk for Injury
	1.6.1.1	Risk for Suffocation
	1.6.1.2	Risk for Poisoning
	1.6.1.3	Risk for Trauma
	1.6.1.4	Risk for Aspiration
	1.6.1.5	Risk for Disuse Syndrome
*	1.6.1.6	Latex Allergy Response
*	1.6.1.7	Risk for Latex Allergy Response
	1.6.2	Altered Protection
#	1.6.2.1	Impaired Tissue Integrity
★	1.6.2.1.1	Altered Oral Mucous Membranes
#	1.6.2.1.2.1	Impaired Skin Integrity
#	1.6.2.1.2.2	Risk for Impaired Skin Integrity
*	1.6.2.1.3	Altered Dentition
	1.7.1	Decreased Adaptive Capacity: Intracranial
	1.8	Energy Field Disturbance

Pattern 2: Communicating

#	2.1.1.1	Impaired Verbal Communication

Pattern 3: Relating

	3.1.1	Impaired Social Interaction
	3.1.2	Social Isolation

Diagnoses revised by small work groups at the 1996 Biennial Conference on the Classification of Nursing Diagnoses; changes approved and added in 1998.

Pattern 4: Valuing

Pattern 5: Choosing

Pattern 6: Moving

★	6.1.1.1	Impaired Physical Mobility
	6.1.1.1.1	Risk for Peripheral Neurovascular Dysfunction
	6.1.1.1.2	Risk for Perioperative Positioning Injury
	6.1.1.1.3	Impaired Walking
	6.1.1.1.4	Impaired Wheelchair Mobility
*	6.1.1.1.5	Impaired Transfer Ability
	6.1.1.1.6	Impaired Bed Mobility
	6.1.1.2	Activity Intolerance
★	6.1.1.2.1	Fatigue
	6.1.1.3	Risk for Activity Intolerance
★	6.2.1	Sleep Pattern Disturbance
	6.2.1.1	Sleep Deprivation
	6.3.1.1	Diversional Activity Deficit
	6.4.1.1	Impaired Home Maintenance Management
	6.4.2	Altered Health Maintenance
	6.4.2.1	Delayed Surgical Recovery
	6.4.2.2	Adult Failure to Thrive
★	6.5.1	Feeding Self-Care Deficit
★	6.5.1.1	Impaired Swallowing
	6.5.1.2	Ineffective Breastfeeding
	6.5.1.2.1	Interrupted Breastfeeding
	6.5.1.3	Effective Breastfeeding
	6.5.1.4	Ineffective Infant Feeding Pattern
★	6.5.2	Bathing/Hygiene Self-Care Deficit
★	6.5.3	Dressing/Grooming Self-Care Deficit
★	6.5.4	Toileting Self-Care Deficit
	6.6	Altered Growth and Development
	6.6.1	Risk for Altered Development
	6.6.2	Risk for Altered Growth
	6.7	Relocation Stress Syndrome
	6.8.1	Risk for Disorganized Infant Behavior
★	6.8.2	Disorganized Infant Behavior
	6.8.3	Potential for Enhanced Organized Infant Behavior

Pattern 7: Perceiving

#	7.1.1	Body Image Disturbance
	7.1.2	Self-Esteem Disturbance
	7.1.2.1	Chronic Low Self-Esteem
	7.1.2.2	Situational Low Self-Esteem
	7.1.3	Personal Identity Disturbance

#	7.2	Sensory/Perceptual Alterations (specify: Visual, Auditory, Kinesthetic, Gustatory, Tactile, Olfactory)
	7.2.1.1	Unilateral Neglect
	7.3.1	Hopelessness
	7.3.2	Powerlessness

Pattern 8: Knowing

	8.1.1	Knowledge Deficit (specify)
	8.2.1	Impaired Environmental Interpretation Syndrome
	8.2.2	Acute Confusion
	8.2.3	Chronic Confusion
	8.3	Altered Thought Processes
	8.3.1	Impaired Memory

Pattern 9: Feeling

	9.1.1	Pain
	9.1.1.1	Chronic Pain
*	9.1.2	Nausea
	9.2.1.1	Dysfunctional Grieving
	9.2.1.2	Anticipatory Grieving
*	9.2.1.3	Chronic Sorrow
	9.2.2	Risk for Violence: Directed at Others
	9.2.2.1	Risk for Self-Mutilation
	9.2.2.2	Risk for Violence: Self-Directed
★	9.2.3	Post-Trauma Syndrome
★	9.2.3.1	Rape-Trauma Syndrome
	9.2.3.1.1	Rape-Trauma Syndrome: Compound Reaction
	9.2.3.1.2	Rape-Trauma Syndrome: Silent Reaction
*	9.2.4	Risk for Post-Trauma Syndrome
#	9.3.1	Anxiety
*	9.3.1.1	Death Anxiety
#	9.3.2	Fear

Appendix C

DSM-IV CLASSIFICATION

◆ MULTIAXIAL SYSTEM

Axis I   Clinical disorders
           Other conditions that may be a focus of clinical attention
Axis II   Personality disorders
           Mental retardation
Axis III General medical conditions
Axis IV Psychosocial and environmental problems
Axis V   Global assessment of functioning

           NOS = Not Otherwise Specified.

           An *x* appearing in a diagnostic code indicates that a specific code number is required.

◆ DISORDERS USUALLY FIRST DIAGNOSED IN INFANCY, CHILDHOOD, OR ADOLESCENCE

Mental Retardation

Note: *These are coded on Axis II.*

317	Mild mental retardation
318.0	Moderate mental retardation
318.1	Severe mental retardation
318.2	Profound mental retardation
319	Mental retardation, severity unspecified

Learning Disorders

315.00	Reading disorder
315.1	Mathematics disorder
315.2	Disorder of written expression
315.9	Learning disorder NOS

Adapted from American Psychiatric Association. (1994). Diagnostic and Statistical Manual of Mental Disorders, 4th ed. Washington, DC: American Psychiatric Press, pp. 13–24; reprinted by permission. Copyright 1994 American Psychiatric Association.

Motor Skills Disorder

315.4   Developmental coordination disorder

Communication Disorders

315.31   Expressive language disorder
315.31   Mixed receptive-expressive language disorder
315.39   Phonological disorder
307.0   Stuttering
307.9   Communication disorder NOS

Pervasive Developmental Disorders

299.00   Autistic disorder
299.80   Rett's disorder
299.10   Childhood disintegrative disorder
299.80   Asperger's disorder
299.80   Pervasive developmental disorder NOS

Attention-Deficit and Disruptive Behavior Disorders

314.xx   Attention-deficit/hyperactivity disorder
   .01   Combined type
   .00   Predominantly inattentive type
   .01   Predominantly hyperactive-impulsive type
314.9   Attention-deficit/hyperactivity disorder NOS
312.8   Conduct disorder
313.81   Oppositional defiant disorder
312.9   Disruptive behavior disorder NOS

Feeding and Eating Disorders of Infancy or Early Childhood

307.52   Pica
307.53   Rumination disorder
307.59   Feeding disorder of infancy or early childhood

Tic Disorders

307.23   Tourette's disorder
307.22   Chronic motor or vocal tic disorder
307.21   Transient tic disorder
           Specify if: single episode/recurrent
307.20   Tic disorder NOS

Elimination Disorders

—.—	Encopresis
787.6	With constipation and overflow incontinence
307.7	Without constipation and overflow incontinence
307.6	Enuresis (not due to a general medical condition)

Other Disorders of Infancy, Childhood, or Adolescence

309.21	Separation anxiety disorder
313.23	Selective mutism
313.89	Reactive attachment disorder of infancy or early childhood
307.3	Stereotypic movement disorder
313.9	Disorder of infancy, childhood, or adolescence NOS

◆ DELIRIUM, DEMENTIA, AND AMNESTIC AND OTHER COGNITIVE DISORDERS

Delirium

293.0	Delirium due to . . . *[indicate the general medical condition]*
—.—	Substance intoxication delirium *(refer to Substance-Related Disorders for substance-specific codes)*
—.—	Substance withdrawal delirium *(refer to Substance-Related Disorders for substance-specific codes)*
—.—	Delirium due to multiple etiologies *(code each of the specific etiologies)*
780.09	Delirium NOS

Dementia

290.xx	Dementia of the Alzheimer's type, with early onset *(also code on Axis III)*
.10	Uncomplicated
.11	With delirium
.12	With delusions
.13	With depressed mood
290.xx	Dementia of the Alzheimer's type, with late onset *(also code on Axis III)*
.0	Uncomplicated
.3	With delirium
.20	With delusions
.21	With depressed mood

290.xx	Vascular dementia
.40	Uncomplicated
.41	With delirium
.42	With delusions
.43	With depressed mood
294.9	Dementia due to HIV disease *(also code HIV affecting central nervous system on Axis III)*
294.1	Dementia due to head trauma *(also code on Axis III)*
294.1	Dementia due to Parkinson's disease *(also code on Axis III)*
294.1	Dementia due to Huntington's disease *(also code on Axis III)*
290.10	Dementia due to Pick's disease *(also code on Axis III)*
290.10	Dementia due to Creutzfeldt-Jakob disease *(also code on Axis III)*
294.1	Dementia due to . . . *[indicate the general medical condition not listed above] (also code the general medical condition on Axis III)*
—.—	Substance induced persisting dementia
—.—	Dementia due to multiple etiologies
294.8	Dementia NOS

Amnestic Disorders

294.0	Amnestic disorder due to . . . *[indicate the general medical condition]* *Specify if*: transient-chronic
—.—	Substance-induced persisting amnestic disorder
294.8	Amnestic disorder NOS

Other Cognitive Disorder

294.9	Cognitive disorder NOS

◆ MENTAL DISORDERS DUE TO A GENERAL MEDICAL CONDITION NOT ELSEWHERE CLASSIFIED

239.89	Catatonic disorder due to . . . *[indicate the general medical condition]*
310.1	Personality change due to . . . *[indicate the general medical condition]*
293.9	Mental disorder NOS due to . . . *[indicate the general medical condition]*

◆ SUBSTANCE-RELATED DISORDERS

Alcohol-Related Disorders

Alcohol Use Disorders

303.9	Alcohol dependence[a]
305.00	Alcohol abuse

Alcohol-Induced Disorders

303.00	Alcohol intoxication
291.8	Alcohol withdrawal
291.0	Alcohol intoxication delirium
291.0	Alcohol withdrawal delirium
291.2	Alcohol-induced persisting dementia
291.1	Alcohol-induced persisting amnestic disorder
291.x	Alcohol-induced psychotic disorder
.5	With delusions
.3	With hallucinations
291.8	Alcohol-induced mood disorder
291.8	Alcohol-induced anxiety disorder
291.8	Alcohol-induced sexual dysfunction
291.8	Alcohol-induced sleep disorder
291.9	Alcohol-related disorder NOS

Amphetamine (or Amphetamine-Like)–Related Disorders

Amphetamine Use Disorders

304.40	Amphetamine dependence[a]
305.70	Amphetamine abuse

Amphetamine-Induced Disorders

292.89	Amphetamine intoxication
292.0	Amphetamine withdrawal
292.81	Amphetamine intoxication delirium

---

[a]*The following specifiers may be applied to Substance Dependence*:
With physiological dependence/without physiological dependence
Early full remission/early partial remission
Sustained full remission/sustained partial remission
On agonist therapy/in a controlled environment

292.xx	Amphetamine-induced psychotic disorder
.11	With delusions[I]
.12	With hallucinations[I]
292.84	Amphetamine-induced mood disorder
292.89	Amphetamine-induced anxiety disorder
292.89	Amphetamine-induced sexual dysfunction
292.89	Amphetamine-induced sleep disorder
292.9	Amphetamine-related disorder NOS

Caffeine-Related Disorders

Caffeine-Induced Disorders

305.90	Caffeine intoxication
292.89	Caffeine-induced anxiety disorder[I]
292.89	Caffeine-induced sleep disorder[I]
292.9	Caffeine-related disorder NOS

Cannabis-Related Disorders

Cannabis Use Disorders

| 304.30 | Cannabis dependence |
| 305.20 | Cannabis abuse |

Cannabis-Induced Disorders

292.89	Cannabis intoxication
292.81	Cannabis intoxication delirium
292.xx	Cannabis-induced psychotic disorder
.11	With delusions[I]
.12	With hallucinations[I]
292.89	Cannabis-induced anxiety disorder[I]
292.9	Cannabis-related disorder NOS

Cocaine-Related Disorders

Cocaine Use Disorders

| 304.20 | Cocaine dependence[a] |
| 305.60 | Cocaine abuse |

Cocaine-Induced Disorders

292.89	Cocaine intoxication
	Specify if: with perceptual disturbances
292.0	Cocaine withdrawal
292.81	Cocaine intoxication delirium

292.xx   Cocaine-induced psychotic disorder
.11   With delusions[I]
.12   With hallucinations[I]
292.84   Cocaine-induced mood disorder
292.89   Cocaine-induced anxiety disorder
292.89   Cocaine-induced sexual dysfunction[I]
292.89   Cocaine-induced sleep disorder
292.90   Cocaine-related disorder NOS

Hallucinogen-Related Disorders

Hallucinogen Use Disorders

304.50   Hallucinogen dependence[a]
305.30   Hallucinogen abuse

Hallucinogen-Induced Disorders

292.89   Hallucinogen intoxication
292.89   Hallucinogen persisting perception disorder
         (flashbacks)
292.81   Hallucinogen intoxication delirium
292.xx   Hallucinogen-induced psychotic disorder
.11   With delusions[I]
.12   With hallucinations[I]
292.84   Hallucinogen-induced mood disorder[I]
292.89   Hallucinogen-induced anxiety disorder[I]
292.9   Hallucinogen-related disorder NOS

Inhalant-Related Disorders

Inhalant Use Disorders

304.60   Inhalant dependence[a]
305.90   Inhalant abuse

Inhalant-Induced Disorders

292.89   Inhalant intoxication
292.81   Inhalant intoxication delirium
292.82   Inhalant-induced persisting dementia
292.xx   Inhalant-induced psychotic disorder
.11   With delusions[I]
.12   With hallucinations[I]
292.84   Inhalant-induced mood disorder[I]
292.89   Inhalant-induced anxiety disorder[I]
292.9   Inhalant-related disorder NOS

Nicotine-Related Disorders

Nicotine Use Disorder

305.10	Nicotine dependence[a]

Nicotine-Induced Disorders

292.0	Nicotine withdrawal
292.9	Nicotine-related disorder NOS

Opioid-Related Disorders

Opioid Use Disorders

304.00	Opioid dependence[a]
305.50	Opioid abuse

Opioid-Induced Disorders

292.89	Opioid intoxication
292.0	Opioid withdrawal
292.81	Opioid intoxication delirium
292.xx	Opioid-induced psychotic disorder
.11	With delusions[I]
.12	With hallucinations[I]
292.84	Opioid-induced mood disorder[I]
292.89	Opioid-induced sexual dysfunction[I]
292.89	Opioid-induced sleep disorder
292.9	Opioid-related disorder NOS

Phencyclidine (or Phencyclidine-Like)–Related Disorders

Phencyclidine Use Disorders

304.90	Phencyclidine dependence[a]
305.90	Phencyclidine abuse

Phencyclidine-Induced Disorders

292.89	Phencyclidine intoxication
292.81	Phencyclidine intoxication delirium
292.xx	Phencyclidine-induced psychotic disorder
.11	With delusions[I]
.12	With hallucinations[I]
292.84	Phencyclidine-induced mood disorder[I]
292.89	Phencyclidine-induced anxiety disorder[I]
292.9	Phencyclidine-related disorder NOS

Sedative-, Hypnotic-, or Anxiolytic-Related Disorders

Sedative, Hypnotic, or Anxiolytic Use Disorders

304.10	Sedative, hypnotic, or anxiolytic dependence[a]
305.40	Sedative, hypnotic, or anxiolytic abuse

Sedative-, Hypnotic-, or Anxiolytic-Induced Disorders

292.89	Sedative, hypnotic, or anxiolytic intoxication
292.0	Sedative, hypnotic, or anxiolytic withdrawal *Specify if*: with perceptual disturbances
292.81	Sedative, hypnotic, or anxiolytic intoxication delirium
292.81	Sedative, hypnotic, or anxiolytic withdrawal delirium
292.82	Sedative-, hypnotic-, or anxiolytic-induced persisting dementia
292.83	Sedative-, hypnotic-, or anxiolytic-induced persisting amnestic disorder
292.xx	Sedative-, hypnotic-, or anxiolytic-induced psychotic disorder
.11	With delusions
.12	With hallucinations
292.84	Sedative-, hypnotic-, or anxiolytic-induced mood disorder[I,W]
292.89	Sedative-, hypnotic-, or anxiolytic-induced anxiety disorder[W]
292.89	Sedative-, hypnotic-, or anxiolytic-induced sexual dysfunction[I]
292.89	Sedative-, hypnotic-, or anxiolytic-induced sleep disorder[I,W]
292.9	Sedative-, hypnotic-, or anxiolytic-related disorder NOS

Polysubstance-Related Disorder

304.80	Polysubstance dependence[a]

Other (or Unknown) Substance-Related Disorders

Other (or Unknown) Substance Use Disorders

304.90	Other (or unknown) substance dependence[a]
305.90	Other (or unknown) substance abuse

Other (or Unknown) Substance-Induced Disorders

292.89	Other (or unknown) substance intoxication
292.0	Other (or unknown) substance withdrawal
292.81	Other (or unknown) substance-induced delirium
292.82	Other (or unknown) substance-induced persisting dementia
292.83	Other (or unknown) substance-induced persisting amnestic disorder
292.xx	Other (or unknown) substance-induced psychotic disorder
.11	With delusions[I,W]
.12	With hallucinations[I,W]
292.84	Other (or unknown) substance-induced mood disorder[I,W]
292.89	Other (or unknown) substance-induced anxiety disorder[I,W]
292.89	Other (or unknown) substance-induced sexual dysfunction[I]
292.89	Other (or unknown) substance-induced sleep disorder[I,W]
292.9	Other (or unknown) substance-related disorder NOS

◆ SCHIZOPHRENIA AND OTHER PSYCHOTIC DISORDERS

295.xx	Schizophrenia

The following Classification of Longitudinal Course applies to all subtypes of Schizophrenia:

Episodic with interepisode residual symptoms (*specify if*: with prominent negative symptoms)/episodic with no interepisode residual symptoms/continuous (*specify if*: with prominent negative symptoms)

Single episode in partial remission (*specify if*: with prominent negative symptoms)/single episode in full remission

Other or unspecified pattern

.30	Paranoid type
.10	Disorganized type
.20	Catatonic type
.90	Undifferentiated type
.60	Residual type
295.40	Schizophreniform disorder
	Specify if: without good prognostic features/with good prognostic features

295.70	Schizoaffective disorder
	Specify type: bipolar type/depressive type
297.1	Delusional disorder
	Specify type: erotomanic type/grandiose type/jealous type/persecutory type/somatic type/mixed type/ unspecified type
298.8	Brief psychotic disorder
	Specify if: with marked stressor(s)/without marked stressor(s)/with postpartum onset
297.3	Shared psychotic disorder
293.xx	Psychotic disorder due to . . . *[indicate the general medical condition]*
.81	With delusions
.82	With hallucinations
—.—	Substance-induced psychotic disorder
	Specify if: with onset during intoxication/with onset during withdrawal
298.9	Psychotic disorder NOS

◆ MOOD DISORDERS

Code current state of major depressive disorder or bipolar I disorder in fifth digit:

1 = Mild
2 = Moderate
3 = Severe without psychotic features
4 = Severe with psychotic features
   Specify: Mood-congruent psychotic features/mood-incongruent psychotic features
5 = In partial remission
6 = In full remission
0 = Unspecified

Depressive Disorders

296.xx	Major depressive disorder
.2x	Single episode
.3x	Recurrent
300.4	Dysthymic disorder
	Specify if: early onset/late onset
	Specify: with atypical features
311	Depressive disorder NOS

Bipolar Disorders

296.xx	Bipolar I disorder
.0x	Single manic episode
.40	Most recent episode hypomanic
.4x	Most recent episode manic
.6x	Most recent episode mixed
.5x	Most recent episode depressed
.7	Most recent episode unspecified
296.89	Bipolar II disorder
	Specify (current or most recent episode): hypomanic/depressed
301.13	Cyclothymic disorder
296.80	Bipolar disorder NOS
293.83	Mood disorder due to . . . *[indicate the general medical condition]*
	Specify type: with depressive features/with major depressive-like episode/with manic features/with mixed features
——.—	Substance-induced mood disorder
	Specify type: with depressive features/with manic features/with mixed features
	Specify if: with onset during intoxication/with onset during withdrawal
296.90	Mood disorder NOS

◆ ANXIETY DISORDERS

300.01	Panic disorder without agoraphobia
300.21	Panic disorder with agoraphobia
300.22	Agoraphobia without history of panic disorder
300.29	Specific phobia
	Specify type: animal type/natural environment type/blood-injection-injury type/situational type/other type
300.23	Social phobia
	Specify if: generalized
300.3	Obsessive-compulsive disorder
	Specify if: with poor insight
309.81	Posttraumatic stress disorder
	Specify if: acute/chronic
	Specify if: with delayed onset
308.3	Acute stress disorder
300.02	Generalized anxiety disorder
293.89	Anxiety disorder due to . . . *[indicate the general medical condition]*

Specify if: with generalized anxiety/with panic attacks/with obsessive-compulsive symptoms

——.—— Substance-induced anxiety disorder
Specify if: with generalized anxiety/with panic attacks/with obsessive-compulsive symptoms/with phobic symptoms
Specify if: with onset during intoxication/with onset during withdrawal

300.00 Anxiety disorder NOS

◆ SOMATOFORM DISORDERS

300.81 Somatization disorder
300.81 Undifferentiated somatoform disorder
300.11 Conversion disorder
Specify type: with motor symptom or deficit/with sensory symptom or deficit/with seizures or convulsions/with mixed presentation
307.xx Pain disorder
.80 Associated with psychological factors
.89 Associated with both psychological factors and a general medical condition
Specify if: acute/chronic
300.7 Hypochondriasis
Specify if: with poor insight
300.7 Body dysmorphic disorder
300.81 Somatoform disorder NOS

◆ FACTITIOUS DISORDERS

300.xx Factitious disorders
.16 With predominantly psychological signs and symptoms
.19 With predominantly physical signs and symptoms
.19 With combined psychological and physical signs and symptoms
300.19 Factitious disorder NOS

◆ DISSOCIATIVE DISORDERS

300.12 Dissociative amnesia
300.13 Dissociative fugue
300.14 Dissociative identity disorder
300.6 Depersonalization disorder
300.15 Dissociative disorder NOS

◆ SEXUAL AND GENDER IDENTITY DISORDERS

Sexual Dysfunctions

The following specifiers apply to all primary Sexual Dysfunctions:

Lifelong type/acquired type/generalized type/situational type
due to psychological factors/due to combined factors

Sexual Desire Disorders

302.71   Hypoactive sexual desire disorder
302.79   Sexual aversion disorder

Sexual Arousal Disorders

302.72   Female sexual arousal disorder
302.72   Male erectile disorder

Orgasmic Disorders

302.73   Female orgasmic disorder
302.74   Male orgasmic disorder
302.75   Premature ejaculation

Sexual Pain Disorders

302.76   Dyspareunia (not due to a general medical
          condition)
306.51   Vaginismus (not due to a general medical condition)

Sexual Dysfunction Due to a General Medical Condition

625.8   Female hypoactive sexual desire disorder due to . . .
          [indicate the general medical condition]
608.89   Male hypoactive sexual desire disorder due to . . .
          [indicate the general medical condition]
607.84   Male erectile disorder due to . . . *[indicate the
          general medical condition]*
625.0   Female dyspareunia due to . . . *[indicate the general
          medical condition]*
608.89   Male dyspareunia due to . . . *[indicate the general
          medical condition]*
625.8   Other female sexual dysfunction due to . . . *[indicate
          the general medical condition]*
608.89   Other male sexual dysfunction due to . . . *[indicate
          the general medical condition]*
——.——   Substance-induced sexual dysfunction
302.70   Sexual dysfunction NOS

Paraphilias

302.4	Exhibitionism
302.81	Fetishism
302.89	Frotteurism
302.2	Pedophilia
302.83	Sexual masochism
302.84	Sexual sadism
302.3	Transvestic fetishism
302.82	Voyeurism
302.9	Paraphilia NOS

Gender Identity Disorders

302.xx   Gender identity disorder
.6   in children
.85   in adolescents or adults
Specify if: sexually attracted to males/sexually attracted to females/sexually attracted to both/ sexually attracted to neither
302.6   Gender identity disorder NOS
302.9   Sexual disorder NOS

◆ EATING DISORDERS

307.1   Anorexia nervosa
Specify type: restricting type; binge-eating/purging type
307.51   Bulimia nervosa
Specify type: purging type/nonpurging type
307.50   Eating disorder NOS

◆ SLEEP DISORDERS

Primary Sleep Disorders

Dyssomnias

307.42	Primary insomnia
307.44	Primary hypersomnia
	Specify if: recurrent
347	Narcolepsy
780.59	Breathing-related sleep disorder
307.45	Circadian rhythm sleep disorder
307.47	Dyssomnia NOS

Parasomnias

307.47	Nightmare disorder
307.46	Sleep terror disorder
307.46	Sleepwalking disorder
307.47	Parasomnia NOS

Sleep Disorders Related to Another Mental Disorder

307.42	Insomnia related to . . . *[indicate the disorder]*
307.44	Hypersomnia related to . . . *[indicate the disorder]*

Other Sleep Disorders

780.xx	Sleep disorders due to . . . *[indicate the general medical condition]*
.52	Insomnia type
.54	Hypersomnia type
.59	Parasomnia type
.59	Mixed type
——.—	Substance-induced sleep disorder

Specify type: insomnia type/hypersomnia type/parasomnia type/mixed type

Specify if: with onset during intoxication/with onset during withdrawal

◆ IMPULSE-CONTROL DISORDERS NOT ELSEWHERE CLASSIFIED

312.34	Intermittent explosive disorder
312.32	Kleptomania
312.33	Pyromania
312.31	Pathological gambling
312.39	Trichotillomania
312.30	Impulse-control disorder NOS

◆ ADJUSTMENT DISORDERS

309.xx	Adjustment disorder
.0	With depressed mood
.24	With anxiety
.28	With mixed anxiety and depressed mood
.3	With disturbance of conduct
.4	With mixed disturbance of emotions and conduct

.9   Unspecified
            Specify if: acute/chronic

◆ PERSONALITY DISORDERS

Note: *These are coded on Axis II.*

301.0   Paranoid personality disorder
301.20   Schizoid personality disorder
301.22   Schizotypal personality disorder
301.7   Antisocial personality disorder
301.83   Borderline personality disorder
301.50   Histrionic personality disorder
301.81   Narcissistic personality disorder
301.82   Avoidant personality disorder
301.6   Dependent personality disorder
301.4   Obsessive-compulsive personality disorder
301.9   Personality disorder NOS

◆ OTHER CONDITIONS THAT MAY BE A FOCUS OF CLINICAL ATTENTION

Psychological Factors Affecting Medical Condition

316   . . . *[Specified psychological factor]* affecting . . .
            [indicate the general medical condition]
            Choose name based on nature of factors:
            Mental disorder affecting medical condition
            Psychological symptoms affecting medical condition
            Personality traits or coping style affecting medical
                condition
            Maladaptive health behaviors affecting medical
                condition
            Stress-related physiological response affecting
                medical condition
            Other or unspecified psychological factors affecting
                medical condition

Medication-Induced Movement Disorders

332.1   Neuroleptic-induced parkinsonism
333.92   Neuroleptic malignant syndrome
333.7   Neuroleptic-induced acute dystonia
333.99   Neuroleptic-induced acute akathisia
333.82   Neuroleptic-induced tardive dyskinesia

| 333.1 | Medication-induced postural tremor |
| 333.9 | Medication-induced movement disorder NOS |

Other Medication-Induced Disorder

| 995.2 | Adverse effects of medication NOS |

Relational Problems

V61.9	Relational problem related to a mental disorder or general medical condition
V61.20	Parent-child relational problem
V61.1	Partner relational problem
V61.8	Sibling relational problem
V62.81	Relational problem NOS

Problems Related to Abuse or Neglect

V61.21	Physical abuse of child
V61.21	Sexual abuse of child
V61.21	Neglect of child
V61.1	Physical abuse of adult
V61.1	Sexual abuse of Adult

Additional Conditions That May Be a Focus of Clinical Attention

V15.81	Noncompliance with treatment
V65.2	Malingering
V71.01	Adult antisocial behavior
V71.02	Child or adolescent antisocial behavior
V62.89	Borderline intellectual functioning
	Note: *This is coded on Axis II.*
780.9	Age-related cognitive decline
V62.82	Bereavement
V62.3	Academic problem
V62.2	Occupational problem
313.82	Identity problem
V62.89	Religious or spiritual problem
V62.4	Acculturation problem
V62.89	Phase of life problem

Appendix D

MEDICATION CARDS

◆ BENZTROPINE MESYLATE

Category: Antiparkinsonian
Trade Name: Cogentin

Uses

1. Treating Parkinson's disease
2. Treatment of extrapyramidal symptoms (except tardive dyskinesia) caused by use of neuroleptic/antipsychotic medications

Action

Cogentin is an anticholinergic agent. This drug increases and prolongs the dopamine activity in the central nervous system (CNS), thereby correcting neurotransmitter imbalances and minimizing involuntary movements.

Dosages and Routes

Adult

0.5–1 mg/day PO initially; gradually increase to 4–6 mg/day
For drug-induced extrapyramidal symptoms: 1–4 mg IM/PO
1–2 times daily
For acute dystonic reactions: 0.5–2 mg IM or IV

Elderly

Use lower doses

Contraindications

Narrow-angle glaucoma, pyloric or duodenal obstruction, peptic ulcers, prostatic hypertrophy, obstructions of the bladder neck, myasthenia gravis, and in children under 3 years of age. Rarely indicated for children.

Cautions

The elderly and clients with cardiac, liver, or kidney disease or hypertension. Also used with caution in clients taking barbiturates or alcohol.

Remarks

The effects of benztropine are cumulative and may not be evident for 2 or 3 days. After 4 to 6 months of long-term maintenance antipsychotic therapy, antiparkinsonian drugs can be used on an as-necessary basis or withdrawn. Some clients respond best to the medication given every day. Others do better with divided doses. Long-term use of benztropine with a neuroleptic can predispose a patient to tardive dyskinesia.

Side Effects

Autonomic: Dry mouth, blurred vision, nausea, restlessness
CNS: Sedation, vertigo, paresthesias
Cardiovascular: Palpitations, tachycardia
Gastrointestinal: Nausea, vomiting, constipation, paralytic ileus
Genitourinary: Dysuria, urinary retention
Ocular: Blurred vision, mydriasis, photophobia
Other: Anhidrosis (abnormal deficiency of sweat)

Adverse Reactions

CNS: CNS depression, mild agitation, hallucinations, delirium, toxic psychosis, muscle weakness, ataxia, numbness of the fingers

Nursing Measures

1. Monitor intake and output. Observe for urinary retention.
2. Give medication after patient voids to reduce possibility of urinary retention.
3. Monitor for constipation; abdominal pain or distention may indicate potential for paralytic ileus.
4. Indications of CNS toxicity (depression or excitement, hallucinations, psychosis, or other) warrant withholding the drug and informing the physician immediately.

Inform Client

1. Avoid driving or operating hazardous equipment if drowsiness or dizziness occurs.
2. Tolerance to heat may be reduced owing to diminished ability to sweat. Plan periods of rest in cool places during the day.
3. Stop taking the medication if CNS toxic effects, or difficulty swallowing or speaking, or vomiting occurs. Inform physician immediately.
4. Monitor urinary output and watch for signs of constipation.
5. Consult with physician before using any medication, prescribed or over the counter, once started on benztropine.

◆ BUSPIRONE HYDROCHLORIDE

Category: Antianxiety agent
Trade Name: BuSpar

Use

Management of anxiety disorders

Action

The exact action of buspirone is not clear. It may exert a potent presynaptic dopamine antagonist effect in the CNS, resulting in increased dopamine at the synapses. It may also have an effect on serotonin receptors.

Dosages and Routes

Adult and Elderly

5 mg PO 2–3 times daily; may increase 5 mg every 3–4 days
Maintenance: 15–30 mg/day in 2–3 divided doses; not to
    exceed 60 mg/day

Contraindications

Severe renal or hepatic impairment, clients on MAOIs

Cautions

Renal or hepatic impairment, pregnant or lactating women, elderly or debilitated clients

Remarks

The advantages of buspirone (BuSpar) are that it is not sedating, tolerance does not develop, and it is not addicting. The drug has a more favorable side effect profile than do the benzodiazepines.

Side Effects

Dizziness, nausea, headache, nervousness, lightheadedness, and excitement, which generally are not major problems. Other less common problems may occur (e.g., blurred vision, tachycardia, palpitations, paresthesia, abdominal distention).

Adverse Reactions

Overdose may produce severe nausea, vomiting, dizziness, drowsiness, abdominal distention, excessive pupil constriction.

Nursing Measures

1. Offer emotional support to anxious clients.
2. Liver and renal function tests and blood counts should be done regularly for clients on long-term therapy.
3. Assist with ambulation and put in place other safety features if dizziness and lightheadedness occur.

Inform Client and Family

1. Teach clients to inform their physicians:
   a. About any medications (prescription or nonprescription), alcohol, or drugs that they are taking
   b. If they are now or plan to get pregnant
   c. If they are breast-feeding an infant
2. Do not drive a car or operate potentially dangerous machinery until you experience how this medication will affect you.
3. Notify physician of difficulty breathing, change in vision, sweating, flushing, or cardiac problems.
4. Improvement may be noted in 7 to 10 days, but it may take 3 to 4 weeks or longer to note therapeutic effects.

◆ CARBAMAZEPINE

Categories: Anticonvulsant, antineuralgic, bipolar disorder
Trade Names: Tegretol, Epitol, Mazepine

Uses

1. Management of generalized tonic-clonic seizures (grand mal) and psychomotor seizures
2. Trigeminal neuralgia
3. Potential mood stabilizer, particularly in acute mania. Used clinically, but not Food and Drug Administration (FDA) approved at present for this use.

Action

Reduces post-tetanic potentiation at the synapse, preventing repetitive discharge.

Dosages and Routes

For seizures: PO only (tablets, suspension, and chewable tablets)

Adult

100–200 mg twice daily, gradually increase until response is attained
Maintenance: 800–1200 mg/day

Child (6–12)

15–30 mg/kg/day administered in divided doses.
Note: Oral suspensions produce higher peak concentrations. Going from tablets to suspension, give in smaller and more frequent doses.

Contraindications

History of bone marrow depression, history of hypersensitivity to tricyclic antidepressants (TCAs)

Cautions

Impaired cardiac, hepatic, and renal function; pregnancy or lactation (crosses placenta, appears in breast milk, accumulates in fetal tissues)
Administer with meals to reduce gastric irritation

Remarks

Monitoring drug levels has increased the safety of anticonvulsant therapy.

Side Effects

Frequent: Drowsiness, dizziness, nausea and vomiting
Infrequent: Lethargy, visual abnormalities (spots before the eyes, difficulty focusing), dry mouth, headache, urinary frequency or retention, rash

Adverse Reactions

Hematologic: Blood dyscrasias (e.g., aplastic anemia, agranulocytosis, thrombocytopenia, leukopenia, bone marrow depression)
Hepatic: Abnormal hepatic function test results; jaundice may be noticed; hepatitis
Cardiovascular: Congestive heart failure, edema, aggravation of coronary artery disease, arrhythmias and atrioventricular block,

primary thrombophlebitis. Some complications have resulted in fatalities.

CNS: Abrupt withdrawal may precipitate status epilepticus.

Nursing Measures

1. Monitor for therapeutic serum level (3–12 µg/ml).
2. Assess for clinical evidence of early toxic signs (fever, sore throat, mouth ulcerations, easy bruising, unusual bleeding, joint pain).
3. Observe frequently for recurrence of seizure activity.

Inform Client and Family

1. Blood tests should be repeated frequently during the first 3 months of therapy and at monthly intervals thereafter for 2 to 3 years.
2. Do *not* abruptly withdraw medications following long-term use (may precipitate seizures).
3. Avoid tasks that require alertness until response to drug is established.
4. Report visual abnormalities.

◆ CHLORPROMAZINE

Categories: Antipsychotic/neuroleptic; phenothiazine
Trade Names: Thorazine, Chlorazine

Uses

1. Management of acute psychotic disorders (schizophrenia, manic phase of a bipolar disorder) and to maintain remission of these psychotic disorders
2. Management of severe behavioral disturbances in (a) children or (b) clients with organic mental disorders
3. Other: Intractable hiccups, acute intermittent porphyria, tetanus, preoperatively, or to control nausea and vomiting

Action

Blocks postsynaptic dopamine receptors in the cerebral cortex basal ganglia, hypothalamus, limbic system, brain stem, and medulla. Therefore, there is inhibition or alteration of dopamine release, which is thought to be related to the suppression of the clinical manifestations of schizophrenia.

Dosages and Routes

Hospitalized: Acute Psychotic Disorders
Adult

PO: Gradually increase over several days to maximum of 400 mg q4–6h

25 mg IM; may give an additional 25–50 mg in 1 hour if needed

Outpatient: Maintenance Dose
Adult

25 mg tid gradually increased (usual maintenance dose is 400 mg/day)

25–50 mg IM 1–4 times daily

50–100 mg rectal suppository 3–4 times daily

Child

0.5 mg/kg PO q4–6h

Elderly (Debilitated)

25 mg PO daily gradually increased up to 25 mg tid

Contraindications

Comatose states, alcohol or barbiturate withdrawal states, bone marrow depression, pregnancy, lactation

Cautions

Seizure disorders, diabetes, hepatic disease, cardiac disease, glaucoma, prostatic hypertrophy, asthma

Remarks

A "low-potency" neuroleptic—low neurological symptoms (extrapyramidal symptoms [EPS])—but with high sedation and autonomic side effects (e.g., hypotension, cardiac, allergic). Food or antacids decrease absorption. Liquid preparation is more rapidly absorbed.

Side Effects

Autonomic: Dry mouth, nasal congestion, constipation or diarrhea, urinary retention or urinary frequency, inhibition of ejaculation and impotence in men

CNS: *EPS* (pseudoparkinsonism, akathisia, dystonia). Possible vertigo or insomnia.

Cardiovascular: Orthostatic hypotension, hypertension, vertigo, electroencephalogram (EEG) changes
Endocrine: Changes in libido, galactorrhea in women, gynecomastia in men
Ocular: Photophobia, blurred vision, aggravation of glaucoma
Other: Weight gain, allergic reactions such as eczema and skin rashes

Adverse Reactions

CNS: *Acute dystonias* (e.g., painful neck spasms, torticollis, oculogyric crisis, convulsions). *Tardive dyskinesia* (choreiform movements of the tongue, face, mouth, jaw, and possibly extremities). The elderly and those on the drug for extended periods of time are more susceptible; often the condition is irreversible.
Hematologic: Agranulocytosis—stop drug immediately.
Hepatic: Jaundice; clinical picture resembles hepatitis.
Neuroleptic Malignant Syndrome (NMS): Rare life-threatening syndrome. Includes severe rigidity, fever, increased white blood cell (WBC) count, unstable BP, renal failure, tachycardia, tachypnea. Hold all drugs. Immediate administration of dantrolene sodium and bromocriptine is the most successful somatic prescription.

Nursing Measures

1. Take BP lying and standing (withhold if systolic is 90 mm Hg or below) and notify physician.
2. Hold dose with EPS or jaundice.
3. Check frequently for urinary retention.
4. Check for constipation (avoid impaction).
5. Observe for fever, sore throat, and malaise, and monitor complete blood count, indicating a blood dyscrasia.

Inform Client

1. Rise slowly to a sitting position and dangle the legs 5 minutes before standing to minimize orthostatic hypotension.
2. Avoid sun. Use sunscreen when in direct light to avoid skin blotching. Wear long sleeves and hats. Client may experience severe photosensitivity. Advise wearing sunglasses to minimize photophobia.
3. Avoid use of alcoholic beverages because they enhance CNS depression.
4. Do not operate machinery if drowsiness occurs.

◆ **CLOZAPINE**

Categories: Antipsychotic/neuroleptic; tricyclic dibenzodiazepine derivative
Trade Name: Clozaril

Use

Management of severely ill schizophrenic patients who fail to respond to other antipsychotic therapy

Action

May involve antagonism of dopaminergic, serotoninergic, adrenergic, and cholinergic neurotransmitter systems. Exact action unknown.

Dosages and Routes

Adult

PO only: initially, 25 mg 1-2 times daily; may increase by 25–50 mg/day over 2 weeks until 300–450 mg/day achieved; range 200–600 mg/day; not to exceed 900 gm/day

---

Contraindications

Clients who are hypersensitive to tricyclics, have a history of severe granulocytopenia; concurrent administration with other drugs having potential to suppress bone marrow function; clients who are CNS depressed or comatose or have myeloproliferative disorders

Cautions

Clients with a history of seizures; cardiovascular disease; impaired respiratory, hepatic, or renal function; alcohol withdrawal; urinary retention. Drug has potent anticholinergic effects, and extreme caution is advised for clients with prostatic enlargement or narrow-angle glaucoma. Also use with caution in pregnant or lactating women.

Remarks

May take 2 to 4 weeks for therapeutic effects or as long as 3 to 6 months. Because 1% to 2% of people on clozapine develop agranulocytosis, weekly WBC counts must be done.

Side Effects

Frequent: Sedation, salivation, tachycardia, dizziness, constipation (in order of frequency)
Occasional: Hypotension or hypertension, gastrointestinal upset, nausea and vomiting, sweating, dry mouth, weight gain
Rare: Visual disturbances, diarrhea, rash, urinary abnormalities

Adverse Reactions

Hematologic: One per cent to 2% of clients develop agranulocytosis; mild leukopenia may develop.
CNS: *Seizures:* Develop in about 5% of patients on Clozaril and up to 15% of patients on dosages over 550 mg/day.
NMS: Has been reported when clozapine is used concurrently with lithium or other CNS-active agents.
Other: Dizziness or vertigo, drowsiness, restlessness, akinesia, agitation.
Cardiovascular: Severe orthostatic hypotension (with or without syncope); marked tachycardia may occur in 25% of clients.

Nursing Measures

1. Check baseline WBC count before initiating treatment.
2. Check weekly WBC count; hold drug if the count falls below 3000/mm^3 and notify physician.
3. Check BP lying and standing to assess for potential orthostatic hypotension.
4. Observe for signs of agranulocytosis (e.g., sore throat, fever, malaise).
5. Make baseline assessment of behavior, appearance, emotional status, response to environment, speech pattern, and thought content.

Inform Client and Family

1. Teach about the side effects and toxic effects of the drug and the need for a weekly WBC count.
2. Avoid the use of over-the-counter medications, alcohol, or CNS medication because of potential and severe drug interactions.
3. Report immediately the appearance of lethargy, weakness, fever, sore throat, malaise, mucous membrane ulceration, or other possible signs of infection.
4. Refrain from operating machinery, driving, and other tasks that require alertness until response to the drug is established.

5. Inform the physician if pregnancy occurs.
6. Do not breast-feed an infant if Clozaril is being taken

◆ DIAZEPAM

Categories: Anxiolytic (antianxiety agent); benzodiazepe
Trade Name: Valium

Uses

1. Management of anxiety disorders, for short-term relief of anxiety symptoms
2. Presurgical sedation to allay anxiety and tension
3. Alcohol withdrawal
4. Seizure disorders
5. Anticonvulsant
6. Relief of skeletal muscle spasticity

Action

One action of the benzodiazepines is to increase the ction of gamma-aminobutyric acid (GABA). The benzodiazepes help GABA open a chloride channel in the postsynaptic menrane of many neurons, thereby reducing the neuron's excitabilit

---

Dosages and Routes

Adult

Anxiety: 2–10 mg PO 2–4 times daily
2–10 mg IM/IV 2–4 times daily
Muscle relaxant: 2–10 mg PO 2–4 times daily
5–10 mg IM/IV 13–4h
Convulsions: 2–10 mg PO 2–4 times daily
5–10 mg IM/IV at 10-min intervals
Alcohol withdrawal: 10 mg PO 3–4 times daily
10 mg IM/IV initially, followed b
5–10 mg q3–4h

Elderly

2.5 mg PO bid
Convulsions: 2–5 mg IM/IV (increase gradually as need)

Contraindications

Acute narrow-angle glaucoma, untreated open-angle glaucoma, during or within 14 days of MAOI therapy, depressed or psychotic patients in the absence of anxiety, first-trimester pregnancy, breast-feeding, shock, coma, acute alcohol intoxication

Cautions

Epilepsy, myasthenia gravis, impaired hepatic or renal function, drug abuse, addiction-prone individuals. Injectable diazepam is used with extreme caution in the elderly, the very ill, and people with chronic obstructive pulmonary disease. May elicit rage reactions in some clients.

Remarks

The benzodiazepines can produce psychological and physical habituation, dependence, and withdrawal. Therefore, they are recommended for short-term therapy (2 to 4 weeks). These drugs need to be used with caution in individuals who have histories of addiction. Withdrawal from these drugs should be gradual in order to minimize withdrawal symptoms.

Side Effects

CNS: Sedation, vertigo, weakness, ataxia, decreased motor performance, confusion
Ocular: Double or blurred vision
Skin: Urticaria, rash, photosensitivity
Gastrointestinal: Change in weight, dry mouth, constipation

Adverse Effects

CNS: Benzodiazepines are CNS depressants. They are fairly safe when used on their own, but when used in combination with other CNS depressants, they can cause death.
Cardiovascular: Tachycardia to cardiovascular collapse
Metabolic: Changes in liver or renal function test results
Injection Sites: Can cause venous thrombosis or phlebitis at injection sites

Nursing Measures

1. Obtain drug history of prescribed and over-the-counter medications.

2. Periodically monitor blood cell count and liver function test results during prolonged therapy.
3. Assess for unexplained bleeding, petechiae, fever, and so forth.
4. Intramuscular therapy: Aspirate back, administer deep into large muscle mass; inject slowly; rotate injection sites.

Inform Client

1. Avoid alcohol or any other CNS depressants (anticonvulsants, antidepressants) while taking a benzodiazepine—can lead to respiratory depression. Check with physician before taking.
2. Avoid driving or operating hazardous machinery if drowsiness or confusion occurs.
3. Avoid abrupt withdrawal of benzodiazepine.

◆ DISULFIRAM

Categories: Alcohol deterrent; aldehyde dehydrogenase inhibitor
Trade Name: Antabuse

Uses

Adjunct treatment for selected clients with chronic alcoholism who want to remain in a state of enforced sobriety. A form of aversion therapy.

Action

Inhibits hepatic enzymes from normal metabolic breakdown of alcohol, resulting in high levels.

Dosages and Routes

Adult
PO only: initially, a maximum of 250–500 mg daily given as a
single dose for 1–2 weeks
Maintenance: 250 mg daily; not to exceed 500 mg daily

Contraindications

Severe heart disease, psychosis, and hypersensitivity to disulfiram

Cautions

Diabetes, hypothyroidism, epilepsy, cerebral damage, nephritis, hepatic disease, pregnancy

Remarks

Clients must abstain from alcohol intake for at least 12 hours before the initial dose of drug is administered.

Side Effects

Common side effects experienced during the first 2 weeks of therapy include mild drowsiness, fatigue, headache, metallic or garlic aftertaste, allergic dermatitis, and acne eruptions. Symptoms disappear spontaneously with continued therapy of reduced dosage.

Adverse Reactions

Disulfiram-Alcohol Reaction: Flushing or throbbing in head and neck, throbbing headache, nausea, copious vomiting, diaphoresis, dyspnea, hyperventilation, tachycardia, hypotension, marked uneasiness, vertigo, blurred vision, confusion. Can cause death.

Nursing Measures

1. Client must be able to demonstrate sobriety.
2. Client must be fully aware of drug's action when taken along with alcohol before treatment commences.
3. In severe disulfiram-alcohol reactions, supportive measures to restore BP and treat for shock in a medical facility are vital.

Inform Client and Family

1. Avoid any substances that contain alcohol:
   a. *Ingestion*: Elixirs, cough syrups, vinegars, vitamin/mineral tonics; be aware that some sauces, soups, ciders, and flavor extracts (vanilla, cherry) and some desserts (flaming, and some cakes and pies) are made with alcohol.
   b. *Topical*: Mouthwash, body lotions, liniments, shaving lotion
   c. *Inhalation*: Avoid inhaling fumes from substances that may contain alcohol, such as paints, wood stains, varnishes, and "stripping" compounds.
2. Carry a card stating that, if found disoriented or unconscious, he or she may be having a disulfiram-alcohol reaction and telling the finder whom to contact for medical care.
3. A disulfiram-alcohol reaction can occur within 5 to 10 minutes after ingestion of alcohol and can last 30 to 60 minutes or longer.
4. Reaction may occur with alcohol up to 14 days after ingesting disulfiram.

◆ DONEPEZIL HYDROCHLORIDE

Category: Cholinesterase inhibitor
Trade Name: Aricept

Use

Treatment of mild to moderate dementia of the Alzheimer's type

Action

The cholinergic system deteriorates in Alzheimer's disease. Donepezil inhibits the breakdown of endogenously released acetylcholine.

Dosages and Routes

Adults and Elderly

Start with 5 mg PO daily dose. After 6 weeks may increase to 10 mg daily.

Contraindications

Hypersensitivity to donepezil or piperidine derivatives

Cautions

Cholinesterase inhibitors may increase gastric acid secretion. Therefore, clients should be monitored for gastrointestinal bleeding, especially those at increased risk of developing ulcers (e.g., history of ulcer disease, taking nonsteroidal anti-inflammatory medication). Use with caution in clients who have a history of seizures. Prescribe with care to clients with asthma or obstructive pulmonary disease.

Side Effects

Frequent: Nausea, vomiting, diarrhea, insomnia, muscle cramps, fatigue, and anorexia

Adverse Reactions

Syncopal episodes have been reported in association with the use of this drug.

Nursing Measures

1. Ascertain what other drugs client is taking because donepezil has the potential to interfere with the activity of anticholinergic medications.
2. Discuss with family/friend who is to administer the medication to client, to prevent dosage errors.

Inform Client and Family

1. Take drug in evening before retiring.
2. Drug may be taken with food.
3. In case of accidental overdose, call a poison control center to determine the latest recommendations for management.

◆ FLUOXETINE HYDROCHLORIDE

Category: Antidepressant
Trade Name: Prozac

Uses

1. Prozac is an atypical antidepressant medication that is chemically unrelated to TCAs or MAOIs.
2. Has been found effective in clients with bulimia and obsessive-compulsive disorder (OCD).

Action

A potent selective serotonin reuptake inhibitor (SSRI) whose use results in an increase in the amount of active serotonin within the synaptic cleft and at the serotonin receptor site. Increased serotonin in these areas appears to modify affective and behavioral disorders.

Dosages and Routes

Adult

20 mg/day PO; may reach 40–60 mg in divided doses; do not exceed 80 mg daily

Elderly

Same as for adults

Child

No dosage for children as yet established.

Contraindications

Not to be taken within 14 days of an MAOI. Also, client must wait 5 weeks when going from fluoxetine to an MAOI.

Cautions

Use with clients with concomitant systemic illness has not been studied extensively. Caution should be used with pregnant women or women who are breast-feeding, children, and the elderly. Caution should also be used with clients with liver disease or renal impairment or in a client who has had a recent myocardial infarction.

Remarks

Fluoxetine, like the TCAs and MAOIs, takes from 2 to 5 weeks to produce an elevation of mood. Advantages of this drug are fewer anticholinergic side effects and a low incidence of cardiovascular effects. However, fluoxetine may impair judgment, thinking, and motor skills.

Side Effects

General: The most common side effects reported with fluoxetine hydrochloride are nausea, nervousness and anxiety, insomnia, and vertigo. When these side effects are severe, the drug is discontinued. If a rash or urticaria or both develop, the drug should be discontinued. Anorexia may appear in some people.

Adverse Reactions

See Side Effects.

Nursing Measures

1. Fluoxetine hydrochloride is given in the early morning without consideration to meals.
2. Clients who are potentially suicidal are assessed for suicidal thoughts or actions. Carefully observe taking of medication.
3. If client is underweight and experiences anorexia, the physician should be alerted to re-evaluate continuation of medication.

Inform Client

1. If rash or urticaria appears, notify physician immediately.
2. Do not drive or operate machinery if drowsiness occurs.
3. Avoid alcoholic beverages.

◆ FLUVOXAMINE MALEATE

Category: Antidepressant
Trade Name: Luvox

Uses

Treatment of OCD; treatment of depression

Action

Selectively inhibits serotonin neuronal uptake in CNS, producing an antidepressant affect

---

Dosages and Routes

Adult

50 mg PO at bedtime; increase by 50 mg every 4–7 days to a maximum of 300 mg/day. Give doses over 100 mg in 2 divided doses.

Children (8–17)

25 mg PO at bedtime; increase by 25 mg every 4–7 days up to a maximum of 200 mg/day

---

Contraindications

Do not take within 14 days of MAOI ingestion; concurrent astemizole or terfenadine therapy.

Cautions

History of seizures, heart disease, kidney disease, liver disease, or allergies. This drug should be used only if clearly needed during pregnancy. This medication appears in breast milk.

Remarks

This drug may interact with a variety of other medications both prescribed and over the counter (e.g., lithium, all antidepressants [SSRIs and others], dexfenfluramine, warfarin, phenytoin, benzodiazepines, carbamazepine, clozapine, methadone, propranolol, any MAOI, haloperidol). A careful drug history is warranted for anyone going on this medication.

Side Effects

Frequent: Nausea, vomiting, constipation, upset stomach, delayed ejaculation, decreased libido, urinary frequency, drowsiness, headache, anxiety, tremors, trouble sleeping, dry mouth

Infrequent: Dizziness, fatigue, constipation, rash, pruritis, back pain, visual disturbances

Adverse Reactions

Cardiac: Rapid, pounding, or irregular heart beat; chest pain

CNS: Confusion, disorientation, unusual uncontrolled movements, especially around the face

Hematological: Bruising or bleeding

General: Flu-like symptoms (fever, chills)

Nursing Measures

1. For clients on long-term therapy, baseline liver/renal function test and baseline blood counts need to be done and repeated periodically throughout treatment.
2. Perform a suicide assessment and evaluate risk factors. Does client's history include past suicidal behavior or threats? Identify client's support system.
3. Obtain a drug history from client as to over-the-counter, prescription (especially psychoactive medications and cardiac and many other), and recreational drugs client currently takes. How much and how often does client use alcohol? Be sure there is good documentation made in client's chart, and prescribing health care worker is well informed.

Inform Client and Family

1. Drug may take up to 4 weeks before improvement is noted.
2. Helpful interventions for common side effects include:
   a. Sunglasses for photosensitivity.
   b. Sugarless gum and sips of water for dry mouth.
   c. Rise and move slowly to avoid hypotensive effects.
   d. Avoid tasks that require motor skills (driving a car) until response to drug is established.
3. Because of drug interactions, client should avoid alcohol.

◆ GABAPENTIN

Category: Anticonvulsant

Trade Name: Neurontin

Uses

1. Adjunctive therapy in the treatment of partial seizures with and without secondary generalization in adults with epilepsy. Neuropathic pain.
2. *Used experimentally with selected refractory bipolar clients.*

Action

May be related to increased GABA synthesis rate, increased GABA accumulation, or binding to as-yet undefined receptor sites in the brain to produce anticonvulsant activity. Exact mechanism is not known.

Dosage and Routes

PO: 100-, 300-, 400-mg capsules

Adult

Effective dose is 900–1800 mg given in divided doses (tid). Titration to an effective dose can take place rapidly, giving 300 mg on day 1 (hs), 300 mg bid (q12h) on day 2, and 300 mg tid (q8h) on day 3; continue increasing dose up to 1800 mg when indicated.

Elderly

In elderly clients with compromised renal function, dose needs to be adjusted.

Contraindications

Clients who have demonstrated hyperactivity to the drug or its ingredients

Cautions

In clients with renal impairment, dose needs to be modified. Use with caution in pregnant women. Safety and effectiveness has not been established in children under 12.

Side Effects

Frequent: Fatigue, somnolence, dizziness, ataxia, nystagmus, tremor, diplopia, rhinitis, hypertension
Infrequent: Weight gain, dyspepsia, myalgia, nervousness, dysarthria, pharyngitis, diplopia, nausea and vomiting

Adverse Reactions

Difficulty breathing or tightening of the throat, swelling of lips or tongue, rash, slurred speech, drowsiness, diarrhea

Nursing Measures

1. Review history of seizure disorder (type, onset, intensity, frequency, duration, level of consciousness).
2. Assess for seizure activity. Provide safety measures as needed.
3. Obtain baseline assessment, including vital signs.
4. Obtain information on all other medications (prescription, nonprescription, nutritional supplements, or herbal products) that client is taking.
5. Obtain history of alcohol frequency and amount. Identify any recreational drugs that client is taking. These may affect the way the medication will work.

Inform Client and Family

1. Drug should not be abruptly discontinued because of the possibility of increasing seizure activity.
2. Drug should be taken as prescribed.
3. Gabapentin may cause dizziness, somnolence, and other symptoms of CNS depression; therefore, clients should be advised to refrain from driving a car or operating complex machinery.
4. Client should tell physician if she:
   a. Is about to become pregnant
   b. Is breast-feeding

◆ HALOPERIDOL

Categories: Antipsychotic/neuroleptic; butyrophenone
Trade Name: Haldol

Uses

1. Management of psychotic disorders
2. Helps control remissions in schizophrenia
3. Controversial use for children with combative, explosive hyperexcitability
4. Control of tic and vocal utterances of Tourette's syndrome
5. Useful in acute mania and acute and chronic organic psychosis
6. Management of drug-induced (LSD) psychosis

Action

Blocks the binding of dopamine to the postsynaptic dopamine receptors in the brain

---

Dosages and Routes

Adult

1.0–2.0 mg 2–3 times daily up to 4.0–6.0 mg 2–3 times daily (30–40 mg daily may be necessary)
(Severe) 3–5 mg IM q1–8h to control symptoms, then give PO

Child

Not for children under 3 years; for children 3–12 years, 0.05–0.15 mg/kg/day PO in 2–3 divided doses

Elderly

PO: Elderly or debilitated clients may require smaller doses than adults

---

Contraindications

Hypersensitivity, Parkinson's disease, depression, seizures, coma, alcoholism, during lithium therapy

Cautions

The elderly; clients on anticoagulant therapy; clients with glaucoma, prostatic hypertrophy, urinary retention, asthma, or pregnancy/lactation

Remarks

A "high-potency" neuroleptic; higher incidence of EPS but lower incidence of sedation and orthostatic hypotension. Haldol Decanoate E or D given intramuscularly can have lasting effects from 1 to 3 weeks.

Side Effects

Autonomic: Dry mouth, nasal congestion, constipation or diarrhea, urinary retention or urinary frequency, inhibition of ejaculation and impotence in men
CNS: EPS (pseudoparkinsonism, akathisia, dystonia), vertigo, insomnia, headache

Cardiovascular: Orthostatic hypotension, hypertension, dizziness, EEG changes

Endocrine: Changes in libido, galactorrhea in women, gynecomastia in men

Ocular: Photophobia, blurred vision, aggravation of glaucoma

Other: Weight gain, allergic reactions such as eczema and skin rashes

Adverse Reactions

CNS: *Acute Dystonias* (e.g., painful neck spasms, torticollis, oculogyric crisis, convulsions). *Tardive dyskinesia* (choreiform movements of the tongue, face, mouth, jaw, and possibly extremities). The elderly and those on the drug for extended periods are more susceptible; often irreversible.

Hematologic: Agranulocytosis—drug immediately stopped.

Hepatic: Jaundice; clinical picture resembles hepatitis.

NMS: Occurs within 24 to 72 hours. Fever, rigidity, renal failure, arrhythmias, and more. Hold drug and give dantrolene sodium or bromocriptine immediately.

Nursing Measures

1. Check for signs of tardive dyskinesia (protrusion of tongue, puffing of cheeks, chewing or pucking of the mouth) and report them to physician immediately.
2. Observe for other signs of EPS and jaundice.
3. Check for orthostatic hypotension (take BP laying and standing). Withhold if systolic is 80 mm Hg or below.
4. Check frequently for urinary retention.
5. Check for constipation (avoid impaction).
6. Observe for fever, sore throat, and malaise, and monitor complete blood count, indicating a blood dyscrasia.
7. Monitor renal function during long-term therapy.
8. Monitor blood levels every week.

Inform Client

1. Rise slowly to a sitting position and dangle the legs 5 minutes before standing to minimize orthostatic hypotension.
2. Use sunscreen when in direct light to avoid skin blotching, and wear sunglasses to prevent photophobia.
3. Avoid the use of alcoholic beverages because they enhance CNS depression.
4. Refrain from operating machinery if drowsiness occurs.

◆ IMIPRAMINE HYDROCHLORIDE

Category: Tricyclic antidepressant
Trade Name: Tofranil

Uses

1. The principal indication for TCAs is the treatment of depression (major, bipolar, or dysthymia).
2. Imipramine is effective in some organic affective disorders and OCD.
3. Imipramine is used as adjunctive treatment in childhood enuresis and in bulimia.
4. Found useful in the treatment of agoraphobia with panic attacks and generalized anxiety disorder.

Action

TCAs block the reuptake of norepinephrine and serotonin into their presynaptic neurons.

Dosages and Routes

Adult

50 mg/day PO to start, given in 1–4 divided doses up to 200 mg daily for outpatients. Maintenance level 50–150 mg/day.
IM: Do not exceed 100 mg/day in divided doses.

Child

Childhood enuresis: 25 mg PO before bedtime
Depression in children over *12 years*: 30–40 mg PO daily initially

Elderly

PO: Used with caution—usually start at lower dose. Geriatric clients start on 30–40 mg daily in divided doses initially

---

Contraindications

Recent myocardial infarction or cardiac disease, severe renal or hepatic impairment. Death may occur if used with an MAOI; however, the two may be cautiously used together in cases of refractory depression. TCAs may also cause fatal cardiac arrhythmias in clients with hyperthroidism. Use with caution in children and adolescents. Special cautions for the elderly, especially those with cardiac, respiratory, cardiovascular, hepatic, or gastrointestinal diseases.

Cautions

Renal or hepatic disease, narrow-angle glaucoma. The potential for suicide must be assessed. TCAs lower the seizure threshold: Any client with a seizure disorder needs careful monitoring.

Remarks

1. Before receiving TCAs, clients need a thorough physical and cardiac work-up.
2. Patients need to know that mood elevation may not occur for 2 to 4 weeks.

Side Effects

Anticholinergic: Dry mouth and nasal passages, constipation, urinary hesitancy, esophageal reflux, blurred vision
Cardiovascular: Orthostatic hypotension, hypertension, palpitations
CNS: Tachycardia, vertigo, tinnitus, numbness and tingling of extremities, stimulation
Endocrine: Galactorrhea, increased or decreased libido, ejaculatory and erectile disturbances, delayed orgasm
Other: Weight gain and impotence, cholestatic jaundice, fatigue

Adverse Reactions

Autonomic: Intracardiac conduction slowing
Cardiovascular: Myocardial infarction, congestive heart failure, arrhythmias, heart block, cardiotoxicity; cerebrovascular accident, shock
CNS: Ataxia, neuropathy, EPS, lowered seizure threshold, delirium
Hematologic: Bone marrow depression, agranulocytosis
Psychiatric: Hallucinations, shift to hypomania, mania, exacerbation of psychosis

Nursing Measures

1. Monitor BP (both lying and standing) every 2 to 6 hours when initiating therapy.

2. Observe suicidal clients closely during initial therapy.
3. Supervise drug ingestion to prevent hoarding of drug.
4. Assess for urinary retention.
5. Monitor liver function test results and complete blood count (assess for signs of cholestatic jaundice and agranulocytosis).
6. Small amount of drugs should be dispensed if client is to be discharged.
7. Diabetic clients should be closely monitored, especially during early therapy, because hypo- or hyperglycemia may occur in some clients.
8. All clients on TCAs need to be observed for the occurrence of hypomania or manic episodes, urinary retention, orthostatic hypotension, and seizure activity.

Inform Client

1. Rise slowly to prevent hypotensive effects.
2. Do not drive or use hazardous machinery if drowsiness or vertigo occurs.
3. Do not use over-the-counter drugs in conjunction with a TCA without a physician's approval.
4. The effects of alcohol and imipramine are potentiated when used together, and alcohol use should be discussed with a physician before taking the drug.
5. One to 4 weeks may pass before therapeutic effects are experienced.

◆ LAMOTRIGINE

Category: Anticonvulsant (antiepileptic drug [AED] of the phenyltriazine class)
Trade Name: Lamictal

Uses

1. Adjunctive treatment of partial seizures in adults with epilepsy.
2. *Used experimentally in the treatment of refractory bipolar depression.*

Action

The precise mechanism by which lamotrigine exerts its anticonvulsant action is unknown. It is thought to be related to the drug's effect on sodium channels.

Dosages and Routes

PO: 25-, 100-, 150-, 200-mg tablets

Adult, Elderly, Children Over 16

If receiving enzyme-inducing AEDs but not valproate; recommend as add-on therapy

50 mg qd for 2 weeks, followed by 100 mg/day in 2 divided
doses for 2 weeks

Maintenance dose: Dose may be increased by 100 mg/day
every week up to 300–500 mg in 2 divided doses.

If receiving combination therapy of valproic acid and enzyme-inducing AEDs

25 mg every other day for 2 weeks followed by 25 mg qd for
2 weeks

Maintenance dose: Dose may be increased by 25–50 mg/day
every 1–2 weeks up to 150 mg/day in 2 divided doses.

Children 16 or Under

**NOT approved for children under 16 years of age
(see contraindications).**

Contraindications

Children Under 16 Years of Age: The incidence of severe, potentially life-threatening rash in pediatric clients is very much higher than that reported in adults using lamotrigine (1:50 to 1:100 pediatric clients).

Cautions

Renal impairment, hepatic function impairment, cardiac function impairment. Can reduce fetal weight; delayed ossification noted in animals. Pregnancy Category C. Breast-feeding not recommended.

Side Effects

Frequent: Dizziness, double vision, headache, ataxia (muscular incoordination), nausea, blurred vision, somnolence, and rhinitis
Occasional: Pharyngitis, vomiting, cough, flu-like syndrome, diarrhea, dysmenorrhea, fever, insomnia, and dyspepsia
Infrequent: Constipation, tremor, anxiety, pruritis, and vaginitis

Adverse Reaction

Warning: Potentially life-threatening rashes have been reported in association with the use of lamotrigine. The rashes occur in approximately 1 in every 1000 adults.

Nursing Measures

1. Review history of seizure disorder (type, onset, intensity, frequency, duration, and level of consciousness).
2. Identify what prescription and over-the-counter medications the client is taking.
3. Identify amount and frequency of alcohol intake. Identify any other recreational drugs client is taking.
4. Identify other medical conditions, particularly renal or hepatic impairment.
5. Obtain baseline vital signs.
6. Report promptly any rash. May herald a life-threatening medical event.
7. Assess for dizziness or ataxia, and provide safety measures.
8. Assess for clinical improvement (decrease in intensity/frequency of seizures).

Inform Client and Family

1. Prior to initiation of treatment with lamotrigine, the client and family should be instructed that a rash or other signs or symptoms of hypersensitivity (e.g., fever, lymphadenopathy, facial swelling) may herald a serious medical event. The client should report any such occurrence to a physician **immediately.**
2. Report first signs of a rash to the physician.
3. EDs should not be abruptly discontinued because of the possibility of increasing seizure frequency, unless safety concerns (*rash*) require a rapid withdrawal.
4. Carry identification card; wear bracelet to note anticonvulsant therapy.
5. Avoid alcohol—lowers seizure threshold.

◆ LITHIUM CARBONATE/CITRATE

Category: Antimanic
Trade Names: Carbolith, Eskalith, Lithane, Lithizine, Lithonate, Lithobid

Uses

1. Primarily used to control, prevent, or diminish manic episodes in people with bipolar depression (manic-depressive psychosis).
2. Used *experimentally* in alcoholism, premenstrual syndrome, drug abuse, phobias, eating disorders, and rage reactions.

Action

Lithium is an alkali metal salt that behaves in the body much like a sodium ion. Lithium acts to lower concentrations of norepinephrine and serotonin by inhibiting their release and enhancing their reuptake by neurons. The therapeutic effects, as well as the side effects and toxic effects, of lithium are thought to be related to the partial replacement of sodium by lithium in membrane action.

Dosages and Routes

Adult

Acute mania: 600 mg PO 3 times daily
Maintenance dose: 300 mg PO 3 times daily or 4 times daily

Child

Not labeled for pediatric use

Elderly

Starting dose of 300 mg/day. Serum levels of 0.4–0.6 mEq/L are usually effective in elderly clients.

Contraindications

Pregnancy, nursing mothers, significant cardiovascular or renal disease, schizophrenia, severe debilitation, dehydration, sodium depletion

Cautions

The elderly, thyroid disease, epilepsy, concomitant use with haloperidol or other antipsychotics, parkinsonism, severe infections, urinary retention, diabetes

Remarks

Serum lithium levels must be monitored during drug therapy. The therapeutic range is very narrow, and the potential for toxic effects is high if blood levels are not monitored. During the acute stage, blood levels are raised to 1.0 to 1.4 mEq/L. Maintenance therapy blood levels run from 0.8 to 1.2 mEq/L. Side effects and toxic effects are common at higher doses (1.5 mEq/L or more). Before a patient is started on lithium, blood urea nitrogen, thyroxine, triiodothyronine, and thyroid-stimulating hormone levels should be measured, and an electrocardiogram should be done.

Side Effects

The major long-term risks of lithium therapy are hypothyroidism and impairment of the kidney's ability to concentrate urine.
Below 1.5 mEq/L: Polyuria, polydipsia, lethargy, fatigue, muscle weakness, headache, mild nausea, fine hand tremor, and inability to concentrate. May experience ankle edema. Symptoms disappear during continued therapy.

Adverse and Toxic Effects

1.5 to 2.0 mEq/L: Vomiting, diarrhea, muscle weakness, ataxia, dizziness, slurred speech, confusion
2.0 to 2.5 mEq/L: Blurred vision, muscle twitching, severe hypotension, persistent nausea and vomiting. Thyroid toxicity is common.
2.5 to 3.0 mEq/L or more: Urinary and fecal incontinence, seizures, cardiac arrhythmias, peripheral vascular collapse, death

Nursing Measures

1. If serum lithium levels are above 1.5 mEq/L or if client has persistent diarrhea, vomiting, excessive sweating in hot weather, infection, or fever, check with physician before giving dose.
2. Check urine specific gravity periodically and teach patient to do so at home (normal: 1.005 to 1.025).
3. Administer lithium with meals.
4. Ensure that client is well hydrated.

Inform Client

1. Drink plenty of liquids (2 to 3 L/day) during initial therapy and 1 to 1.5 L/day during remainder of therapy.
2. Know the side effects and toxic effects of lithium therapy and seek out physician immediately if problems arise.
3. Have blood lithium levels measured at regular intervals as directed in order to regulate dosage and prevent toxicity.
4. Maintain a regular diet, thus maintaining average salt intake (6 to 8 g) required to keep the serum lithium level in the therapeutic range.
5. Avoid alcohol.
6. Be aware that antibiotics (metronidazole and tetracycline) and nonsteroidal anti-inflammatory agents (indomethacin) can increase lithium levels.
7. Know that caffeine can lower lithium levels.

◆ LORAZEPAM

Categories: Antianxiety agent; benzodiazepine
Trade Name: Ativan

Uses

1. Treatment of anxiety disorders associated with depression
2. Preoperative sedation
3. Nausea and vomiting associated with chemotherapy for cancer

Action

CNS depressant, especially the limbic system and reticular formation. Enhances action of inhibitory neurotransmitter GABA, producing a calming effect. Can suppress spread of seizure activity and can directly depress motor nerve and muscle function, creating some muscle relaxation.

Dosages and Routes

Adult
Anxiety: 2–3 mg PO daily in 2–3 doses
Insomnia: 2–4 mg PO at bedtime

Elderly
Anxiety: 0.5–1 mg PO daily (may increase gradually)
Insomnia: 0.5–1 mg PO at bedtime

Contraindications

Acute narrow-angle glaucoma and alcohol intoxication, pregnant clients or lactating mothers, children under 12

Cautions

Clients with renal or hepatic dysfunction, elderly or debilitated clients, clients with a history of drug abuse/additions. People taking other *CNS depressants (narcotics, barbiturates, alcohol)* may have a synergistic effect, increasing CNS depression. May reduce *digoxin* excretion, increasing the potential for toxicity.

Side Effects

Frequent: Drowsiness, fatigue, dizziness, incoordination
Occasional: Blurred vision, slurred speech, hypotension, headache

Rare: Paradoxical CNS restlessness, excitement in elderly/debilitated

Adverse Reactions

Can have pronounced withdrawal symptoms (seizures, pronounced restlessness, insomnia, abdominal/muscle cramps) with abrupt withdrawal from the drug.

Nursing Measures

1. Assess for history of glaucoma, substance abuse, allergies, past reactions to benzodiazepines, and current list of medications.
2. Before long-term therapy, assess complete blood count and liver function tests in collaboration with physician.
3. Make sure client has written information about medications covering side effects, doses, precautions, and other information.

Inform Client and Family

1. Avoid tasks that require alertness or motor skills (driving, operating machinery).
2. Do not take over-the-counter medications or new medications without approval from your physician.
3. Do not drink alcohol or take other CNS depressants while taking this medication.
4. Do not stop medication abruptly.

◆ METHYLPHENIDATE

Category: CNS stimulant
Trade Name: Ritalin

Uses

Attention deficit disorder (children 6 years and older), narcolepsy, and occasionally for depression in the elderly

Action

Direct release of catecholamines into synaptic clefts and thus onto postsynaptic receptor sites; blocks reuptake of catecholamines, thus prolonging their actions; serves as false neurotransmitter.

Dosages and Routes

Children 6 Years and Older

Usual starting dose is 5 mg PO twice daily (breakfast and lunch). Most children are maintained on 60 mg/day and should be monitored regularly by prescribing physician.

Adults

Doses may start at 5 mg PO 2–3 times daily. Dose range for adults is 10 mg/day to not more than 60 mg/day (20–40 mg/day is usual).

Elderly

Elderly clients using Ritalin for depression usually are maintained on 2.5–20 mg/day PO.

Contraindications

Glaucoma, hypertension, heart problems, or a history of Tourette's syndrome. People with a history of seizure disorders may experience an increase in number, duration, or severity of seizures.

Cautions

Can cause growth delay in children. Can interact with other medications (e.g., alcohol, antidepressants [MAOIs and TCAs], some over-the-counter medications, health food products containing *ma huang*). Serious problems can also develop if clients are taking any other amphetamine-type or diet drugs.

Side Effects

Frequent: Nervousness and sleeplessness are most common. Other reactions are loss of appetite, weight loss, nausea, dizziness, heart palpitations, increases in blood pressure, stomach upset, and growth delay in children with prolonged therapy
Occasional: Dizziness, dysphoria, joint pain, fever

Adverse Reactions

Can increase frequency of seizures in people with seizure disorders; chest pain, dysrhythmias. Can have serious interactions with other medications and over-the-counter preparations.

Nursing Measures

1. Take a careful inventory of any other medications client is taking, prescribed and over-the-counter or health food products. Check with pharmacy if there might be a problem with compatibility.
2. Medications are best taken shortly before meals, and not after 12:00 noon or 1:00 PM for children or 6:00 PM for adults, because stimulant effect may keep people awake.

Inform Client and Family

1. Suggest to parents to discuss drug holidays, which can help avoid the side effect of growth delay, with their prescribing health care agent (physician, nurse, therapist).
2. Caution client and family that drug may have serious side effects when mixed with other substances. Have client or family check with physician before taking any over-the-counter medications or other drugs or health food products from other sources.
3. If the child must take this medication during school hours, ask your pharmacist to provide an empty labeled container and place no more than 1 week's worth of medication in the bottle. Be sure the medication is secured with a school official.
4. Once client is stabilized on a dose, Ritalin can be given in extended-release form. These tablets are to be swallowed whole, *never crushed or chewed.*
5. Keep tablets dry, tightly capped, away from direct heat.
6. Keep out of reach of children and pets.

◆ NEFAZODONE

Categories: Antidepressant; selective serotonin/norepinephrine reuptake inhibitor
Trade Name: Serzone

Use

Treatment of depression

Action

Nefazodone and one of its active metabolites exert dual effects on serotoninergic neurotransmission through blockade of serotonin

(5-hydroxytryptamine) type 2 (5-HT$_2$) receptors and inhibition of serotonin uptake. The parent compound (NEF) and another active metabolite also exhibit affinity for the 5-HT$_{1C}$ receptor. Nefazodone lacks anticholinergic or antihistaminic effects but exhibits some affinity for alpha$_1$-adrenergic receptors.

Dosages and Routes

Adult

Start on 100–200 mg/day PO (50–100 mg twice daily)
Maintenance dose: 300–500 mg/day (150–200 mg twice daily)

Elderly

Start on 50–100 mg/day PO (25–50 mg twice daily)
Maintenance dose: 150–250 mg daily (75–175 mg twice daily)

Cautions

During pregnancy this drug should be used only if clearly needed. Lactating women should not nurse their infants while receiving nefazodone. Caution should be used when nefazodone is initiated in people with pre-existing hypotension or a labile circulation. Nefazodone should be used with caution on anyone with pre-existing liver, kidney, or heart disease or a history of seizures or allergies. As with all antidepressants, a suicide assessment is needed and prescriptions should be written for the smallest quantity of tablets consistent with good client management.

Contraindications

To avoid potentially life-threatening cardiotoxicity, the nonsedating antihistamines *terfenadine (Seldane)* and *astemizole (Hismanal)* should not be taken by clients on nefazodone. Drugs such as *alprazolam (Xanax)* and *triazolam (Halcion)* require dosage reductions when used concomitantly. As with the SSRIs and venlafaxine, nefazodone should not be used in combination with MAOIs or within 2 weeks of terminating treatment with MAOIs. MAOIs should not be introduced until at least 2 weeks after the cessation of nefazodone therapy. Contraindicated in clients with known hypersensitivity to nefazodone and components of the formulation, or other phenylpiperazine antidepressants.

Side Effects

Frequent: Sleepiness, dry mouth, nausea, dizziness (especially when standing), constipation, confusion, incoordination, blurred vision or changes in vision
Infrequent: Irregular heartbeat or skin rash

Adverse Reactions

Cardiovascular: Sinus bradycardia and first-degree atrioventricular block
Genitourinary: Nefazodone is structurally related to trazodone, which has been associated with priapism. *No cases have been reported*; however, a client who presents with a prolonged or inappropriate erection should discontinue therapy immediately and consult a physician right away.

Nursing Measures

1. The drug is given twice daily in divided doses.
2. Clients who are suicidal are observed for suicidal actions if hospitalized; if in the community, they are given the smallest number of tablets consistent with good management.
3. Teach measures for combating orthostatic hypotension in case the client experiences dizziness upon rising.

Inform Client

1. Do not drive or operate machinery if drowsiness occurs.
2. Drug may take 2 to 3 weeks before therapeutic effects are noted.
3. Excessive sedation may occur during initial therapy.

◆ OLANZAPINE

Category: Atypical antipsychotic
Trade Name: Zyprexa

Uses

1. First-line treatment for schizophrenia, targeting both the positive and negative symptoms
2. Other psychotic illness

Action

Olanzapine blocks various serotonin ($5-HT_{2A}$) receptors and dopamine (D_2) receptors. It also antagonizes dopamine D_1 through

D_4 receptors, serotonin 5-HT_{2C} and 5-HT_3 receptors, and the alpha$_1$-adrenergic and H_1 histamine receptors.

Dosages and Routes

Adult

Given in 5- to 10-mg doses qd, with a target of 10 mg/day (15 mg/day *does not* seem to be more effective than 10 mg/day). Range 5–20 mg/day.
PO: 5-, 7.5-, and 10-mg tablets.

Contraindications

Client is pregnant or nursing; is hypersensitive to olanzapine.

Cautions

Olanzapine seems to have a good side effect profile and low potential interactions. *Carbamazepine* may increase olanzapine clearance by 50% at a dose of 200 mg twice daily, and *nicotine* may increase olanzapine clearance by 40% in smokers. Alcohol may potentiate the CNS effects; olanzapine may potentiate some antihypertensive agents.

Side Effects

Frequent: Psychomotor slowing (somnolence, asthenia), psychomotor activation (agitation, nervousness, insomnia, hostility), and dizziness. Weight gain.
Infrequent: At higher doses, anticholinergic effects (constipation, dry mouth, increased appetite). Mild transient dose-related increases in hepatic transaminase and prolactin levels resolve spontaneously and do not require discontinuation of the drug.

Nursing Measures

Monitor blood pressure. Educate patient on how to minimize postural hypertension. Caution client that alcohol or benzodiazepines may potentiate hypertension.

◆ PHENELZINE SULFATE

Categories: Antidepressant; MAOI
Trade Name: Nardil

Uses

1. MAOIs are used primarily for depression that is refractory to TCA therapy.
2. MAOIs are particularly effective in atypical depression, agoraphobia, or hypochondriasis.
3. Panic disorders

Action

Antidepressant effect thought to be due to irreversible inhibition of MAO, thereby increasing the concentration of epinephrine, norepinephrine, serotonin, and dopamine within the presynaptic neurons and at the receptor site.

Dosages and Routes

Adult

15 mg PO 3 times daily; increase rapidly to 60 mg daily until therapeutic level is noted.

Elderly

Are prone to side effects; in adults older than 60 may be contraindicated.

Child

Not used with children.

Contraindications

MAOIs can cause untoward interactions with certain foodstuffs or cold remedies, which may produce hypertensive crises, cerebrovascular accident, or hyperpyrexia states that can lead to coma or death. Therefore, a confused or noncompliant client is at risk with an MAOI.

Other contraindications include people with congestive heart failure, cardiovascular or cerebrovascular disease, impaired renal function, glaucoma, history of severe headaches, or liver disease; elderly or debilitated patients; and people who are pregnant or who have paranoid schizophrenia.

Cautions

Depression accompanying alcoholism or drug addiction, manic-depressive states, suicidal tendencies, agitated clients, and people with chronic brain syndromes or a history of angina pectoris

Remarks

Because of the severe interactions of some foodstuffs and medication, clients need comprehensive teaching, teaching aids, and supervision.

High-Tyramine Foods: Include beer, red wine, aged cheese, dry sausage, fava beans (Italian green beans), brewer's yeast, smoked fish, any kind of liver, avocados, and bologna. Chocolate and coffee should be used in moderation.

Drugs: Those causing severe medication interactions include meperidine (Demerol), epinephrine, local anesthetics, decongestants, cough medications, diet pills, and most over-the-counter medications.

Side Effects

General: Constipation, dry mouth, vertigo, orthostatic hypotension, drowsiness or insomnia, weakness, fatigue, weight gain, hypomania, mania, blurred vision, skin rash. Muscle twitching is common.

Adverse Reactions

Hypertensive Crisis: Intense occipital headache, palpitation, stiff neck, fever, chest pain, bradycardia or tachycardia, intracranial bleeding

Hepatic: Jaundice, malaise, right upper quadrant pain, change in color or consistency of stools

Nursing Measures

1. Monitor BP for orthostatic hypotension every 2 to 4 hours during initial therapy.
2. Assess for other potential signs of hypertensive crises.
3. Observe for marked changes in mood (e.g., hypomania, mania).
4. Monitor intake and output and frequency of stools.
5. Have client dangle legs 5 minutes before standing.
6. Depressed persons are at risk for suicide; continue to monitor and observe for potential suicidal behaviors.

Inform Client

1. Inform client and family clearly and carefully about foodstuffs and medications to avoid. REVIEW IN DETAIL.
2. Instruct clients taking MAOIs to wear a medical identification tag or bracelet.

3. Caution clients to avoid all over-the-counter drugs unless a physician's approval has been obtained.
4. Caution clients to avoid all alcohol.
5. Encourage clients and their families to go to the emergency room immediately if signs and symptoms of hypertensive crises are suspected. Phentolamine (Regitine) can be given for hypertensive crises.

◆ QUETIAPINE

Category: Antipsychotic (dibenzothiazepine derivative)
Trade Name: Seroquel

Use

Management of the manifestation of both positive and negative symptoms of schizophrenia

Action

Interacts with multiple neurotransmitter receptors, including serotonin, dopamine, and histamine. Exact mechanism is unknown.

Dosages and Routes

PO: 25-, 100-, or 200-mg tablets

Adults

Initially, 25 mg bid, then 25–50 mg qd up to a target dose of 300 mg/day given **bid** within 4–7 days

Elderly

Because plasma clearance is reduced by 30%–50% in elderly individuals, the rate of dose titration may need to be slower, and the daily therapeutic target dose lower.

Contraindications

Known hypersensitivity to this medication or any of its ingredients

Cautions

In clients with pre-existing hepatic disorders, in clients who are being treated with potentially hepatotoxic drugs, or if treatment-emergent signs or symptoms of hepatic impairment appear. Liver function test should be done periodically.

Side Effects

Frequent: Headache, somnolence, postural hypotension, dizziness, tachycardia, agitation, insomnia, dry mouth. May cause sedation and impair motor skills during initial dose titration period.
Infrequent: Back pain, fever, palpitations, weight gain, hyperthyroidism, rhinitis, leukopenia, ear pain

Adverse Reactions

Cardiac: Elevated aspartate transaminase levels
Hepatic: Elevated alanine transaminase (ALT) levels
Hematological: Leukopenia
Hormonal: Reduction of thyroxine levels usually during first 2 to 4 weeks of treatment

Nursing Measures

1. Always monitor clients on antipsychotics for signs of:
   a. Tardive dyskinesia
   b. NMS
2. Assess for orthostatic hypotension, dizziness, and possible syncope during initial dose titration. Take necessary measures to prevent injury.
3. If client has a history of seizures or a condition associated with lowered seizure threshold, take necessary precautions.
4. For clients who have a known or suspected abnormal hepatic function or clients who develop any signs or symptoms suggestive of new-onset liver disorder during quetiapine therapy, initial assessment and then periodic clinical assessment with transaminase levels is recommended.

Inform Client and Family

1. Client should inform physician:
   a. If she is about to become pregnant
   b. If she is breast-feeding a baby
   c. About over-the-counter and any prescription drugs he or she is taking (especially antihypertensive drugs)
   d. About any and all alcohol and recreational drug consumption
2. Teach client to dangle feet before getting out of bed to prevent dizziness.

3. Because drug may slow cognitive function and motor skills initially, inform client to refrain from performing activities requiring mental alertness (driving, using hazardous machinery) until it is certain that the drug does not adversely affect cognitive function.
4. Alcoholic beverages should be avoided while taking quetiapine because both the cognitive and motor effects of alcohol consumption are potentiated with quetiapine.

◆ RISPERIDONE

Category: Atypical antipsychotic
Trade Name: Risperdal

Use

Potent antipsychotic agent, targets negative (withdrawal, apathy, negativism) as well as positive symptoms (hallucinations, delusions, paranoia, hostility) of schizophrenia.

Action

A potent antagonist at $5\text{-}HT_{2A}$ and D_2 receptors (serotonin and dopamine)

Dosages and Routes

PO: tablets only
Adults
Start with 1 mg bid, increase to 2 mg bid on second day and 3 mg bid on third day.
Elderly
Start at 0.5 mg bid, titrate up to maximum of 3 mg/day.

Contraindication

Hypersensitivity to risperidone

Cautions

Can cause orthostatic hypotension and tachycardia. Because of these reactions, it should be started at low doses (e.g., 0.5 mg in the elderly and 1.0 for adults). Risperidone is associated with dose-related EPS, although often minimal in therapeutic range. Use with caution in clients with a history of seizures.

Side Effects

Frequent: Sedation, insomnia, rhinitis, coughing, back or chest pain, erectile problems in men, weight gain, and decreased sexual interest. Initial dosing especially may cause orthostatic hypotension and tachycardia or syncope. Some clients report anorexia, polyuria/polydipsia, and/or an increase in dream activity.

Occasional

EPS; increases in plasma prolactin can lead to galactorrhea and menstrual disturbances in some women.

Adverse Reactions

A number of cases of NMS have been reported. Rare cases of priapism have been reported.

Nursing Measures

1. Client should know what the medication can do and what it cannot do. This drug can target some of the negative symptoms, and that should be included in client teaching about the drug.
2. Client needs a list of the possible expected side effects and those reactions that would warrant contacting the prescribing nurse, physician, or therapist (e.g., palpitations, erectile problems, or sexual disinterest problems that might threaten compliance; palpitations; dizziness).
3. Teach clients initially to sit on the side of the bed before getting up in the morning, to avoid dizziness when getting up and potential falls.
4. Check to see if client has had seizures in the past.

Inform Client and Family

1. When starting medication, be careful driving cars, working around machinery, and crossing streets. Medication can make people sleepy and perhaps dizzy, especially initially.
2. Do not suddenly stop taking medication even if there is no immediate return of symptoms. Relapse is a very high risk in the weeks and months after medications have been stopped.

3. Client or family member should notify the doctor if the client is having a sore throat during the first several months of treatment, if NMS appears (client should have a fact sheet on NMS) or if client is going to have general or dental surgery or is experiencing chest pain or tachycardia/palpitations.

◆ SERTRALINE HYDROCHLORIDE

Categories: Antidepressant; SSRI
Trade Name: Zoloft

Uses

1. Major depression
2. OCD

Action

Enhances serotoninergic activity in the CNS by blocking reuptake of serotonin in neuronal presynaptic membranes. Has only a very weak effect on dopamine and norepinephrine reuptake.

Dosages and Routes

Adults

Initially 50 mg PO once daily with morning or evening meal. May be increased no sooner than every week up to a maximum of 200 mg/day.

Elderly

Initially 25 mg/day PO once daily as above. May increase 25 mg every 2–3 days.

Contraindications

Use within 2 weeks of MAOI. The safety for children and in pregnancy has not been established. Anyone with hypersensitivity to the drug.

Cautions

Severe hepatic or renal insufficiency, elderly and debilitated clients, suicidal clients, and clients with a history of seizures or mania.

Drug Interactions

Cimetidine can increase sertraline concentrations. Other drug interactions with sertraline include an increase in diazepam concentrations, a decrease in tolbutamide, and increased bleeding for clients taking warfarin.

Side Effects

Frequent: Dizziness, headache, tremor, insomnia, somnolence, fatigue, agitation, nausea, dry mouth, loose stools/constipation, sexual dysfunction
Occasional: Increased sweating, dyspepsia, anorexia, nervousness, rhinitis, abnormal vision
Rare: Rash, vomiting, frequent urination, palpitations, paresthesia, twitching

Nursing Measures

1. Zoloft is best given in the morning.
2. If hospitalized, watch for signs of *cheeking* of medications (i.e., instead of swallowing medications, holding them under the tongue or in the cheek for the purpose of saving them and taking an overdose later).

Inform Client and Family

1. Medication may have to be taken 1 to 3 weeks before improvement is noticed, but often the time is much shorter.
2. If client is extremely depressed, client should be given only 1 week's supply at a time.
3. Caution client about premature discontinuation of therapy, which can result in a relapse. In general, medication should continue for at least 6 months to 1 year after symptoms have subsided.
4. Have client and family assess for signs of improvement in symptoms, especially in areas such as depressed mood and loss of interest or pleasure in usual activities.
5. Have client and family watch for signs of suicidal ideation.

◆ TACRINE

Category: Reversible cholinesterase inhibitor
Trade Name: Cognex

Use

Can help mild to moderate dementia in people with Alzheimer's disease. Appears to reverse 6 months of dementia progression.

Action

Cholinergic system deteriorates in Alzheimer's dementia. Tacrine inhibits breakdown of endogenously released acetylcholine.

Dosages and Routes

Adults

40 mg/day PO (more improvement noticed with 80–160 mg/day). Because of 2- to 4-hour half-life, needs qid dosing.
Start at 10 mg qid (40 mg) and continue 6 weeks if tolerated. Every 6 weeks increase *each dose* by 10 mg qid. If tolerated, go to 160 mg daily.

Contraindication

Can be hepatoxic to some clients.

Cautions

Because of elevation in liver enzymes, clients need frequent liver function testing. Other drugs can alter (raise or lower) tacrine levels. Anticholinergic agents can reverse tacrine's effects. Tacrine increases risk of cholinergic agent toxicity. Smoking can lower tacrine levels.

Side Effects

Frequent: Flu-like symptoms without fever; gastrointestinal symptoms (nausea, diarrhea, dyspepsia, anorexia, vomiting)

Adverse Reactions

Elevation of ALT. Liver function tests must be done and ALT levels monitored weekly for 6 weeks after each dose increase. Most common reason for dropouts.

Nursing Measures

Check for other medications (and smoking) that can alter tacrine levels. Be sure that client has informed prescribing physician and nurse of all medications client is taking.

Inform Client and Family

1. Clients taking tacrine need to have serum transaminases monitored monthly.
2. Remind family to let physician know of any and all medications client is taking, because tacrine levels are easily altered by some medications.
3. This drug is not a panacea but can be very useful in the early stages of dementia.

◆ ZOLPIDEM

Category: Nonbenzodiazepine sedative-hypnotic
Trade Name: Ambien

Use

Short-term treatment of insomnia

Action

Zolpidem is thought to bind to the GABA receptors in the CNS, giving the drug sedative, anticonvulsant, and antianxiety properties.

Dosages and Routes

Adults

10 mg PO immediately before bedtime

Elderly

5 mg PO immediately before bedtime

Contraindications

Safety has not been established for pregnancy, lactation, and children under age 18.

Cautions

People with renal or hepatic dysfunction. Clients with history of drug abuse/addictions or depressed and suicidal clients. Elderly or debilitated clients.

Side Effects

Frequent: Drowsiness, vertigo, double vision, headache, drugged feeling, euphoria, insomnia, and nausea
Occasional: Palpitations, myalgia, sinusitis, rash

Adverse Reactions

Rarely, doses over 10 mg have been associated with psychotic reactions and amnesia.

Nursing Measures

1. Establish baseline history of sleep pattern.
2. Assess for other medications that the client may be taking that can cause CNS depression, including level of alcohol consumption.
3. Identify other methods client has used to induce sleep.
4. Assess for adverse reactions and side effects.

Inform Client and Family

1. Zolpidem is only for short-term use. Explore other methods of inducing sleep.
2. Do not drive or use machinery once drug has been taken.
3. Take right before sleep.
4. When taking this drug, do not take other medications or over-the-counter medications unless approved by physician.
5. Do not consume alcohol while taking this drug.

INDEX

Page numbers in *italics* refer to figures; page numbers followed by t refer to tables; page numbers followed by b refer to text in boxes.

NURSE, CLIENT, AND FAMILY RESOURCES

National Alliance for the Mentally Ill (NAMI)
(800) 950-6264

Anxiety Disorders

Anxiety Disorder Association of America
(301) 231-9350

Cognitive Disorders

Alzheimer's Association: Information and Referral Service
(800) 272-3900

Alzheimer's Disease and Related Disorders Association
(312) 335-8700

Alzheimer's Disease Education and Referral Center
(800) 438-4380

Crisis

Emotions Anonymous
(612) 647-9712

Workaholics Anonymous
(510) 273-9253

Domestic Violence

Batterers Anonymous
(909) 355-1100

Child Abuse Prevention—Kids Peace
(800) 257-3223

Child Help USA Hotline
(800) 422-4453

Family Violence Sexual Assault Institute (FUSAI)
(903) 595-6600

National Domestic Violence Hotline (NDV Hotline)
(800) 799-SAFE

Rape, Abuse, Incest National Network (RAINN)
(800) 656-HOPE

Runaway Hotline
(800) 231-6946

Survivors of Incest Anonymous (SIA)
(410) 282-3400

Youth Crisis Hotline
(800) HIT-HOME

Eating Disorders

American Anorexia/Bulimia Association
(212) 891-8686

Eating Disorders Awareness and Prevention
(206) 382-3587

National Association of Anorexia Nervosa and Associated Disorders
(ANAD)
(847) 831-3438

National Eating Disorders Organization
(918) 481-4044

Grieving

About Dying
(800) 646-6460